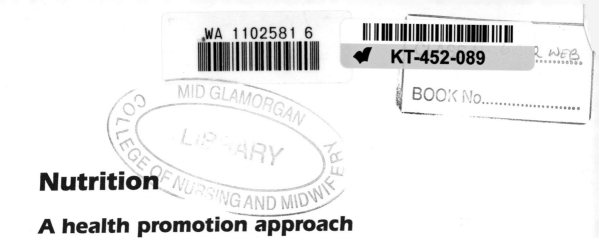

Nutrition

A health promotion approach

Nutrition

A health promotion approach

Geoffrey P. Webb *BSc, MSc, PhD*

Senior Lecturer in Nutrition and Physiology, University of East London, London, UK

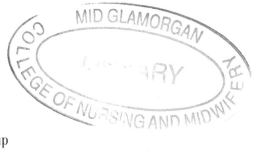

Edward Arnold

A member of the Hodder Headline Group

LONDON   SYDNEY   AUCKLAND

First published in Great Britain in 1995 by
Edward Arnold, a division of Hodder Headline PLC,
338 Euston Road, London NW1 3BH

British Library Cataloguing in Publication Data
A catalogue record for this book is available from the British Library

ISBN 0 340 61027 1

1 2 3 4 5   95 96 97 98 99

Typeset in 10.5/11.5 Plantin by GreenGate Publishing Services, Tonbridge, Kent
Printed and bound in Great Britain by J.W. Arrowsmith Ltd., Bristol

Contents

Preface

This book is essentially a formalised and polished amalgamation of my lecture notes and so the nature of the audiences for my lectures should help to define the intended audience for the book. Various parts of my lecture notes have been used with students ranging in level from those taking sub-degree certificates and diplomas right through to MSc level. My student audiences have also varied greatly in their academic priorities, from those taking professionally-orientated courses like physiotherapy, nursing, health promotion and midwifery through to those taking courses in pure and applied laboratory sciences. Two of the common characteristics of these audiences have been firstly, that most of the students have had almost no previous academic experience of nutrition, and secondly that nutrition is but one aspect of a broader course. The scientific background of the students has also varied enormously, but many have had limited background in the physical and mathematical sciences or in biochemistry. I have therefore tried to produce a book that introduces nutrition to a wide range of students in a way that assumes minimal knowledge of these supporting subjects. The title of the book reflects another major aim, namely to deal with nutrition in a way that reflects the current nutrition education priorities in industrialised countries, with more emphasis on nutrition as a positive means to promoting health and reduced emphasis on dietary inadequacy and avoiding the diseases of undernutrition.

Specialist students of nutrition and dietetics may find the book useful as a readable and thought-provoking overview of the health promotion aspects of their subject. I would also like to think that this book is accessible to the general interest reader who has done some science at school.

The book, like most of my lecture notes, has been written with a primarily British audience in mind. Nevertheless I have tried to make the book accessible to a wider audience, particularly to readers in the USA. To this end, I have given alternative terminology, American standards and American statistical information wherever possible. This broader international perspective should also be of value to British readers, for example: a consistent trend in the two countries indicates that it may be part of a wider pattern common to several industrialised countries; the sometimes widely differing dietary standards in the two countries emphasise that these standards are the judgement of an expert committee and not unarguable fact; and American food labelling legislation provides a working example of the sort of legislation that some Europeans would like to see enacted on this side of the Atlantic. Reading about nutrition from a non US perspective could be of even greater benefit to American readers because several of the excellent, modern introductory nutrition texts deal with nutrition from an almost totally North American viewpoint.

The way I have organised the book, particularly the inclusion of the large Concepts and Principles section, means that some topics will be addressed several times from differing angles; some examples will also be used more than once to illustrate different points. I make no apologies for any apparent repetition: one of the features of a good lecture course is reinforcement of important concepts, facts and principles throughout the course.

I have tried to avoid producing yet another prescriptive guide to healthy eating. Rather I have aimed to discuss current issues in nutrition education in a critical way. These discussions are intended not only to indicate where the current consensus of scientific opinion lies but also to give a flavour of the reasoning and evidence that underpins these opinions and to highlight unresolved issues and alternative opinions. At the end of such discussions, I have tried to indicate realistic, low risk and consistent strategies for promoting health that have a high probability of producing holistic benefit. The book should therefore not be a vehicle just for transmitting factual information, but I hope it will stimulate readers to read further, to think and to criticise, and thus empower them to evaluate alternative views and make independent, rational decisions.

Geoffrey P. Webb

Acknowledgements

Two periods have been instrumental in equipping me even to attempt to write such a wide ranging text as this one. The first was a year's study leave spent in the Nutrition Department of King's College, London in 1986–87 and the second was a semester spent as a visiting professor in the College of Health, University of North Florida (UNF) in 1992. Many of the staff at both of these establishments have unknowingly contributed to this book by giving me the benefit of their knowledge, experience and opinions.

Many of my present colleagues at the University of East London (UEL) have also helped me by advising on topics that are outside my main areas of expertise, by criticising some of the things that I have written and by collaborating with me in nutrition research. Past and present students, both at UNF and UEL, have influenced what is written here by their comments in classes and by what they have written in their essays and dissertations. I should like to mention in particular: Dr Judy Rodriguez and Dr Simin Vaghefi from UNF; Dr Catherine Geissler, Dr Mike Nelson and Professor Donald Naismith from King's; Dr Paul Rogers, Dr Mike Jakobson, Dr Alun Morinan and Dr Dennis Hide from UEL; and Ms J Gatehouse (osteoporosis) and Mr C Taylor (fish oils) two of my project students at UEL.

I am also grateful to Sister Pearl Burnham, a nutrition nurse specialist at Oldchurch Hospital, Romford, Essex, for some useful discussion that gave me a practical insight that proved invaluable in writing Chapter 13. I should like to thank Mr Kevin Head from UEL who drew some of the diagrams and converted all of the rest into a uniform format. Mr Keith Eley from UEL drew several of the original diagrams for my previous papers that are reproduced here. I also gratefully acknowledge the support, encouragement and advice of Mr Richard Holloway from Edward Arnold. I am also grateful to Dr Diane Jakobson for helping to persuade me that I should write a nutrition text.

Several publishers have generously allowed me to reproduce material from their books and journals and these are specifically acknowledged in the text. I should, however, like to mention particularly the *Journal of Biological Education* (*JBE*), which is the source of several tables and figures reproduced from review articles that I have previously published in the journal. The *JBE* has provided me with an outlet for a series of discursive review articles upon which several sections of this text are based.

Finally and especially, I must acknowledge the support and encouragement of my family. My wife and daughter, in particular, have provided me with the will and the opportunity to spend long periods of my spare time writing. They have uncomplainingly made do with a part time father and husband during the preparation of this manuscript.

PART I
CONCEPTS AND PRINCIPLES

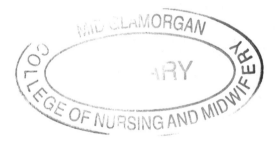

1 Introduction

Historical overview of changing priorities for nutrition education

Traditional priority – Adequacy

Scientific research into food and nutrition was initially directed towards identifying the essential nutrients, those that must be present in our diets if we are to remain healthy. In the first half of this century, many essential nutrients were identified and their ability to cure certain deficiency diseases was recognised, for example:

1 The B vitamin, niacin, was shown to cure the deficiency disease, pellagra, a disease that was so prevalent in some southern states of the USA in the early decades of this century that it was thought to be an infectious disease. Pellagra remained a problem in several southern states of America until the 1940s.

2 At the turn of the century, up to 75% of children in some British industrial cities suffered from the disease rickets, which was shown to be due to lack of vitamin D. Again, it was not until the 1940s that this disease was eradicated in British children.

3 The disease beriberi exacted a heavy toll of death and misery in the rice-eating countries of the Far East, well into the third quarter of this century. It was shown to be cured by thiamin, a B vitamin that is removed from white rice during the milling process.

Several of the Nobel prizes in Physiology and Medicine in this era were awarded for work on the vitamins – the prizes of 1929, 1934, and 1943. It was for the work on thiamin and beriberi, mentioned above, that Eijkman received the 1929 prize.

Such spectacular successes as these may have encouraged a "magic bullet" image of nutrition – the expectation that simple dietary changes may be able to prevent or cure diseases other than those due to nutrient deficiency. This is only true for a few, relatively uncommon, diseases where the symptoms are due to an inborn or acquired intolerance to a specific component of food. In these cases the symptoms can be controlled by avoidance of the offending substance, e.g. phenylketonuria (intolerance to the amino acid phenylalanine), galactosaemia (intolerance to the galactose component of milk sugar) and coeliac disease (intolerance to a protein found in wheat and some other cereals).

The traditional priority in nutrition has been to ensure nutritional adequacy, to ensure that the diet contains adequate amounts of energy and the essential nutrients. To date, well over 30 essential nutrients have been identified as necessary to ensure dietary adequacy, namely:

- energy
- water
- protein and the essential amino acids
- essential fatty acids
- the vitamins
- and, the minerals.

In most cases, not only have these nutrients been identified, but also good estimates of average requirements have been made. Many governments and international agencies use these estimates of requirements to publish lists of dietary standards which can be used as yardsticks to test the adequacy of diets or food supplies. These standards, termed Recommended Dietary Allowances (RDAs) in the US and Dietary Reference Values (DRVs) in the UK are discussed fully in Chapter 3.

Adequacy was the traditional priority in all countries, and it remains the nutritional priority for the majority of the world population. Even today, dietary inadequacy is prevalent in many countries, so that:

- large sections of the world population still suffer from overt starvation
- a quarter of a million Asian children go blind each year due to lack of vitamin A
- many more people, especially children, suffer from less obvious consequences of suboptimal nutrition such as reduced

immunocompetence, impaired growth and development, slow wound healing and reduced strength and work capacity.

Fifty years ago, the quality of a diet would thus have been judged by its ability to supply all of the essential nutrients and to prevent nutritional inadequacy. Nowadays, in the wealthy industrialised countries of North America, Western Europe and Australasia, nutritional adequacy is almost taken for granted. This is because people who satisfy their energy needs and who eat a range of foods also generally satisfy at least their minimum requirements for the essential nutrients. Nutrient deficiencies only become likely if total food intake is restricted or if the range of foods that are available or acceptable is narrowed. In these industrialised countries, there is an almost limitless abundance of food and a year-round variety that would have astounded our ancestors.

Even the poor in these countries should obtain their minimum needs of the essential nutrients. Overt deficiency diseases are very uncommon in industrialised countries and are usually associated with some predisposing medical condition, or with alcoholism or drug addiction, or with extremes of social and economic disadvantage. Overnutrition, manifested most obviously by obesity, is far more common in such countries than all of the diseases of undernutrition.

Is long term adequacy assured in industrialised countries?

The assumption of adequacy in industrialised countries may be much more precarious than many of us fortunate enough to live in them would like to believe. War, for example, can precipitate food shortages and lead to a very rapid re-emergence of the diseases of undernutrition in a previously affluent and well-nourished population. This is strikingly illustrated by recent events in some areas of former Yugoslavia. Economic dislocation is having a similar effect in other parts of Eastern Europe. Wartime mass starvation in Holland and Germany are still recent enough to be within living memory. In Britain, during World War II there were considerable constraints placed upon the food supply by attacks on merchant shipping; paradoxically, because of effective food policy measures, these constraints upon food supply were associated with an apparent improvement in the nutritional health of the British population.

In the both the UK and US, average energy intakes of the population have fallen substantially in recent decades; presumably, this is a reflection of reduced energy expenditure caused by our increasingly sedentary lifestyle. This trend towards reduced energy intake (i.e. total food intake), coupled with a high proportion of energy being obtained from nutrient-depleted sugars, fats and alcoholic drinks, might well increase the likelihood of suboptimal nutrient intakes or perhaps even overt nutrient deficiencies in some groups like the elderly.

Nutrition as a means to health promotion or disease prevention

The priority of nutrition education in industrialised countries is now directed towards changing the "Western diet", with the aim of reducing the toll of diseases like cardiovascular disease, cancer, maturity onset diabetes, osteoporosis and dental disease. These diseases are variously known as the "Western diseases" or the "diseases of affluence/civilisation/industrialisation". As a population becomes more affluent then its life expectancy tends to increase and mortality from the infectious diseases, particularly amongst children, falls. In contrast, these degenerative "diseases of industrialisation" become more prevalent in adults and account for an increasing proportion of death and illness.

There is an almost unanimous assumption that these diseases of industrialisation are environmentally triggered, i.e. due to the "Western lifestyle". This assumption leads to the widespread belief that major improvements in health and longevity can be achieved by simple modifications of lifestyle. Diet is one of the environmental variables that has received much attention in recent years and poor diet has been blamed for contributing to the relatively poor health record of some affluent groups. Of the top ten leading causes of death in the USA, eight have been associated with nutritional causes or excessive alcohol consumption. Numerous expert committees in several industrialised countries have suggested dietary modifications that they consider would reduce or delay mortality and morbidity from these diseases of industrialisation and thus ultimately lead to increases in life expectancy and enhanced health-quality of life. These recommendations usually include advice to reduce consumption of fats, sugar, alcohol and perhaps salt and to replace them with starchy and fibre-rich foods. A good diet today thus not only satisfies the criterion of adequacy but also meets other compositional objectives set by expert committees which are aimed at reducing morbidity and mortality from the diseases of industrialisation.

Dietary intervention for health promotion

Much current nutrition research is directed towards relating individual components of the diet to individual diseases or even disease risk markers like high serum cholesterol and high blood pressure. This approach is justified by the expectation that it will rapidly furnish those involved in promoting health with information about changes in dietary practices that might lead to disease prevention. In the longer term, this is expected to result in reduced morbidity and increased longevity. The practical result of this approach, however, is a profusion of papers in the medical and scientific literature cataloguing a series of suggested associations between individual dietary or other environmental variables and individual causes of mortality, morbidity or disease risk markers. The sheer number of such reported associations is sometimes bewildering, and this bewilderment may be compounded because there are, more often than not, contradictory reports. As an example, a staggering 250 risk markers have been reported for coronary heart disease (McCormick and Skrabanek, 1988).

A major problem that will inevitably confront those involved in health promotion or nutrition education will be to decide whether and how to act upon the latest reported association between a dietary factor (or indeed any other alterable environmental variable) and a disease. These individual associations will also frequently be relayed to the general public through brief summaries, often sensationalised and distorted, prepared by the health correspondents of the media. Health conscious members of the public may then try to decide upon the optimal diet and lifestyle on the basis of such snippets – this is rather like trying to work out the picture on a huge jigsaw puzzle by reading inaccurate and incomplete descriptions of some of the individual pieces.

Quite a number of these individual associations are discussed and evaluated in this book. In such discussions there are two broad aims:

1 to indicate to the reader where the current consensus of scientific opinion lies, to give a flavour of the reasoning and evidence underpinning that position and also to highlight unresolved issues and/or alternative opinions

2 to indicate diet and lifestyle patterns or modifications that are realistic, low risk, consistent and likely to produce overall health benefits.

Are recommendations to alter diet and lifestyle offered too freely?

A drug or a food additive intended for use by vast numbers of apparently healthy people would be subject to an extremely rigorous and highly structured evaluation of both its efficacy and safety. Despite this, mistakes still occur and drugs or additives have to be withdrawn after sometimes many years of use. Compared to this rigorous approval procedure, some dietary and lifestyle interventions seem to be advocated on the basis of incomplete appraisal of either efficacy or safety – perhaps, on occasion, almost casually. Even properly constituted expert committees may make premature judgements based upon incomplete or incorrect evidence. There will also be a plethora of advice from those whose actions are prompted by belief in an untenable theory or myth (quackery), by political or ethical prejudice or even by economic or other self interest.

There are clear legal frameworks regulating the licensing of drugs and food additives, yet there is not, nor can there realistically be, any restrictions on the offering of dietary or lifestyle advice. All that governments and professional bodies can do is to try to ensure that there is some system of registration or accreditation so that those seeking or offered advice have some means of checking the credentials of the would-be adviser.

The author's perception is thus that there is a tendency for dietary or lifestyle intervention to be advocated before rigorous appraisal has been satisfactorily completed. This is probably because of the implicit assumption that such interventions are innocuous and that if they do no good then nor will they do any harm. Intervention, rather than non intervention, therefore becomes almost automatically regarded as the safer option – "If dietary change can't hurt and might help, why not make it?" Hamilton *et al.* (1991).

Simple changes in diet or lifestyle can't do any harm?

The assumption that dietary, or other lifestyle, interventions are inevitably harmless seems logically inconsistent with the notion of diet and lifestyle as major causes of ill-health. If dietary changes are capable of producing large changes in morbidity and mortality then there must be the potential to do harm as well as great good. It should also be borne in mind that even if unjustified intervention does not do direct physiological harm, it may have important social, psychological or economic repercussions. Social and psychological factors have traditionally been the dominant influences on food selection and any ill-considered intervention risks causing anxiety, cultural impoverishment and social and family tensions. It has been suggested that the resources spent on unjustified health education interventions may serve only to induce a morbid preoccupation with death (McCormick and Skrabanek, 1988). Major changes in food selection practices will also have economic repercussions, perhaps disrupting the livelihoods of many people and thus adversely affecting their quality of life.

Repeated changes of mind and shifts of emphasis by health educators are also liable to undermine their credibility and thereby increase public resistance to future campaigns. Even many relatively young consumers in industrialised countries will have noticed marked changes in the dietary advice they are given, away from advice whose priority was to ensure nutritional adequacy and towards using food as a means to wellness or health promotion. These changes in emphasis often reflect changing social conditions and consumption patterns but some may be justifiably perceived as evidence of the inconsistency and thus unreliability of expert advice. The examples below may serve to illustrate this latter point.

1 Obesity was once blamed upon excessive consumption of high carbohydrate foods, like bread and potatoes. These foods would have been strictly regulated in any weight-reducing diet. Bread and potatoes are now viewed much more positively by nutritionists as foods rich in complex carbohydrate and fibre; consumers are recommended to incorporate more of these into their diets to make them bulkier (i.e. to reduce the energy density), which may in turn reduce the likelihood of excessive energy intake and thus of obesity.

2 The weight of scientific opinion supporting nutritional guidelines aimed at lowering serum cholesterol concentrations has now been increasing for more than three decades. Although this cholesterol-lowering objective may have remained constant, there have been several subtle shifts of opinion as to the best dietary means to achieve this goal:

   • reducing dietary cholesterol was once considered an important factor in serum cholesterol-lowering; it is now usually given low priority
   • a wholesale switch from saturated to the omega-6 type of polyunsaturated fats prevalent in many vegetable oils was once advocated, but is no longer
   • monounsaturated fats were once considered neutral in their effects upon serum cholesterol but are now much more positively regarded, accounting for the current healthy image of olive oil and rapeseed (canola) oil
   • the omega-3 type of polyunsaturated fatty acids have also been viewed much more positively in

recent years, especially the long chain acids omega-3 polyunsaturates found predominantly in fish oils

- the current emphasis of both UK and US recommendations is to aim for a reduction in total fat intake, with a proportionately greater reduction in the saturated fraction of dietary fat.

Attitudes to some individual foods could be strongly affected by such changes of emphasis. This is illustrated in Table 1.1; certain fatty foods come out very differently in a "worst" to "best" rank order when cholesterol content, total fat content, saturated fat content or ratio of polyunsaturated to saturated fatty acids (P:S ratio) are used as the criteria. Sunflower oil comes out at the top of the rankings if total fat content is the criterion but at or near the bottom if cholesterol content, P:S ratio or saturated fat content is used. Eggs and liver are worst by the cholesterol criterion but around half way down by all other criteria. Prawns are at the bottom for all criteria except cholesterol content; they are also relatively rich in the now positively regarded long chain, omega-3 polyunsaturated fatty acids.

Examples of past interventions that are now less fashionable

In the light of the above discussion, it would seem prudent to regard any proposed dietary or lifestyle intervention as potentially harmful until this possibility has been actively considered and, as far as possible, eliminated. Below are some examples that may serve to demonstrate that this is a real possibility rather than just a theoretical one.

Prone sleeping position for infants

During the 1970s and much of the 1980s a prone sleeping position for infants was recommended by health professionals in the UK rather than the traditional supine one. This recommendation arose because of observations of benefits in premature babies, especially those with respiratory problems, when they were placed in the prone position. There is now evidence that this prone sleeping position may be associated with increased risk of cot death (Engelberts and de Jonge, 1990; Dwyer *et al.*, 1991) and a return to the traditional supine sleeping position has now been officially

Table 1.1 Rank orders by different fat-related criteria of some foods. Ranks are from 1 "worst" to 14 "best" (after Webb, 1992a)

Food	% energy as fat	% energy sat. fat	cholesterol content	P:S ratio
Liver	11	8	2	8
Lean steak	12	9=	6	4
Cheddar cheese	7	2	7	2=
Butter	1=	1	3	2=
Polyunsaturated margarine	1=	6	10=	13
Low fat spread	1=	4	10=	10
Sunflower oil	1=	11	10=	14
Milk	9=	3	9	1
Human milk	9=	5	8	5
Chicken meat	13	12=	5	7
Avocado	5	12=	10=	9
Peanuts	6	9=	10=	11
Egg	8	7	1	6
Prawns	14	14	4	12

recommended in the UK. In early 1993, the UK Department of Health released figures that showed a dramatic decline in cot deaths in 1992 (Bignall, 1993). This decline has been widely attributed to campaigns aimed at persuading parents to revert to the traditional sleeping position for infants. The authors of an official UK expert report (DH, 1993) concluded that the prone sleeping position is associated with a 3 to 8 fold increase in risk of cot death. A government minister was quoted as claiming that this recent decline in infant deaths illustrated the benefits of health education:

> The figures on cot deaths show that behaviour change can work, can save lives.
> *The Daily Telegraph* 30/3/93

What these figures even more obviously demonstrate, however, are the potential dangers of prematurely advocating changes in lifestyle before the assumption that these changes will promote health has been thoroughly evaluated. The current "success", if indeed it is really attributable to a reversion to the traditional sleeping position, has merely been to reverse the damage done by the earlier, ill-considered and insufficiently tested advice to change the traditional sleeping position.

If one is seeking to justify intervention for a whole population then it is not enough merely to demonstrate that a specific group will benefit from the proposed change. Intervention with a relatively small sample of "high risk" subjects is likely to exaggerate the benefits of intervention for the population as a whole. Such small scale intervention will also only show up the grossest of harmful effects. It may thus fail to show up harmful effects that could be very significant for indiscriminate intervention and which might cancel out or even exceed any benefits of the intervention.

Lowering serum cholesterol concentrations

As already stated, diets containing very large amounts of polyunsaturated fatty acids were widely advocated as a means of lowering serum cholesterol concentrations. Short term experiments had demonstrated very convincingly that switching from high saturated to high polyunsaturated fat diets could reduce serum cholesterol concentrations in young men (e.g. Keys *et al.*, 1959). However, there was no convincing evidence that, in the long term, such a wholesale switch from saturated to polyunsaturated fat produced any increase in life expectancy, even in studies using "high risk" subjects. There have recently been suggestions that very high intakes of polyunsaturated fatty acids may be associated with increased cancer risk and may have some adverse effects on blood lipoprotein profiles (see Chapter 9 for details).

Britons are currently advised to limit their individual intakes of omega-6 polyunsaturated fatty acids to no more than 10% of energy, with a population average of 6% (COMA, 1991).

Reducing a symptomless risk marker, such as serum cholesterol concentration, cannot, in itself, be taken as evidence of benefit. There must be evidence that such reduction in the risk marker will lead to the predicted decrease in disease risk and also that there will not be an accompanying increase in some other risk.

Protein deficiency

In the 1950s and 1960s, protein deficiency was thought to be the most prevalent and serious form of worldwide malnutrition. It was considered likely that "in many parts of the world the majority of young children suffer some protein malnutrition" (Trowell, 1959). Very considerable efforts and resources were committed to alleviating this perceived problem. However, as estimates of human protein requirements were revised downwards, it then seemed probable that primary protein deficiency was likely to be uncommon and thus that the resources committed to alleviating widespread protein deficiency were largely wasted (Webb, 1989). See Chapter 8 for further discussion.

Even though the provision of extra protein was probably not, in itself, harmful, scarce resources were committed to a non-beneficial measure and other, more real, problems deprived of resources. In the current edition of both the US (NRC, 1989a), and UK dietary standards (COMA, 1991), the possibility that high intakes of protein might even be directly harmful is acknowledged and an upper limit of twice the dietary standard is advised.

Resources for research, development, international aid and educational programmes are always finite. If these resources are diverted into unnecessary measures or programmes based upon false theories, then, inevitably, worthwhile projects will be deprived of funding.

Iron supplements

These were once routinely and almost universally prescribed for pregnant women in the UK. These supplements were considered necessary because of the perception that the risks of anaemia in pregnancy were very high, a perception that was compounded by the misinterpretation of the normal decline in blood haemoglobin concentration during pregnancy as pathological. In the UK, routine iron supplements in pregnancy are now thought to be unnecessary. The UK panel on Dietary Reference Values (COMA, 1991) suggest that, for most women, the extra iron demands of pregnancy can be met by utilisation of maternal stores and physiological adaptation.

Iron supplements are well known as causing unpleasant short term gastrointestinal side-effects, although there is no evidence that they cause any lasting harm to mothers or babies. Note, however, that iron poisoning was the second most common cause of accidental poisoning in children in the UK. One indirect side effect of this intervention was increased exposure of children to risk of accidental poisoning.

Note that in the latest US dietary standards (NRC, 1989a) universal iron supplementation is still recommended for pregnant women.

Vitamin K

It has been common practice in many maternity units in the UK routinely to inject newborn babies with vitamin K. This vitamin K reduces the risk of postnatal brain haemorrhage that affects some babies, particularly premature babies. The measured vitamin K status of newborn babies has also been found to be low. The recent report of the UK panel on Dietary Reference Values (COMA, 1991) supported the proposition that vitamin K should be given prophylactically to all newborn babies. However, there has recently been a cautious, but highly publicised, suggestion that these vitamin K injections may be associated with a doubling of the risk of childhood cancer (Golding et al., 1992).

In an editorial in the *British Medical Journal* (Hull, 1992) it was suggested that this reported association between vitamin K and childhood cancer should be investigated more thoroughly before current practice is changed. Sometimes such commendable caution seems to be less obvious when the *status quo* is non intervention rather than intervention. In this work of Golding et al. no association was found between orally administered vitamin K and cancer risk. A recent very large

Swedish survey found no difference in cancer rates in children given vitamin K by the oral or intramuscular routes (Ekelund *et al.*, 1993). The pendulum of evidence appears to have swung back to the safety of vitamin K injections, at least as compared to orally administered vitamin K.

These five examples have been selected to try to illustrate that once very popular dietary or lifestyle interventions may in later years become regarded as unnecessary or perhaps even harmful. The eventual outcome of each debate will not alter their demonstration of how scientific opinion about the value and safety of such interventions fluctuates.

If a holistic view is taken then it is likely that any intervention that produces no benefits will have some detrimental effects even though this may not involve direct physiological harm. Majority support amongst scientists and health professionals for intervention based upon a particular theory is no guarantee that it will continue to be regarded as useful or even safe.

Those involved in health promotion and nutrition education need to be constructively critical of current fashions. They need to be receptive to criticism of current wisdom and objective in the evaluation of such criticism. They need to be cautious about advocating mass intervention especially if there is no convincing, direct evidence of long term benefit or where evidence of benefit is restricted to a relatively small "high risk" group. Any non beneficial intervention should be regarded as almost inevitably detrimental.

Criteria to judge whether intervention is justified (after Webb, 1992a)

Evidence linking diet and disease seldom materialises in complete and unequivocal form overnight. More usually, it accumulates gradually over a period of years, with a high probability that some of the evidence will be conflicting. The problem of deciding when evidence is sufficient to warrant intervention is thus one that will frequently need to be faced. If action is initiated too soon then there is a risk of costly and potentially harmful errors. If action is too slow then the potential benefits of change may be unduly delayed.

There is likely to be intense pressure to take action or to issue guidelines in the light of the latest highly publicised research findings. Below is a set of criteria that might be used to decide whether any particular intervention is justified by available knowledge:

1 Have clear and realistic dietary objectives been set and have all foreseeable aspects of their likely impact considered?
2 Is there strong evidence that a large proportion of the population or target group will gain significant benefits from the proposed change?
3 Has there been active and adequate consideration of whether the intended change, or any consequential change, might have adverse effects on a significant number of people?
4 Have the evaluations of risk and benefit been made holistically?

A reduction in a disease risk marker, or even reduced incidence of a particular disease, are not ends in themselves; the ultimate criterion of success must be a net improvement in the quantity or quality of life, i.e. increased life expectancy or reduced total morbidity. Likewise evaluation of risk should not be confined to possible direct physiological harm but should also include, for example, economic, psychological or social repercussions. It should also include the possibly harmful effects of any consequential changes and consider the damage ineffective intervention might have on the future credibility of nutrition education and health promotion.

5 Has the possibility of targeting intervention to likely gainers been fully explored so as to maximise the benefits to risks ratio?

6 Has consideration been given to how the desired change can be implemented with the minimum intrusion into the chosen lifestyle and cuisine of the target group?

Intervention that precedes satisfactory consideration of the risks and benefits of intervention is experimentation and not health education.

Such criteria are probably not, in themselves, controversial; it is in deciding when these criteria have been satisfactorily fulfilled or even whether they have been properly considered that the controversy arises.

Judging whether these intervention criteria have been fulfilled

There are several levels of critical questioning that should be undertaken and satisfactorily answered before any report of an association between a dietary variable and a disease or disease risk marker can be said to satisfy these criteria and is thus ready to be translated into practical health promotion advice, for example:

- Is the reported association likely to be genuine?
- Is the association likely to represent cause and effect?
- What change in dietary composition is realistically achievable and what magnitude of benefit is this predicted to produce?
- Is this predicted benefit sufficient to warrant intervention – at the population level – at the individual level?
- Are there any foreseeable risks from the proposed compositional change for any group within the target population?
- Are there any foreseeable non-nutritional adverse consequences of these changes?

- What changes in other nutrient intakes are likely to occur as a result of the proposed advice?
- Are there any foreseeable risks from these consequential changes?
- How can the desired compositional change be brought about?

Is the association genuine?

The decision about what weight to attach to any suggested association between diet and disease will depend upon quality assessment of individual reports. It is quite possible that an apparent association may have arisen because of bias in the study or simply by chance. There is often a range of papers reporting conflicting findings; these need to be evaluated and weighted rather than the latest or the majority view being mechanically accepted. It is quite possible that a common logical flaw, incorrect assumption or methodological error is present in all of the papers supporting one side of an argument.

Easterbrook *et al.* (1992) reported that, in clinical research, positive results are more likely to be published than negative findings. This not only means that the literature may not give an entirely balanced view of total research findings, but also encourages authors to highlight positive findings. In another analysis Ravnskov (1992) reported that, when citation rates were determined for papers dealing with cholesterol lowering trials, then those with positive outcomes (i.e. suggesting a beneficial effect on coronary heart disease) were cited six times more frequently than those with negative outcomes. Thus at the author, peer review, editorial selection and citation level there may be bias towards positive over negative findings.

The meaning of statistical significance also needs to be considered; significance at, or below, the 5% level is, by convention, taken as the point at which a scientist can claim that say a correlation or a difference between two means is "statistically significant". Significance at this level means that there is less than a one in 20 probability that the correlation or difference between the means has arisen simply by chance. This statistically significant difference or association may simply reflect flaws or bias in the design of the experiment, in the allocation of subjects or in the measurement of variables. Given a large number of investigators all correlating numerous lifestyle and dietary variables, with many health variables then it is also inevitable that some statistically significant associations will arise simply by chance. Significance at the 5% level is not proof of the underlying theory, merely an indication that any difference or association is unlikely to be due to pure chance – this should be borne in mind when evaluating isolated reports of improbable sounding associations. This may be particularly important if there is an onus upon authors to highlight positive results.

Much dietary advice will be based upon the conclusions of reviewers of the literature or expert committees but, as the examples cited earlier demonstrate, even apparent consensus amongst experts does not guarantee the long term future of a particular position or theory; there was once almost unanimous belief in a crisis of world protein supply but few would support this view today. Scientists are trained to make objective judgements based solely upon experimental and observational evidence. Scientists are also fallible human beings and thus their judgements may, on occasion, perhaps unwittingly, be affected by prejudice, political or peer pressure and self-interest. Reviewers and committee members will often be selected because of their active involvement, and thus expertise, in a particular field of study. This may sometimes hamper their objectivity especially when they are required to evaluate material that questions current wisdom and the *status quo*; their reputation or even their career prospects may be dependent upon that *status quo* being maintained. It is probably unreasonable to expect total objectivity when asking someone to choose between material that may undermine or support their own work and reputation, or to evaluate material that might even jeopardise their own career or research funding. McLaren (1974) tried to identify some of the reasons for the now discredited concept of a world protein crisis or protein gap, and for its persistence. As early as 1966, when this theory was still at its height, he suggested that many scientists had privately expressed sympathy with his opposition to the theory and some of the consequential measures designed to alleviate the perceived crisis. He also claimed that they were unwilling to support him publicly for fear of having their research funding withdrawn. He even suggested that critical discussion of the issues was suppressed.

The health educator will thus need to make his or her own quality judgements about conclusions drawn from data presented in the literature; this requires some basic understanding of research methodology. I have made a conscious decision to include a substantial section on nutrition research methods, even though the bulk of readers are unlikely to be aiming for research careers. Those readers who consider themselves to be interested only in the practice of promoting health and who have little likelihood of being actively involved in research projects may be tempted to regard some of this section devoted to methodology as marginal, or even superfluous, to their needs. But a general appreciation of the research methodology, the strengths, limitations and weaknesses of the various methods, is essential for any critical reading and evaluation of the literature. Anyone who wishes to keep up to date with the literature and to be able to make quality judgements about conflicting evidence, or controversial new reports, will need some basic understanding of the methodology.

Is the association causal?

Epidemiological methods produce evidence of associations between diseases and suggested causes but even strong evidence of association does not necessarily mean that the association is due to a cause and effect relationship; association may be purely coincidental and due to some confounding variable. Changes in exposure to putative risk factors tend not to occur in isolation: often many changes in dietary and other environmental variables occur concurrently. Increasing affluence and industrialisation tend to bring with them numerous changes in diet, lifestyle and environment, as well as major changes in the patterns of morbidity and mortality, i.e. reduced mortality from infectious diseases, increased life expectancy but increased prevalence of the "diseases of industrialisation". An association between one of these diseases of industrialisation and one of the wealth-related environmental variables needs to be treated with extreme caution until there is substantial evidence to support this association being causal. In many epidemiological studies, results will be "corrected" for confounding variables, but there is no statistical magic wand that unfailingly eliminates confounding effects. It is a matter of judgement as to what confounders are corrected for, and the process of adjustment is itself liable to error, particularly if information on the confounding variable is imprecise (Leon, 1993). This problem of confounding variables is discussed more fully in Chapter 3, along with some tests that may be applied to help decide whether any particular association is causal.

Realistically achievable change – magnitude of benefit?

Once one has satisfactorily established that a cause and effect relationship exists between a dietary factor and a disease, then one should be able to predict the general magnitude of benefit that is likely to result from any given change. To take a straightforward example, if it is accepted that there is a direct linear relationship between the average blood pressure of adult populations and their average daily salt consumption then it is relatively easy to predict the reduction in average blood pressure that would result from a specific change in average salt consumption. Then, making certain assumptions, one can go on to predict by how much the incidence of hypertension will fall and thence the beneficial effects on mortality from the hypertension-related diseases (see Chapter 11 for further discussion of this example). It is, however, of limited value to predict huge health gains for a population if the dietary changes necessary to bring them about are, in practice, unrealistic. Thus one might predict that a fall in average UK daily salt consumption from around 10 g to the 1 g seen in Kalahari Bushmen or certain New Guinea highlanders might eradicate hypertension and produce major reductions in mortality from hypertension-related diseases. However, there is, of course, no possible chance that a change of this magnitude can be achieved.

Expert committees on both sides of the Atlantic have concluded that very major health benefits would accrue if the proportion of total energy derived from fat were to be reduced from a population average of around 40% to around 30% (e.g. NACNE, 1983) or less (NRC, 1989b). Whilst such a change may be readily achievable by small numbers of highly motivated and well educated individuals, is it a realistic goal for the population as a whole? According to Passmore and Eastwood (1986), fat provided 38% of total energy in Britain in the period 1934–1938 but, as a result of wartime shortages and rationing, this figure fell gradually in the following years to reach a minimum of 33% in 1947. Passmore and Eastwood discuss the widespread discontent that this relatively small reduction in fat consumption caused. They concluded that although this wartime diet contained much more fat than was strictly necessary, it was, nonetheless, unpalatable to British tastes and did not satisfy the social and cultural demands for fat in the diet.

This is not a good omen for hopes of bringing average fat consumption down to 30% or less of total energy. It is likely to be a difficult task to persuade an unrestricted population voluntarily to consume a diet in peacetime that is even lower in fat than the partly imposed wartime diet that caused so much discontent. Despite the apparent increase in diet consciousness of the British population over the last two decades there has been no significant reduction in the proportion of dietary energy that is derived from fat (COMA, 1984; Chesher, 1989; MAFF, 1993). Experience would further suggest that those most refractory to change are likely to be those perceived to be most likely to benefit from the change. Young women from the upper social groups are more likely to respond than young and middle-aged working class men, and yet, the latter would be predicted to have much more to gain than the former. Thus Gregory *et al.* (1990) found that British women were more likely than men to choose food items with a "healthy image", such as low fat milks, salad vegetables, fruit and wholemeal bread, but less likely than men to choose sausages, meat pies, chips (french fries) and fried white fish. Social class differences in food selection are discussed under economics in Chapter 2.

Is intervention justified? At what level?

Even when there is clear evidence of a causal association between a dietary factor and a disease then it may still be difficult to decide whether this justifies intervention at the population level. Taking the extreme cases: if a minor dietary change could produce a major reduction in the risk of a common fatal disease then the case for intervention would appear strong; if a major dietary change was only predicted to reduce marginally the risk of a relatively uncommon disease then clearly population level intervention would not be justified. In between these extremes, the significance or "cost" of the proposed change will need to be balanced against the predicted reduction in population risk.

Even where likely benefit cannot justify intervention at the population level, if those who are particularly "at risk" or who are particularly susceptible to the causal factor can be identified then this may justify intervention for those high risk groups. The decision as to whether to advocate either individual or population level intervention may not always be clear cut.

There is widespread agreement that, at least for young and middle-aged males, a high serum cholesterol concentration is predictive of an increased risk of premature death from coronary heart disease (CHD). Figure 1.1 shows that for one population of American men, mortality risk for CHD approximately doubles for a doubling of the serum cholesterol concentration. It is widely assumed that lowering of serum cholesterol will result in a corresponding reduction in CHD risk. Figure 1.2 shows that there are relatively few men in this population with very highly elevated serum cholesterol levels, and so restricting cholesterol-lowering efforts to these high risk subjects can only have limited impact upon population mortality from CHD. A major proportion of the population risk of CHD, that is attributed to an elevated serum cholesterol concentration, is accounted for by the very large numbers of individuals whose serum cholesterol, and thus also their individual risk of CHD, is only slightly to moderately elevated. A small reduction in individual risk for this large group is much more significant, in population terms, than a bigger reduction in individual risk for the relatively few men

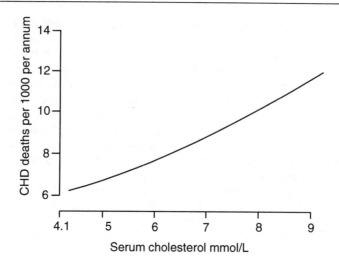

Figure 1.1 The relationship between serum cholesterol concentration and subsequent death rate from coronary heart disease in a sample of American men Source: Webb, G.P. (1992a) *Journal of Biological Education* 26(4), 270. After NACNE (1983)

at the upper extremes of the range. Such arguments have led to the conclusion that if population mortality from CHD is to be significantly reduced then the nutritional guidelines, aimed at cholesterol-lowering, have to be directed at the whole population, with a view to shifting the population distribution for cholesterol (Figure 1.2) downwards. Many individuals are therefore being advised to make major dietary changes despite it being acknowledged that even the theoretical benefits for them (i.e. individual risk reduction) may be calculated as small.

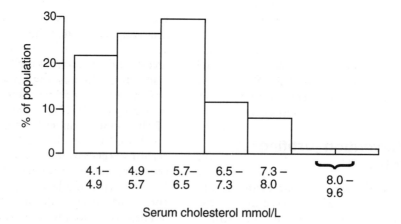

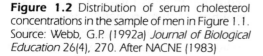

Figure 1.2 Distribution of serum cholesterol concentrations in the sample of men in Figure 1.1. Source: Webb, G.P. (1992a) *Journal of Biological Education* 26(4), 270. After NACNE (1983)

Harmful effects of intervention?

The ultimate aim of dietary intervention is to reduce total morbidity and to increase life expectancy. When considering a dietary intervention aimed at reducing the risk of one disease then the possibility that this may have other deleterious effects has to be actively considered and tested. Simple dietary or lifestyle interventions cannot be assumed to be inevitably risk-free; if such intervention is considered powerful enough to produce major positive changes in health, then clearly the possibility of negative effects must also be real. By analogy, the more potent a drug is then the greater is the likelihood of unwanted side-effects.

Several possible examples of simple dietary or lifestyle interventions having unexpected harmful effects have been discussed earlier in the chapter. Harmful social, psychological, economic or cultural repercussions are likely even where no direct physiological harm results from unjustified intervention. Non beneficial intervention will, at the very least, ultimately undermine the credibility of future nutrition education programmes.

Returning to the decision about cholesterol-lowering guidelines, some recent reports suggest that very low cholesterol levels may be associated with increased total mortality. Coronary heart disease mortality is low in subjects with very low cholesterol levels but there is a rise in mortality from other causes, including most cancers (Neaton *et al.*,1992; Jacobs *et al.*, 1992). One explanation is that a fall in serum cholesterol concentration is an early indication of existing, but undiagnosed disease. The other, more disturbing conclusion, would be that low serum cholesterol levels are causally linked to some of these diseases. If the very low serum cholesterol is simply a marker for existing disease then one would expect the association to diminish and disappear as the duration of follow up was increased. According to Neaton *et al.* (1992), the inverse association between serum cholesterol level and most cancers remained even after a 12 year follow up period.

If low cholesterol level is causally linked to these diseases then cholesterol-lowering interventions that are aimed at the whole population will presumably tend to increase the total mortality of people with low serum cholesterol and also tend to push some individuals into the "danger-zone" at the low end of the range. Hulley *et al.* (1992) argue that this rise in total mortality at low levels of serum cholesterol indicates the need for a change of cholesterol policy in the US. They suggested that, until the association between low blood cholesterol and non coronary heart disease mortality has been clarified, then cholesterol screening and intervention should be limited to that minority of the population for whom the benefits from reduced risk of coronary heart disease clearly predominate over the detraction. They argue against attempts at universal cholesterol-lowering and they specifically warn against cholesterol screening and intervention efforts directed towards children and women because "the overriding ethical obligation is to do no harm".

What are the secondary consequences of change?

Dietary changes almost never occur in isolation. Changing the diet to produce an intended change will almost inevitably affect the intake of other nutrients. When dietary changes are to be advocated then the likely impact of the intended change upon the total diet should be considered. If reduced intake of a particular food or nutrient is advised then how are the intakes of other nutrients likely to be affected and what is likely to replace the missing food? If increased intake of particular foods is advised then what will the preferred foods displace from the existing diet?

For example, if food manufacturers are persuaded to use less salt in processing then what effect will this have on shelf-life and therefore on cost and availability of foods? Will it compromise the microbiological safety of foods? Or, will it lead to increased reliance on other preservatives whose long term safety may also be questioned?

What secondary consequences would be expected from reducing consumption of dairy fats? Will it affect vitamin A intake (present in milk fat)? Will it lead to reduced intake of the non fat components of milk and the associated nutrients, e.g. calcium and riboflavin? Or, will it result in high consumption of "weak" tasting skimmed milk and thus significantly increased protein intake?

How can the desired change be effected?

It is a relatively straightforward matter to devise diets or plan menus that meet any particular set of compositional criteria. It is a much more difficult task to produce diets or menus that are acceptable to the recipients as well as meeting the therapeutic compositional criteria. It is, for example, very easy to produce adequate diets that are low in calories, yet long term dietary treatment of obesity is notoriously unsuccessful. It seems reasonable to expect that diets or dietary recommendations that are devised with due regard to, and in sympathy with, the beliefs, preferences and usual selection practices of the recipients, will fare better than those that ignore the non-nutritional influences on food selection or try to impose the prejudices and preferences of the adviser.

Food has a host of cultural, psychological and social functions in addition to its biological function. It is these non-nutritional uses that have traditionally been the dominant influences upon our food selection. If we lose sight of these functions in the perhaps fruitless pursuit of the optimal chemical diet, then any technical improvements in our nutrition may be outweighed, or at least reduced, by damage to the general emotional health of the population. Miserable, anxious people will probably suffer more illnesses and die younger than happy contented people.

Chapter 2 is devoted to a brief but wide-ranging discussion of some of these non-nutritional influences upon food selection. If one is seeking to effect change in eating behaviour then one must try to understand the reasons and reasoning behind food selection practices. Only then can one endeavour to seek practical measures that will bring about the compositional changes that are considered desirable in a way that is compatible with the overall cultural milieu of the target group. The aim of nutrition education should be to effect the maximum change in the desired direction with the least possible interference, i.e. a cultural conservationist approach. This is the approach most likely to succeed and there are also strong ethical grounds for suggesting such an approach.

Factors influencing the likelihood of dietary change

Fieldhouse (1986) listed certain parameters that will particularly influence the likelihood of dietary change occurring, namely:

- the perceived advantage of change and its observability
- its compatibility with existing beliefs, cultural values and culinary style
- its complexity
- its trialability.

Advantage of change and the observability of that advantage

If one is seeking to persuade someone to change their diet to cure a deficiency disease then the benefits can be demonstrated readily in others who have made the recommended change. The benefits to the individual will also rapidly become apparent once the change has been tried. In such cases, the short term advantages of benefit may be very great, they are readily observable and often the disadvantages of change may be very small.

The benefits of many of the health-promoting dietary changes currently recommended by expert committees are often difficult to demonstrate at the individual level and in the short term. There may also be a significant and vociferous minority of experts who question even the long term beneficial effects of some of these recommendations. Many of the dietary recommendations for health promotion are designed to produce significant long term reductions in the population risk of death and disease, and the individual may only be offered a relatively small reduction in his or her individual risk of suffering from some disease at some seemingly distant date. Most people will also see anecdotal examples of people who have confounded the population level statistics, i.e. flagrant violators of current nutrition education guidelines who have lived long and healthy lives and other who conversely have eaten healthily but died young. The benefits of change, for any individual, are therefore only putative and they are not even readily observable in others.

There may be ways of improving the observability of positive benefits or there may be more short term positive effects of intervention that could be better highlighted by health educators. The benefits of moderating dietary fat intake in reducing the long term risk of cardiovascular disease may be difficult to demonstrate, but reducing fat consumption as an aid to weight control is one possible short term observable benefit that could be highlighted. It might also be argued that feedback could be improved by the regular monitoring of serum cholesterol concentration but, as McCormick and Skrabanek (1988) argue, such focusing upon symptomless risk markers may serve to only to induce an unjustified and morbid pre-occupation with death. Health and fitness promotion is a very positive sounding objective, death delaying has a much more negative ring to it; nutrition education must be presented and implemented in ways that emphasise the former objectives rather than unnecessarily increasing fear of, and preoccupation with, death and disease.

The disadvantages of change may, unlike the benefits of change, be immediately all too apparent. Cholesterol-lowering advice may be perceived as requiring major reductions in the consumption of meat and dairy produce. These are high prestige and high flavour foods that are central to the culinary practices and the food ideology of most Western consumers – they may even be modern examples of "cultural superfoods" (see Chapter 2). Meat may have a particularly strong cultural significance to men because of the masculine image of red meat consumption. Cholesterol-lowering advice is more likely to be widely followed if the apparent costs of change can be reduced by giving advice like: buy leaner cuts of meat; trim off visible fat; grill (broil) rather than fry. Promoting simple modifications of existing practices that involve relatively little "cost" for the consumer may produce more real change than advocating much more ambitious and drastic changes that will be implemented by relatively few people. See the examples in the Appendix.

Compatibility with existing beliefs, cultural values and culinary style

Advice is more likely to be implemented if it is compatible with existing beliefs and practices. Advising Jews or Muslims to eat pork for protein or advising vegetarians to eat liver for iron and B_{12} would be obvious examples of advice that is incompatible. Advising working class British and American men to cut out beef as a means of reducing saturated fat intake may be an example of a piece of advice that, although less obvious, is probably just as incompatible with existing beliefs and practices.

Complexity

The easier it is to understand and implement a proposed change then the more likely it is to be accepted. Advising increased consumption of certain pulses that require quite elaborate processing in order to cook, detoxify and flavour them is likely to have limited impact. Frying in oil instead of lard is a simple measure that has relatively little effect on palatability or convenience – it has thus been widely implemented in the UK, partly accounting for the large rise in the ratio of polyunsaturated to saturated fatty acids in the British diet in recent decades.

Trialling

People are more likely to try something that can be experimented with on a limited basis than they are to try something that initially requires more major commitment. There are many examples of dietary interventions that can readily be tried such as switching from butter to margarine and cooking with vegetable oil rather than animal fats. Fluoridation of water supplies is one obvious example of a change that is not readily trialled. Some factors that may reduce the likelihood of

trialling are: if the change involves significant extra expenditure on ingredients or utensils; if it requires the learning of a new method of preparation or more elaborate preparation; or if the change requires a period of adjustment. People may, for example, get used to food cooked without added salt but in order to adjust to the change they may need an extended trial period. Similarly, increasing fibre intake by say switching from white to wholemeal bread may seem eminently trialable. However, sudden increases in fibre intake may produce transient diarrhoea and abdominal discomfort due to increased gas production – the higher fibre diet may need to be tried for an extended period for the person to adapt to the new diet, or the fibre intake increased slowly over a period of time.

Concluding remarks

If the questions posed in this chapter are fully considered by those making nutrition or other health education recommendations then the likelihood of making changes that ultimately prove to be non-beneficial or harmful will be minimised. If a totally holistic view is taken then any intervention that is non-beneficial can probably be regarded as harmful. Observations upon migrant populations show that, in general, they tend progressively to assume the mortality and morbidity patterns that are characteristic of their new homeland (Barker and Rose, 1990).

This reaffirms the belief that many of the health differences between populations are due to environment rather than genetics and therefore also confirms that there is considerable potential for promoting health by lifestyle intervention. Paradoxically, as each population tends to have its own problem diseases, it also underlines the potential for harm from

ill-considered and insufficiently tested interventions. A narrow pre-occupation with changing diets to reduce the risk of one disease may simply lead to an increase in the risk of another.

Endpiece

At a meeting to celebrate the Golden Jubilee of the Nutrition Society in 1991, I presented a mock paper purporting to be a presentation to the centenary meeting in 2041. In this paper, I envisaged that in the year 2026 a product called Nutribland had been launched:

> Nutribland is an ideal blend of fibre and nutrients prepared from chemically synthesised ingredients. Nutribland is consumed as a thick paste, which is sterile, colourless, odourless and tasteless. It was introduced to simplify the process of optimal diet selection – its composition can be changed each week in response to the latest research. One of the greatest benefits of Nutribland is that because there is no positive sensory reinforcement (pleasure) associated with consuming it then the risk of overeating and consequent obesity is removed.

The author of my mythical paper is surprised that despite the obvious benefits of this method of "nutrification" many people were persisting in the consumption of dead plant and animal remains, even though by 2041 these old-fashioned sources of nutrients are subject to swingeing health taxes. My author even noted that at the centenary dinner of the Nutrition Society most delegates obtained their nutrients from sources other than Nutribland. My author described a 15 year study in which 5000 people were recruited to eat only Nutribland whilst 5000 others bravely agreed to carry on consuming old-fashioned food. Three quarters of the Nutribland group dropped out of the study and the remaining members of this group lived no longer than people in the other group. However, my author concluded that the benefits of Nutribland were clearly proven because the remainder of the Nutribland group were lighter, had lower blood cholesterol levels and blood pressures than the control group and also had slightly lower cardiovascular mortality. My mythical author was amazed that despite such overwhelming benefits, some people were still unconvinced of the benefits of Nutribland. He ended with a quotation from Sherlock Holmes "You see but you do not observe".

My presentation was well received by those present at this session. I wonder how many people who heard the presentation or read the published abstract (Webb, 1991) realised that there was a serious message within this humorous and mythical presentation? How many "heard but did not listen"?

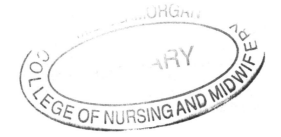

2 Food selection

Contents

Aims and scope of the chapter

The aim of this chapter is to remind readers that nutrient content has traditionally not been a significant factor in food selection. If one is to influence food selection, then some appreciation of the factors that do influence food choices and of the non-nutritional uses of food is essential – "people eat food not nutrients". This brief survey of these non-nutritional influences upon food selection should help the reader to understand why prescribed or recommended dietary changes that seem totally logical from a biological viewpoint may nevertheless have relatively little impact upon actual behaviour.

It is hoped that some discussion of the non-nutritional roles of food will not only encourage health educators to offer advice that is more readily acceptable but also reduce the likelihood that the cost of scientifically better nutrition will be increased anxiety, social tension and cultural impoverishment. It would be impractical in a general text such as this to discuss in depth all of the multitude of non-nutritional factors that affect food selection practices. In this chapter there is a general overview of the factors influencing food selection followed by a more specific discussion of three particular influences, namely: economics; migration; and dietary taboos.

Biological versus consumer models of food

The biological function of food is to provide the body with a sufficient supply of energy and essential nutrients to meet physiological needs. Current research further suggests that, in the longer term, morbidity and mortality from the degenerative diseases of industrialisation may be greatly influenced by diet composition.

The reductionist scientific model of food is thus that it is a complex mixture of macro and micro nutrients that should be combined in optimal proportions to produce an ideal fuel for the body, ensuring not only that it functions efficiently in the short term but also maximising life expectancy and wellbeing. Using such a model of food, then eating is simply the rather flawed and inefficient behavioural mechanism used to select and consume this mixture.

Such paradigms of food and of eating might tempt one to believe that if consumers are given extensive advice about optimal nutrient intakes coupled with full nutritional labelling of food then they will be enabled to select the ideal diet. Increasing information about healthy eating and food composition might be expected to lead to rapid and major "improvements" in the diet of the population.

It is quite obvious, however, that most people do not select their food solely according to biological criteria. In the past, of course, selection on this basis would not have been possible because public awareness, and even scientific awareness, of nutrients and food composition are comparatively recent. Even today, few people would have the skills and knowledge to select food solely on a compositional basis. It has been suggested that biological mechanisms akin to thirst or salt hunger operate for some important nutrients, enabling people to intuitively select a balanced diet. There is little evidence to support such mechanisms but there is some research suggesting that satiation tends to be food specific, i.e. satiation for a particular food develops as that food is consumed but satiation towards other foods is less affected (Rolls *et al.*, 1982). Such a mechanism would tend to increase the range of foods consumed, and dietary deficiencies become less likely if energy needs are fully met and a wide variety of foods consumed. In the circumstances of almost limitless abundance and variety experienced by those in the industrialised countries, such a mechanism might also tend to encourage overconsumption and obesity.

Much current food evangelism seems to be encouraging a trend towards the reductionist scientific models of food and eating, a trend that could greatly impoverish human existence without necessarily extending its duration. Food has numerous social, psychological and cultural functions in addition to its biological role of supplying nutrients. It is the interaction between these sociocultural factors and food availability that has traditionally determined what foods are eaten.

Dietary and cultural prejudice

There is an almost inevitable tendency to regard one's own beliefs and patterns of behaviour as the norm and so preferable to those of other cultures; foreign cultures tend to be regarded as wrong, or irrational, or misguided. The term **ethnocentrism** has been used to describe this tendency. This ethnocentrism is apparent in reactions to alien food habits: there is a widespread tendency to ridicule or even to abhor the food choices or eating habits of others. The intrepid explorer patronisingly accepting some revolting native delicacy to avoid offending his host is a Hollywood cliché. One obvious and widely experienced manifestation of this phenomenon is in the slightly derogatory names used for other races that have their origins in food habits, such as:

- frog, because frog legs are a French delicacy
- kraut, from the traditional fermented cabbage (sauerkraut) associated with German cuisine
- pom, because of the perceived dominance of potatoes or *pomme de terre* in English cuisine
- limey, because of the past practice of providing lime juice to British sailors to prevent scurvy
- even the term Eskimo originates from a disparaging Indian term meaning "eaters of raw flesh".

Ethnocentric-type attitudes need not be confined to "between culture" judgements it is common to hear haughty disapproval and caricaturization of the dietary practices of other regions of one's own country, of other social or religious groups or indeed of anyone who does not share a particular food ideology. For example:

- within the UK, it is not uncommon to hear disparaging comments made about the diets of "northerners" which often implicitly blame northerners for the relatively poor health statistics of the north compared to the south
- vegetarianism is frequently denigrated and ridiculed by meat eaters and conversely some vegetarian propaganda makes very hostile comments about meat eaters
- in recent years, it has been increasingly common to hear disparaging comments exchanged between those who do and those do not consciously attempt to practice healthy eating.

Criticisms of other dietary and cultural practices are often based upon a prejudiced, narrow and inaccurate view of the other group's beliefs and behaviour. Nutritionists and dieticians are not immune to ethnocentrism but one hopes that most enlightened ones would be aware of this tendency and consciously try to avoid it when dealing with an alien culture. They might, however, be more unsuspecting and thus inclined to behave ethnocentrically when dealing with the more familiar behaviour patterns of other groups within their own culture; behaviour patterns that, although familiar, may be quite different from their own. It must be very difficult for a dietician who is a committed vegetarian to give advice to a meat eater that is totally uninfluenced by her own beliefs and, vice versa if the client is vegetarian and the dietician a meat eater.

The opposite of ethnocentrism is **cultural relativism**. An attempt is made to understand and respect other cultural practices they should be accepted as normal no matter how different they are from one's own or how initially bizarre they may seem. Only if practices are clearly and demonstrably dysfunctional should attempts be made to change them. There would be little argument that such an approach was correct if one were dealing with an unique alien culture but more familiar cultural practices may be handled with less sensitivity The American's hamburger, the Briton's fish and chips and even children's sweets or candies have real cultural significance. Nutrition education need not involve attempts to totally blacken the image of such foods but should rather attempt to use them within a diet that, in its entirety, complies with reasonable nutritional guidelines.

It is likely that many practices that are strongly and acutely dysfunctional to a group will have been selected out during the cultural evolution of the group. Changing social conditions, a changed environment or perhaps even simply increased longevity may cause traditional practices to become regarded as dysfunctional. The aim of nutrition educators, under such circumstances, should be to minimise or avoid the dysfunction with the least possible cultural interference – the cultural conservationist approach.

Food classification systems

Biological (food groups and pyramids)

Selecting food solely according to biological criteria requires considerable knowledge of nutrition and food composition. It takes some skill to routinely translate current views on optimal intakes into food portions and yet still eat a varied and palatable diet. Dieticians and nutrition educators have used **food groups** as a means of helping people to select food on a constituent basis. These food group systems were originally developed during the era when adequacy was the nutritional priority. Foods were grouped together based upon the nutrients that they provided – consumers could then be advised that if they consumed specified minimum numbers of portions from each of the groups then nutritional adequacy would be assured, i.e. the diet would be balanced.

A widely used and simple example of this biological food classification system is the **Four Food Group Plan**. Four basic food groups are identified and specified minimum numbers of servings designated, as follows:

1 *The milk group* (milk, cheese and milk products) – These provide good amounts of energy, good quality protein, vitamin A, calcium and riboflavin. On the negative side they are also rich in saturated fat and cholesterol – products within this group such as low fat milk, cottage cheese and low fat yoghurt provide most of the nutrients but have less fat and cholesterol. Adults would be recommended to consume a minimum of two servings daily from this grouping to ensure adequacy (e.g. a serving is a cup of milk or yoghurt, 40–60 g of cheese).

2 *The meat group* (meat, fish, eggs and also meat substitutes such as pulses and nuts) – These provide protein, vitamin A, B vitamins and iron. Some of these foods are also major sources of fat and/or cholesterol. Much of the fat can be avoided by selecting lower fat products, buying lean cuts of meat or white fish and by care in preparation. The fat in oily fish is now much more positively regarded because of the possible anti-thrombotic properties of some of the fatty acids that it contains. Adults would be recommended to take a minimum of two daily servings (e.g. 50–75 g of cooked meat, poultry or fish is a serving).

3 *The fruit and vegetable group* (fruits and those vegetables not classified as meat substitutes) – These provide carotene, vitamin C, folate, riboflavin, potassium and fibre. In their raw state, they usually contain little fat and no cholesterol (avocados are one of the few exceptions to this low fat rule). Many of these foods have a very low energy density (calories per gram) and thus might be particularly useful in low energy, weight-reducing diets. In those that do provide good amounts of energy (e.g. potatoes) that energy is principally in the form of starch; current nutrition education guidelines recommend replacing some of the fat in the Western diet with starch. Note, however that considerable amounts of fat and sugar may be added to these foods during processing. For example, French fried potatoes may absorb considerable amounts of fat during frying, and fruit canned in syrup may contain considerable amounts of added sugar. Adults would be recommended to take at least four daily servings (e.g. an apple or other piece of fruit, half cup of raw or cooked chopped vegetables is a serving).

4 *The bread and cereals group* (bread, rice, pasta, breakfast cereals and products made from flour) – Whole grain cereals are good sources of B vitamins, some minerals and fibre. White flour still provides reasonable amounts of fibre and it is often fortified with vitamins and minerals (in the UK, with iron, calcium and some B vitamins). Many breakfast cereals are also fortified with extra vitamins and minerals. This group provides good amounts of energy which is largely as starch in unsweetened products – high intake from this group tends to reduce the proportion of calories that is derived from fat and also tends to lower the overall energy density of the diet. Adults would be recommended to consume a minimum of four daily servings (e.g. 1 slice of bread, a half cup of rice or pasta, or a small portion of cornflakes is one serving).

A number of foods are not covered by any of these categories (e.g. butter, oil and other fats, sugar, alcoholic drinks etc.) because they provide energy, but few nutrients and thus no minimum portions are recommended; it is merely suggested that they should be used sparingly.

Although originally designed to ensure nutritional adequacy this plan can also be adapted to guide the user towards the modern concept of a healthy diet by, for example, highlighting the low fat/low sugar options within each group. These are the foods with high nutrient density (amount of nutrient per calorie).

Several generations of American school-children and college students have been taught the basic four food group plan since its development in 1955. It would be a classification system familiar to some extent to a large proportion of Americans, although much less familiar to most Britons; note, for example, that in the standard British textbook of nutrition and dietetics there is no reference to food groups in the index (Garrow and James, 1993).

The US Department of Agriculture (USDA, 1992) has recently published a new guide to food selection intended to update and replace the basic four plan. This is the **Food Guide Pyramid** (see Figure 2.1 on the next page). This new food pyramid is still a recognisable development of the basic four food system but it has been designed with the aim of assisting selection of a diet that is not only adequate but meets the nutritional guidelines of the National Research Council (NRC, 1989b).

At the base of the food pyramid are the starchy grain foods which should contribute more servings than any other single group to the ideal diet – six servings for a diet to supply the 1600 kcal needed by some sedentary women and older adults and up to 11 servings for a 2800 kcal diet needed by teenage boys and active men.

At the second level on the pyramid are the fruit group and the vegetable group – the ideal diet should have a combined five to nine servings from these groups depending upon the total calorie requirement.

At the third level on the pyramid are the foods of animal origin and the vegetarian alternatives to meat, the pulses and nuts – the ideal diet should contain two to three servings from each of the two categories at this third level, the milk and meat groups of the basic four food plan.

At the top of the pyramid are the fats, oils and sweets – foods such as salad dressings, cream, butter, margarine, soft drinks, sweets (candies), sweet desserts and alcoholic drinks. These foods at the top of the pyramid provide few nutrients but do contain calories in the form of sugars and fats and thus should be used sparingly in the ideal diet, especially for those seeking to lose weight.

A triangle symbol is distributed lightly within the cereal, fruit and milk groups to show that some foods from these categories may contain added sugars, e.g. sweetened breakfast cereals, fruit canned in syrup, some flavoured yoghurts, milk

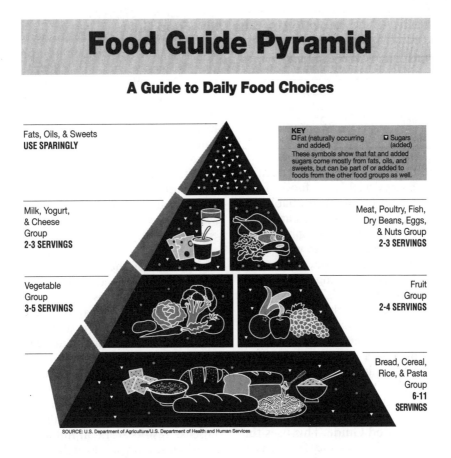

Food Guide Pyramid

A Guide to Daily Food Choices

Fats, Oils, & Sweets
USE SPARINGLY

KEY
□ Fat (naturally occurring and added)   ◨ Sugars (added)
These symbols show that fat and added sugars come mostly from fats, oils, and sweets, but can be part of or added to foods from the other food groups as well.

Milk, Yogurt, & Cheese Group
2-3 SERVINGS

Meat, Poultry, Fish, Dry Beans, Eggs, & Nuts Group
2-3 SERVINGS

Vegetable Group
3-5 SERVINGS

Fruit Group
2-4 SERVINGS

Bread, Cereal, Rice, & Pasta Group
6-11 SERVINGS

SOURCE: U.S. Department of Agriculture/U.S. Department of Health and Human Services

Use the Food Guide Pyramid to help you eat better every day. . .the Dietary Guidelines way. Start with plenty of Breads, Cereals, Rice, and Pasta; Vegetables; and Fruits. Add two to three servings from the Milk group and two to three servings from the Meat group.

Each of these food groups provides some, but not all, of the nutrients you need. No one food group is more important than another — for good health you need them all. Go easy on fats, oils, and sweets, the foods in the small tip of the Pyramid.

Figure 2.1 The food guide pyramid.
Source: US Department of Agriculture/US Department of Health and Human Services

shake and ice cream. A circle symbol is distributed lightly throughout the cereal and vegetable groups to show that these may contain added fats and more densely in the meat and milk groups to show that many of the foods in these groups contain substantial amounts of naturally occurring fat. The top layer of the pyramid contains a high density of both triangles and circles to emphasise its role as a major contributor of fats and added sugar to the diet.

The food pyramid thus indicates a general dietary structure that should ensure adequacy and yet at the same time make it more likely that other nutrition education guidelines will be followed. Highlighting, in a visual way, the likely sources of fat and added sugars in the diet should assist the consumer in making choices that reduce intakes of fat and added sugars.

It is interesting to compare the pyramid in Figure 2.1 with the distribution of the average UK household budget for food and drink between the various tiers of this pyramid (from MAFF, 1993):

layer	% of household food budget
top layer	22%
third layer	42.5%
second layer	20%
base layer	16%

Given the big differences in the relative costs and energy yields of foods from different categories, it is probably an unfair, perhaps even naïve, comparison to make. It is nonetheless striking how very top heavy the pyramid has now become.

Since writing this section, the author has received a poster showing "The British Healthy Eating Pyramid". This pyramid, in all its essentials, is the same as the American version shown in Figure 2.1. In this British version, the fruits and vegetables are shown as a single group with a combined five to nine servings and potatoes are included in the cereal group.

The UK Health Education Authority (HEA, 1994) has also just published a new National Food Guide. This uses the visual image of a plate, various fractions of this plate are occupied by each of five food groups:

- fruit and vegetables occupy approximately 30% of the plate
- bread, cereals and potatoes also about 30%
- meat, fish and alternatives (pulses) about 15%
- milk and dairy foods also about 15%
- fatty and sugary foods about 10%.

The general diet structure being suggested by this image is essentially that being indicated by the Food Guide Pyramid. This guide avoids specific recommendations about portions. The guide does include advice to choose: low fat alternatives from the meat and milk groups; high fibre varieties from the cereal group; and, a wide variety from the fruit and vegetable group.

Consumer classifications

Consumers also classify foods, but such classification systems do not usually have any theoretical basis in scientific nutrition. Such classification systems may, nevertheless, have evolved rules that produce good practical diets despite their lack of a scientific framework and sometimes even though they have a theoretical framework that seems incompatible with nutrition theory. Those seeking to induce health promoting dietary change should seek to understand such classification systems and to offer advice that is consistent with such beliefs.

One of the best known and most widespread of the traditional classification systems is the **hot and cold** classification that is found in various forms in Latin America, India and China. The general principle is that good health results from a state of balance and thus to maintain or restore good health there must be a balance between hot and cold. Foods are classified as hot or cold and foods should be selected and mixed to produce or maintain the balanced state. Disease results from an imbalance. Certain diseases and phases of the reproductive cycle are hot or cold and therefore certain foods will be more or less appropriate in these different circumstances. Thus in the Chinese system a sore throat is a hot disease and might be treated by a cold food such as watermelon to try to restore balance. Hot foods, such as beef, dates or chilli are considered detrimental in such hot conditions (Yeung *et al.*, 1973). Surveys of Chinese families living in London (Wheeler and Tan, 1983) and Toronto (Yeung *et al.*, 1973) both found that the traditional hot and cold system was still widely adhered to and practised despite Western cultural influences.

Wheeler and Tan (1983) concluded that, despite the use of such a non science-based food classification system, the dietary pattern of the London Chinese families in their survey was varied and nutritionally excellent. Any programme designed to increase the science-based nutrition and food composition knowledge of these Chinese families would seem initially more likely to cause confusion and worsening of the diet than to lead to improved nutrition. Such a programme might also be damaging to the cultural security of these families. English people living in the same area would probably have had more science-based nutrition knowledge but these authors would probably have judged that, by their criteria, the English diet was inferior to that of the Chinese. Knowledge of food and nutrition is perhaps more loosely correlated with good dietetic practice than many nutrition educators would like to think.

Most Western consumers do not use such a formal and overtly structured classification system but this does not mean that they do not also classify foods. In any cultural group there is clearly a classification of potentially edible material into food and non food. Except under conditions of extreme deprivation, any cultural group will only eat some of the substances around them that would comply with any biological definition of potential food. In the UK, there are numerous plants, animals, birds, fish and insects that are edible but are rarely if ever eaten by Britons. They are simply not viewed as potential foods and are classified as non food. In many cases, the idea of eating such items would be repellent to most Britons.

The traditional main course of a British dinner (or lunch if that is the main meal of the day) consists of a meat or meat product, potatoes, one or more extra vegetables with sauce or gravy. Very few Britons would, however, consider eating such a meal or even many of the individual foods for breakfast. Clearly some foods are seen, or classified, as more appropriate for particular meals. These classifications of edible material into food or non food and into foods appropriate for particular meals or occasions varies

considerably even within the peoples of Western Europe. In Britain, horsemeat is not classified as food and yet is widely eaten in France; many Britons would not consider cheese and spicy cold meats as suitable breakfast foods, yet in some other European countries they would be typical breakfast fare.

Schutz *et al.* (1975) conducted a survey of 200 female, mainly white and mainly middle class consumers distributed between four American cities. They used a questionnaire in which these consumers were asked to rate 56 different foods in terms of their appropriateness for a total of 48 food-use situations; they used a 7 point scale from 1 "never appropriate" to 7 "always appropriate". Their aim was to allow the respondents to generate classifications of foods based upon their appropriateness ratings. The authors identified five food categories based upon consumer usage rather than upon biological criteria. These were as follows:

1 *High calorie treats* – such as wine, cakes and pies which were considered especially suitable for social occasions and for offering to guests. The foods in this category tended to be rated towards the inappropriate end of the scale for questions relating to healthfulness, e.g. inappropriate when "needing to lose weight" or when "not feeling well". Healthy, wholesome foods seem to be considered more suitable for everyday eating and eating alone than for parties and entertaining.

2 *Speciality meal items* – foods considered suitable only for special occasions and circumstances. The authors offer liver and chilli as examples of this category. The foods in this category were notable for the number of food-use situations for which they were rated as never appropriate.

3 *Common meal items* – foods that were suitable for all occasions and all ages and would be served at main meals, e.g. meats, fish and some vegetable items.

They were generally rated as inappropriate "for breakfast" and not surprisingly "for dessert".

4 *Refreshing healthy foods* – which were considered to be nutritious but not viewed as suitable for a main course, e.g. milk, orange juice, cottage cheese and jello (jelly). These scored highly on the questions concerned with health ("nutritious", "easy to digest") but were rated low in spiciness. Perhaps spiciness/flavour and healthy foods are not generally considered to be compatible.

5 *Inexpensive filling foods* – which were considered cheap and filling as well as fattening, e.g. bread, peanut butter, potato chips (crisps) and candy bars. These were not considered appropriate for those trying to lose weight, but were foods that could be used to assuage hunger between meals and appropriate for hungry teenagers.

This is, of course, just one group of investigators' interpretation of the comments expressed by one group of consumers. It does, however, highlight how even Western consumers, despite not having a formal cultural food classification system like the Chinese hot and cold system, do nonetheless have clear and, within a group, fairly consistent views on the appropriateness of different foods in different situations. They may use quite elaborate classification systems for food, even though such classification may be informal or even subconscious.

If it is to be effective, then clearly any dietary advice or any prescribed diet must recognise such views on the appropriateness of particular foods for particular occasions and situations. It will also only be likely to succeed if it uses foods that are classified as appropriate for the individual. Many cultural groups might classify milk as a food for babies and therefore not suitable for adults; some Western consumers might only grudgingly concede that some pulses or salads are suitable for working men. The enlightened nutrition educator seeks to identify and understand such cultural views on the appropriate uses of particular foods and then tries to frame advice that is compatible with them rather than trying to impose his own classification upon the client.

Anthropological classification

There have been several attempts to devise food categorisation systems that could be used across cultures. These are useful not only for the anthropologist seeking to describe the diets and the uses made of foods in particular cultures but they could also be of great use to the nutrition educator seeking to identify the most appropriate and effective ways of trying to bring about nutritional improvement.

One of the earliest and simplest of these systems was developed by Passim and Bennet (1943) who divided foods up into three categories:

1 *Core foods* – foods that are regularly and universally consumed within the community. In developing countries, these are likely to be starchy staple foods (e.g. bread, rice, millet or cassava). In industrialised countries, like Britain and the US, milk, potatoes, bread and meats would probably fit into this category.

2 *Secondary foods* – foods that have widespread but not universal use. Most fruits and vegetables would probably be classified as secondary foods in the UK.

3 *Peripheral foods* – the least widely and frequently used of the foods. It is in this category that the most individual variation would be expected. Most shellfish and a number of fish would probably be in this category in the UK.

Such categorisation would almost certainly be easier in societies whose range of available foods is relatively restricted and most difficult in countries, like the US and UK, which have a vast array of foods available to an affluent population. This enables consumers to express much more individuality in their diet structure.

Any particular food may be classified differently for different cultures; it may be classified differently for different social classes within a culture and foods may change categories over time. Rice is clearly a core food for the Japanese but for most British groups would probably be classified as secondary. A few decades ago, rice (except pudding rice) would probably have been classified as peripheral for most social groups in Britain; prior to 1960 many working class Britons would almost never have eaten a savoury rice dish. Chinese and Indian restaurants, takeaway outlets and foreign holidays have transformed this situation so that there may now be some groups, even within the indigenous population, for whom rice might be approaching the status of a core food.

A nutritionist trying to effect change in the diet of any community might expect to find most resistance to change in the core foods, more ready acceptance in the secondary foods and the most flexibility in the peripheral foods.

Some foods have acquired a cultural status beyond their purely dietary and nutritional significance: they play an integral part in the cultural life of the community and they have been termed **cultural superfoods**, e.g. rice in Japan and bread in many European cultures.

Rice has maintained a particular emotional and cultural status for the Japanese despite a marked fall in consumption since World War II and a corresponding increase in bread consumption. For example:

- the emperor still cultivates a symbolic crop of rice
- in the Japanese language, the same word can mean either food or rice
- rice plays a part in all Japanese rituals
- in the past, the Japanese calendar was geared to the cycle of rice production,

rice was used as a medium for taxation and some units of measurement were based upon the amount of rice necessary to feed a man for a year.

Bread has declined in its cultural significance in some European countries, but television scenes of people in Eastern Europe queuing for bread strike a particularly poignant chord. If the bread supply is threatened then the situation is perceived as that much more desperate than if other foods are in short supply.

There are numerous reminders of the past importance of bread in the UK, for example:

- bread and dough are both used as slang terms for money
- in Christian communion, bread is used to symbolically represent the body of Christ
- in the Lord's Prayer, Christians pray for their daily bread.

When considering the means of effecting nutritional improvement, the nutrition educator would be well advised to understand and respect the cultural significance of such foods. Insensitive denigration of a cultural superfood by an alien nutritionist is likely to provoke incredulity or even hostility and may reduce the chances of any of the advice being taken seriously. The cultural importance of meat to many Western men has been mentioned in Chapter 1 and it has probably, in the past, even been reinforced by nutrition education that presented meat as a high protein food and suggested that high protein supply was a key requirement of good nutrition. Unnecessary attempts by current nutrition educators to persuade such men that red meat and a healthy diet are now incompatible may simply persuade them that, in that case, the price for a healthy diet is too high and they will thus ignore all dietary advice. As a postscript to the first chapter of Davidson and Passmore's classic nutrition text (Passmore and Eastwood, 1986) a passage is quoted which describes the African's craving for meat as:

> the strongest and most fraternal bond that the continent had in common. It was a dream, a longing, an aspiration that never ceased, a physiological cry of the body, stronger and more torturing than the sexual instinct.
>
> Gary, R. 1958 *The roots of heaven.* London: Michael Joseph.

The speaker goes on to assume that this need for meat is a universal craving for all men. If there is even a grain of truth in this assertion then nutrition education must not suggest that the only option for healthy eating is one that would require unreasonable sacrifice. To use a more recent example from closer to home, chips (French fries) are a traditional and important element in British cuisine and culture. The following quotation from a serious national newspaper emphasises the importance that some Britons attach to their chips:

> According to the Chip Census, one person in 10 would rather give up sex, alcohol and smoking than chips!
>
> *The Independent* 2/3/94

Once again if healthy eating appears to require total avoidance of chips then the chances of acceptance by a high proportion of the British population is probably doomed. Moderate amounts of chips can be included in a diet that meets current nutritional guidelines, especially if attention is paid to advice about their method of preparation and the foods that they most appropriately complement.

Cultural superfood is just one of five food categories described by Jelliffe (1967) in a food classification system that he thought had universal application, both in developing and industrialised countries. The five categories in this system are:

1 *Cultural superfoods* – These are discussed above. Considered by Schutz *et al.* (1975) to correspond to "common meal item" in their consumer classification.

2 *Prestige foods* – These are reserved for important occasions or important people. According to Jelliffe, foods within this category are usually high in protein, often animal protein. They are also usually difficult to obtain because of their scarcity, high cost, or difficult preparation. Truffles and venison would be clearly in this category in the UK; salmon would have been in this category until the ready availability of cheap farmed salmon reduced its scarcity and price.

3 *Body image foods* – These are foods considered to promote wellbeing. Jelliffe lists food that contribute to maintaining or restoring hot/cold balance as an example from developing countries. High fibre foods would be an example in the UK. Schutz *et al.* (1975) considered that their "refreshing healthy foods" might be an example of this category.

4 *Sympathetic magic foods* – These foods are considered to have some special properties that they impart to the consumer. Jelliffe offers, as an example from developing countries, eggs, which are avoided by many women in East African countries because they are thought to cause infertility. He suggests, as an example from an industrialised country, underdone steak used in the training of athletes because it symbolised vigour, masculinity and energy.

5 *Physiologic group foods* – These are foods reserved for or forbidden to certain physiologic groups. Examples are taboos against certain foods for pregnant women, lactating women or for young children. Breast milk, infant formula and certain cereal preparations are normally only consumed by infants and young children and are therefore clear examples of this category.

Non-nutritional uses of food

The biological roles of food are to nourish the body and sometimes to treat particular illnesses for which dietary therapy has an accepted scientific rationale. Fieldhouse (1986) lists almost 20 further non-nutritional functions of food. Below are some examples of these non-nutritional uses of food.

Religion, morality and ethics

- Food and drink are used in the rituals and ceremonies of many religions.
- Adherence to the dietary rules of a religion acts as a common bond for adherents and serves to differentiate them from non believers.
- Adhering to dietary rules is an outward symbol of a person's piety and self-discipline.
- Policing of dietary rules provides a mechanism for religious leaders to exert control over their followers and to demonstrate their authority.
- People may avoid certain foods to demonstrate their disapproval of animal cruelty or their ecological awareness.
- People may boycott food from particular countries or companies to express their moral disapproval of human rights abuses, exploitation of workers or other perceived moral transgressions.

Thus:

- bread and wine are used in Christian communion to symbolise the body and blood of Christ
- adherence to the dietary rules of the Torah certainly helps to set orthodox Jews apart from gentiles
- the strict penalties for alcohol consumption, even for non believers, underlines the primacy of Islam and the mullahs in some countries

- boycotts against food from South Africa, tuna caught in drift nets and food produced by companies that "push" powdered infant foods in Third World countries are all examples of the use of food to make ethical statements.

Status and wealth

- Expensive and exotic foods can be used to demonstrate one's wealth and sophistication.
- Serving elaborate and expensive meals can be used to demonstrate esteem for guests.
- People's social status may be defined by whom they eat with and where they eat.
- Unusual food choices may be used to express a person's individuality.

Thus:

- many companies have different dining areas for workers of different status
- different Hindu castes do not eat together
- serving very expensive but essentially rather bland caviar as a snack can be used to symbolise financial success and high social status.

Interpersonal relationships

- Offerings of food and drink are commonly used to initiate and maintain personal and business relationships.
- Giving of food can be a demonstration of love and withdrawal or failure to offer food can be used to signal disapproval or even to punish.
- Food and drink may provide a focus for social gatherings.

Thus:

- offering new neighbours a drink or food is primarily a gesture of welcome and warmth rather than an attempt to satisfy any perceived nutritional need

– offering a box of chocolates can be a reward, a gesture of affection or a gesture of apology; the nutritional impact is incidental.

Political

● Control of the food supply and the price of foodstuffs can be a very potent method of exerting political control or of gaining political favour.

Thus:

– some would argue that food aid may have purposes beyond its obvious humanitarian one: it may salve the consciences of wealthy donor nations; foster dependence and subservience in the recipients; and, it may be useful in bolstering the political or diplomatic fortunes of the donor government.

Folk medicine

● Diet is an element in many traditional treatments of disease.

Thus:

– in the traditional hot and cold system, cold foods may be used to treat hot diseases.

This list is not definitive, it is merely intended to illustrate the enormous diversity and range of potential non-nutritional uses of food. The relative importance of any particular influence may be quite different in different groups, even within the same local environment. Take, for example, the influence of religion on food choice in the UK or USA, this would have a major influence upon strictly orthodox Jews or Seventh Day Adventists but minimal influence upon equally devout Anglicans or Episcopalians.

The orthodox Jew would, for example:

● avoid all pigmeat and meat from any animal that does not have cloven hooves and chew the cud

● not eat the hind quarters of animals or unbled meat
● not eat flightless birds, shellfish or other fish without fins and scales
● not eat meat and dairy produce together
● not prepare food on the Sabbath.

It would be difficult to identify any specifically religious influences on the diets of the two protestant groups – perhaps, the occasional communion bread and wine and perhaps a voluntary and self-selected abstinence during Lent.

The priority attached to the various biological and non-biological factors influencing food selection are likely to change as one moves from a situation of gross deprivation or scarcity to one of almost limitless abundance. Maslow (1943) suggested that human needs could be arranged into a hierarchy of motivation, needs lower down the hierarchy must be at least partially satisfied before the higher up needs become significantly motivating factors. This hierarchy is summarised in Figure 2:2.

In conditions of extreme deprivation, survival is the priority and people may resort to eating almost anything that is remotely edible, perhaps even breaking one of the strongest and most widespread of all dietary taboos, that against the consumption of human flesh. After survival, the need to ensure future security and safety then become motivating. Potentially edible material is classified into food and non-food and ensuring future needs will be a priority. Food hoarding, perhaps even obesity, might be outward manifestations of this desire for security – obesity in some cultures has been sought after and admired rather than dreaded and despised as it usually is in the UK and US. Once security of food supply is relatively assured, the need for love and belongingness then become motivating influences on food selection. This would be manifested in the extensive use of food to demonstrate group membership and

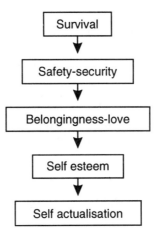

Figure 2.2 Maslow's hierarchy of human needs – a theory of human motivation (after Maslow, 1943). Lower level needs must be at least partially satisfied before higher level needs become significant motivating factors

affection. Then comes the need for self-esteem. This might be manifested in the selection of high cost, prestige foods to demonstrate one's wealth and success. At the pinnacle of Maslow's hierarchy, the need for self actualisation becomes motivating. Selection of food to demonstrate one's individuality or uniqueness becomes prominent, and this may be manifested in experimentation with new foods, new recipes and non-conforming patterns of selection.

The current penchant for the simple peasant foods of the East by some educated, affluent "Westerners" may be one manifestation of this need for self actualisation; the partial replacement of these traditional foods with a more "Western diet" by some in the East may be symbolising their need to demonstrate their new wealth and self esteem. In many Third World countries bottle feeds for infants are promoted as the modern and sophisticated Western alternative to "primitive" breastfeeding – yet in many affluent countries, like the US and UK, breastfeeding predominates in the upper social classes (e.g. White *et al.*, 1992).

There may be some disagreement over the details of Maslow's hierarchy, as applied to food selection, but the underlying principle seems unquestionable – that the priority attached to different influences will change with increasing affluence and food availability. The range of factors influencing selection will tend to be greater in affluent than in poor populations, and the relative prominence of these differing factors will also change with increasing affluence. One might expect the more physiological/biological drives to become less important in the affluent.

Models of food selection

Several workers have attempted to organise and integrate the various and disparate factors influencing food selection into a unified model. Such a model should assist the nutrition educator in attempts to influence food selection practices. Availability of a food is clearly a pre requisite for selection. Wheeler (1992) suggested that various constraints act to limit the range of foods that is, in practice, available to the individual. In effect, the image of the affluent Western consumer having almost limitless theoretical choice of food may be, in practice, partly an illusion. The individual's limited practical availability may greatly limit the scope of the nutrition educator for effecting change. Wheeler envisaged a hierarchy of constraints limiting food choices, in many ways analogous to Maslow's hierarchy of human needs discussed above.

Figure 2.3 shows a simple model for food selection based upon the concept of a hierarchy of availabilities.

Physical availability

There will be absolute limitations on the range of potentially edible materials that are available in any particular local environment. Physical and geographical factors are key determinants of food availability, factors such as climate, soil type, storage facilities, water supply, and quality of transportation links. The range and amounts of food available in an isolated and arid region may be severely

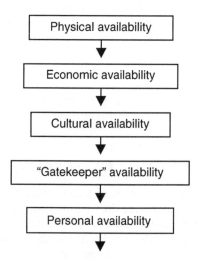

Selection from foods that are "really" available

Figure 2.3 A model of food selection based upon the concept of a hierarchy of constraints upon food availability

limited by such factors. Even within affluent countries, some foods will only be available seasonally and some foods may be unavailable locally because of lack of sufficient demand. Shops will only stock foods that they expect to sell, e.g. Kosher foods may be difficult to obtain in areas where few Jews live. Small local stores will inevitably stock a more limited range than large supermarkets, and there may even be quite marked differences in the range of products stocked by shops in poor and affluent areas.

Economic availability

Monetary means for the purchase of food may exert a variable limiting influence on the availability of foods. In some circumstances, lack of money may have an absolute effect in limiting availability of particular foods or even of food in general. This is very clear in some Third World countries, where having enough money may mean the difference between relative comfort and starvation. Even in affluent countries, economic influences can have a very restricting influence upon the range of foods available – in the UK and US, there are quite marked differences between the food choices of the richest and poorest, and this is partly due to differences in purchasing power (discussed at length later in the chapter).

Cultural availability

Except under extreme conditions, only things that are culturally recognised as foods and only those things that are classified as acceptable for the meal or occasion are likely to be selected. Beef might be physically and economically available to devout Hindus in the UK but, in practice, religious conviction makes it unavailable. The cultural acceptability of a food may be greatly affected by changes in its physical availability – the foods of immigrants may be initially regarded with suspicion and even distaste by the indigenous population but, with time, they become more familiar and maybe acceptable. Likewise, immigrants tend, over time, to adopt at least some of the foods and dietary practices of the indigenous population. Exposure to alien foods through foreign travel may have a similar effect.

"Gatekeeper" limitations on availability

The housewife has traditionally been regarded as the family **gatekeeper,** regulating the availability of food to her family. If most food is eaten within formal family meals and if food purchasing and meal construction are largely the province of the housewife, then she has the potential to impose limitations on the availability of foods to other family members. Personal beliefs and preferences may greatly affect the choices of the gatekeeper and thus the diet of her family; a vegetarian gatekeeper may effectively impose vegetarianism on other family members, or, conversely, a non-vegetarian gatekeeper might refuse to provide a vegetarian alternative to a family member who would wish to be vegetarian.

Convenience of preparation may affect the choices of the gatekeeper. Appreciation or criticisms by other family members will feedback and also be an important influence on her future choices. Changing social patterns have tended to diminish the traditional gatekeeping influence of wives and mothers: more food tends to be eaten outside the home or is purchased by the individual consuming it; ready made versions of dishes that have traditionally been home made shifts control over composition from the housewife to the food manufacturer; other family members are more likely to participate in the shopping and food preparation; even within the home, there is more snacking or "grazing" upon self-selected foods available in the larder or refrigerator and fewer formal family meals.

Despite a diminution in this gatekeeping role of the mother, even within a traditional two parent family, it may still be quite considerable. Certainly much food advertising is still directed towards the gatekeeper housewife. Advertisers stress factors like the convenience of foods to a busy housewife and provide images of wives and mothers who have served the promoted food receiving acclaim from an appreciative and, therefore, loving family. Advertisers also recognise that over-stressing convenience can be a double-edged sword and reduce appeal to the gatekeeper – a food that requires little or no preparation may diminish the satisfaction and credit due to the provider. It is, for example, possible to produce cake mixes that merely require re-hydration, but, if they require the addition of an egg as well, then this gives the final product more claim to be a home baked cake.

Catering managers may exert a considerable gatekeeping influence over those living in institutions such as hospitals, prisons, retirement homes, boarding schools, and, to a lesser extent, those taking lunches at school or work place. Older people living at home, or those receiving welfare may have some food provided or even whole meals delivered to them. In the UK, "meals on wheels" supply inexpensive weekday main meals to some elderly people.

If someone is subject to the gatekeeping influences of someone from a different cultural background, then they may effectively be subject to a double dose of limitation due to cultural availability. The gatekeeper may only offer foods that are culturally available to them and only some of these may be culturally available to the consumer. Unless caterers make special provision for cultural/ethnic minorities, then this may severely restrict the real choices of such people, e.g. hospital patients from minority groups.

Even those people seemingly immune to the influence of gatekeepers such as the affluent person living alone may still use staff dining facilities in the workplace. They may have limited time available for food preparation or low incentive to cook just for themselves. They may thus rely heavily upon commercially pre-prepared meals or restaurants.

Personal availability

Foods that have overcome all of the previous barriers to their availability may still not be consumed. Individual dislike for a food; avoidance for reasons of individual belief or because of physiological intolerance may, in practice, make it unavailable. People who are, or who believe that they are, allergic to fish will be effectively prevented from consuming fish. Someone revolted by the taste or texture of broccoli will not eat it and meat will not be available to someone revolted by the idea of eating the flesh of dead animals.

These availabilities are not usually absolute "all or nothing" phenomena. Availability can be a continuum varying from one extreme, absolute unavailability to high desirability and availability. There can be both positive and negative influences upon the availability of foods at each level of the hierarchy, for example:

- subsidy would increase economic availability, but tax would reduce it
- high prestige would increase cultural, gatekeeper or personal availability while low prestige would reduce it
- the proportion of retail outlets stocking an item, and the geographical location of those outlets would influence its physical availability
- advertising might seek to enhance availability at the cultural, gatekeeper or personal level.

Much current nutrition education is geared towards partly reversing some of the dietary changes that accompany affluence. In some populations and groups, lack of economic availability limits consumption of highly prized sugars and animal foods but affluence removes that constraint upon foods that may be very culturally and personally available because of their high prestige and palatability. Nutrition education is, in part, trying to introduce constraints higher up the hierarchy as indicated in Figure 2.3 to compensate for the lessening of economic and physical restraints at the base of the hierarchy.

Nutrition educators must recognise that, even if an individual understands and accepts any proffered advice, there may still be barriers, sometimes beyond one's control, that prevent or limit the implementation of change. Clearly nutrition educators can take account of at least some of these factors: they can make sure that any suggested change is culturally acceptable to the individual or targeted group; they can ensure that they do not recommend changes that are beyond the economic means of their clients; caterers can be persuaded to provide options that enable their clients to make healthier choices; diets or recommendations constructed for individuals can allow for the personal preferences of that person. Generally, when dealing with populations or groups, then the more options that can be offered the more people who will be enabled to take up some of the options – there are, for example, many relatively minor changes in food uses and selection that can contribute to a reduction in total fat intake or reduce its saturation, at least some of these changes will be available to most people (see Appendix).

Economic influences upon food selection

In the wealthy industrialised countries, health and longevity are strongly and positively correlated with higher socio-economic status. It is difficult to quantify the relative importance of nutritional factors in this association but, given the high priority currently attached to diet as a precipitating factor for ill health, then these factors are generally considered to be significant. It is ironic that the diseases of industrialisation that are internationally strongly and positively correlated with increasing affluence, are, within the industrialised countries, associated with relative poverty.

International trends

If one looks worldwide at the influence of economic status upon food "selection", then some very general trends emerge. Increasing affluence leads initially to increases in total energy intake and this is followed by a switch away from starchy staples to other higher prestige and more palatable foods including fats, meats, dairy produce and sugars. Poleman (1975) suggests that the percentage of calories provided by starchy staples provides a very simple economic ranking of diets.

At very low income levels, then increased wealth leads to increased calorie intake, usually based upon local starchy staples. Excepting times of acute famine, it is poverty rather than inadequate physical availability of food that is the dominant cause of undernutrition. Wealthy countries with inadequate indigenous agriculture do not go hungry, and wealthy people within poor countries do not usually go hungry either. In India in 1975, there was an 18 million ton surplus of grain which caused great storage problems, and yet many people went hungry because they did not have enough money to buy grain. Poleman (1975) presents the results of a survey of the effects of income upon diet and nutrient intake in Sri Lanka. At the lowest income level, calorific value of food purchases was around 2100 calories per head per day, which, if one allows the standard 15% for wastage, implies a 200-calorie daily deficit compared to estimated minimum energy needs; this group represented 43% of the population. In the next lowest income group, the sole change in diet was in quantity; an increase of 200 calories per day but no change in diet composition. Only in the top 20% by income were there qualitative changes in the diet composition of the type outlined below.

Calculations of worldwide production of primary foods (mainly cereals) indicate that sufficient is produced to meet the estimated nutritional needs of the world population. Yet in some poor countries there is starvation and in other richer countries there are "mountains" and "lakes" of surplus food. Poleman (1975) estimated that in the US, *per capita* grain consumption was 1800 pounds per year but less than 100 pounds of this was directly consumed, with almost all of the rest being used as animal feed. An animal consumes between 3 and 10 pounds of grain to produce one pound of meat.

The image of rapid world population growth outstripping growth in food production and being entirely responsible for creating current food shortages is also not entirely accurate. Wortman (1976) suggests that, in developed countries, rates of food production between 1961 and 1975 rose by almost 40% on a *per capita* basis; even in developing countries, population growth did not quite wipe out the substantial increases in absolute food production when they were expressed on a *per capita* basis. Sanderson (1975) suggested that even though population growth had exceeded even the most pessimistic forecasts, worldwide grain production had increased by enough to theoretically allow a 1% annual improvement in worldwide *per capita* consumption. Wortman (1976) also gave projections of future growth in food production and population and concluded that world food production was likely to keep up with population growth for some time to come. Thus the primary cause of worldwide undernutrition is not inadequate food production *per se* but an imbalance in the way this food is distributed between the peoples of the world. Differences in wealth are the key determinant of this uneven distribution.

Once income level has risen beyond the point where energy needs can be satisfied, then increasing affluence tends to be associated with changes in the nature and quality of diet. There is a tendency to replace the local starchy staple with higher prestige rice or wheat; there is an increasing tendency to reduce consumption of starchy staples and to replace them with fattier foods and simple sugars. In the USA in 1875 starchy staples made up 55% of total energy intake whereas a century later this figure had dropped to around 20% (Poleman, 1975); maize was a sufficiently dominant component of the diets of some poor Southerners to trigger epidemics of pellagra (see Chapter 10) in some southern states in the early decades of this century.

In some Third World countries, fat accounts for less than 10% of total calorie intake and carbohydrate more than 75%. In some affluent countries, like the UK and US, fat will account for around 40% of calories and carbohydrate considerably less than 50%. In the poorer countries almost all of the carbohydrate calories are likely to be starches, whereas in richer countries close to half of the carbohydrate calories may be in the form of simple sugars. Improved palatability, higher prestige and simple increases in physical availability all compound to persuade those with the economic means to make changes in this general direction.

Paralleling these changes in food selection practices there will be changes in the general pattern of mortality and morbidity. Child mortality will fall due largely to a general reduction in mortality from infectious diseases. Undernutrition and deficiency diseases will all but disappear, life expectancy will increase but degenerative diseases of adults, the diseases of industrialisation, will account for an increasing proportion of deaths and will be an increasing cause of illness and disabil-

ity. Many of the nutritional guidelines for health promotion in the industrialised countries are directed towards partially reversing some of these wealth-related changes in dietary habits.

Effects of income upon food selection in industrialised countries

Even within industrialised countries, the food choices of the wealthiest and the poorest may vary quite considerably. Table 2.1 on the next page shows a comparison, from the UK National Food Survey (MAFF, 1993), of the household food consumption of families in the highest (A) and lowest (D) income groups of those in employment. The survey only records details of food purchased for home consumption but it does record that those in group A take almost twice as many meals outside the home as those in group D; retired and unemployed people take even fewer meals away from the home. Those in group D purchase significantly more meat than those in group A, but those in group A spend considerably more on their meat – those in group D tend to buy cheaper cuts and more bulky and lower quality meat products. Fresh fish purchases are considerably higher in group A than group D but the difference is proportionately less when all other fish and fish products are included; once again those in the higher income group spend considerably more on their fish, indicating higher quality, or at least higher prestige, purchases. Total milk and cream purchases are almost equal in the two groups but more of the richer group's milk is low fat. Purchases of sugar and preserves, potatoes and bread are all considerably higher in the poorer group. Consumption of wholemeal bread, green vegetables and fruit are all markedly higher in the more affluent group. The richer group purchases more alcoholic drinks, more soft drinks (soda) and more

Table 2.1 Household food purchases of richest and poorest UK families with at least one adult in employment. In group A the head of household earns more than £520 p.w. ($780) and group D less than £140 ($210). Values are per person per week or per day (pppw/pppd). Data source MAFF (1993)

	Group A	Group D
Number outside meals (pppw)	4.1	2.4
Foods (all pppw)		
Fresh meat and poultry (ounces)	16	16
Total meat (ounces)	30	32
Total meat (pence)	368	290
Fresh fish (ounces)	1.3	0.7
All fish and products (ounces)	5.1	4.1
All fish and products (pence)	88	50
Sugar and preserves (ounces)	5.0	7.7
Sugar only (ounces)	3.5	6.3
Potatoes (ounces)	21	36
Green and other fresh veg (ounces)	28	22
Fruit and fruit juice (ounces)	46	24
All bread (ounces)	22	29
Wholemeal bread (ounces)	4.5	3.4
Total milk and cream (pints)	3.9	3.9
Low fat milk (pints)	2.1	1.5
Drinks and confectionary (pppw)		
Alcoholic drinks (centilitres)	42	22
Confectionary/candy (grams)	52	44
Soft drinks/soda (fluid ounces)	29	23
Low calorie soft drinks	9.5	4.4
Nutrient intakes (pppd)		
Energy – kcal (MJ)	1750 (7.33)	1870 (7.83)
Fat (grams)	81	86
Fat (% energy)	42	41
Saturated fat (grams)	32	33
Saturated fat (% energy)	17	16
Polyunsaturated fat (grams)	14	15
Ratio of polyunsaturated:saturated	0.38	0.40
Vitamin C (mg)	62	44
Carbohydrate (% energy)	44	45
Total food expenditure (£/pppw)	**15.4**	**11.1**
Total including food, drink, sweets	**17.8**	**12.2**

confectionery (candy) than the poorer group; a much higher proportion of the soft drinks are low calorie in the richer group. The poorer group spends less on food than the richer group, but this expenditure represents a much higher proportion of the poorer group's total income. The poorer group gets significantly more calories for considerably less money than the richer group.

When one compares the nutritional value of the household food of different socio-economic groups then one finds that, if one allows for meals eaten outside the home, then all groups comfortably obtain or exceed the standards of adequacy for the major nutrients (MAFF, 1993). Thus the previously assumed adequacy of the diets of all groups within industrialised countries seems to be broadly confirmed. However, within any particular income group, the average weekly *per capita* expenditure on food falls with increasing numbers of children in the household. This is, perhaps, to be expected given the lower needs of children and the economies of scale possible in larger families. Nevertheless, the rate of decline in *per capita* expenditure is considerably steeper in poorer than richer families; the highest weekly average was for "adults only" households in group A and this was more than treble that in households in group D with four children or more; the latter group's expenditure was also more than 40% less than the average for group D. Groom (1993) suggests that the poorest UK families may spend more than a third of their income on food compared with a national average of around 12%. Apparently satisfactory overall averages may hide considerable variation in the diets of individual families. Poor families with several children are a likely high risk group.

When expressed as a percentage of total calories, the diet of the poorer group is marginally lower in total fat, saturated fat while having a slightly higher ratio of polyunsaturated to saturated fats. The high intake of fruits and vegetables in group A means that this group has considerably higher intakes of vitamin C and carotene (although total vitamin A is higher in group D). Carbohydrate consumption is higher in the poorer group and also makes up a slightly higher proportion of those people's total calorie intake (45% as compared to 44% in group A). The poorer group also purchases close to twice as much refined sugar as does group A.

This restricted comparison of the foods purchased by these two groups, suggests that socio-economic status has pronounced effects upon food choice. This will be partly due to differences in economic availability but will also be influenced by other factors such as education. Even in an affluent country, like the UK, food choice is still measurably affected by income. When one compares the two diets in terms of current nutrition education guidelines, then the results are rather mixed. The recommendations with respect to fat are currently the focus of nutrition education. In this respect, the diet of the poorer group D appears to be very similar to that of group A and may even be marginally better. Of course these figures only reflect food purchases and are restricted to household food. There may be major differences in preparation and practices at the table which are not allowed for in the National Food Survey such as, trimming fat from meat, relative use of grilling (broiling) and frying or the general amount of food wastage. The survey also only covers household food known to the record keeper, the contribution from food and drink consumed outside the home or purchased and consumed directly by other family members may be quite different in different social groups. In terms of current nutrition education guidelines and issues, the areas where the richer group's diet appears to be better are: higher consumption of fresh fish; higher consumption of fruit and green vegetables and thus of antioxidant vitamins (see Chapter 10); lower consumption of refined sugar; and a general tendency to use bread made from higher extraction flour (30% of bread in group A is standard white compared to almost 60% in group D). The higher use of low fat milk, wholemeal bread and low calorie soft drinks in the richer group suggests a higher level of health consciousness in food selection and an active attempt to make selections that are considered healthier. This general awareness of, and active attempt to make, healthy choices probably permeates into many other facets of diet and lifestyle.

Gregory *et al.* (1990) found that in a survey of British adults, measured intakes of fibre, many vitamins, many minerals and sugars tended to be higher in higher social groups (I and II) than in lower social groups. Biochemical indices of antioxidant vitamin status were also higher in the upper social classes. Overweight and obesity amongst women they found to be more prevalent in the lower than the upper social classes. Gregory and her colleagues found that a dietary pattern they described as "health conscious" was more likely to be associated with the higher social classes whereas one they described as "a traditional meat and vegetable diet" with a tendency to high energy and alcohol consumption was more likely to be found amongst the manual social classes.

The hierarchy of human needs (Figure 2.2) suggests that biological needs become increasingly significant determinants of food selection at lower income levels. If one also assumes that even the poorest groups in an industrialised country should receive at least minimum subsistence level income from welfare payments, then one might expect poverty to have relatively small adverse effect upon nutritional adequacy. The National Food Survey does seem to broadly support this proposition. Despite this, there may be some wide variations that are partly obscured by taking averages, and there will inevitably be individuals or groups who fall through the welfare safety net, e.g. homeless single people and large, low income families.

Welfare payments in the UK have traditionally been calculated on the basis that enough money should be provided to allow purchase of the essentials of life but not enough to allow the purchase of luxuries. The same underlying philosophy governs the welfare systems of most industrialised countries, although there are considerable differences in the generosity of its application. The aim of such a strategy is to prevent those dependent upon welfare from starving or being deprived of basic shelter and clothing whilst at the same time not making their situation so comfortable as to discourage them from seeking employment or to encourage others to voluntarily live off of the state. A more cynical Marxist interpretation of this principle would be that enough money is provided to prevent social unrest but not enough to reduce the competition for jobs and thus risk increasing the cost of labour. Pressures on public expenditure may encourage governments to economise by reducing the purchasing power of those dependant upon welfare payments.

Calculation of minimum subsistence levels of income will be difficult. There is a host of factors which will produce wide variations in the quality of life that different families can achieve with the same level of income. At the physiological level, apparently matched adults performing the same amounts of physical activity may vary considerably in their energy and nutrient requirements. Regional and individual variations in housing, transport and fuel costs may make it difficult to produce a single welfare figure for a nation. Differences in cultural and personal preferences will affect the size of the required food budget. A minimally adequate income may make it difficult to live at maximum economic efficiency. The poorest may be forced to buy in small expensive quantities; they may be unable to stock up when a seasonal food is cheap or when special offers are made; they may not have the transportation or personal mobility to enable shopping at the most economic places. For a variety of reasons such as these, it may well be accurate to say: "the poor pay more".

Other demands upon the household budget may greatly restrain food expenditure for some individuals or families. When financial resources are restricted, especially if there is a sudden decline in income (e.g. through loss of employment, retirement or long term illness), then expenditure on food may be sacrificed in order to maintain spending upon other essentials such as housing, loan repayments, clothing or fuel. Food expenditure may be sacrificed to allow purchase or retention of some prestigious item or activity that helps maintain self esteem, e.g. Christmas presents for children, a car, a colour television, tobacco or going to the pub. Considerable savings can often be made in the food budget without obvious acute hardship, e.g. by switching to cheaper brands or varieties, by reducing wastage and by using cheaper alternatives like margarine for butter or lower quality meat and fish products for fresh meat and fish.

To subsist on a minimum income is likely to be considerably facilitated by a degree of budget management skill. Unfortunately those with the least of these skills may often be those most likely to be required to exercise them – poor educational attainment and poor socio-economic status are strongly correlated. Strictly theoretical calculations of minimum subsistence levels cannot allow for food choices that appear irrational or even irresponsible using strictly biological criteria. People whose self-esteem has been dented by unemployment, disability or social deprivation may buy foods to boost their spirits and self esteem rather than out of strict scientific necessity. In *The road to Wigan pier* George Orwell gives an example of an adequate but dull and low prestige diet that in 1937 could be obtained for twenty pence (30 cents). He also gives an example of the real expenditure of an unemployed miner's family at the time. This real family spent only fourpence each week on green vegetables and sweetened condensed milk, nothing at all on fruit, but 9 pence on sugar (representing 4 kg of sugar), five pence on tea and three pence on jam. Clearly white bread spread with margarine and jam and washed down with sweet tea was an important part of this family's daily diet. Orwell describes this mixture as being almost devoid of nutritional value, and it certainly was low in several micronutrients.

When you are unemployed, which is to say when you are underfed, harassed, bored and miserable, you don't want to eat dull wholesome food. You want something a little bit tasty ....Unemployment is an endless misery that has got to be constantly palliated, and especially with tea, the Englishman's opium. A cup of tea or even an aspirin is much better as a temporary stimulant than a crust of brown bread.

George Orwell (1937)
The road to Wigan Pier

Today, tobacco might be described as the poor "Englishman's opium". Despite health education campaigns and very large increases in taxation, smoking amongst many of the poorest groups is still the rule rather than the exception. Using taxation to discourage smoking probably only serves to make the poor still poorer and shock campaigns that highlight the dangers of smoking or its social unacceptability probably serve only to increase fear, guilt and the social isolation of the poor smoker.

Orwell goes on to describe the poor people of a British industrial city as being small of stature and having universally bad or missing teeth – he suggests that it was rare to see a working class person with good natural teeth. He suggests that the death rate and infant mortality rate of the poorest area of any city was always at least double that in the wealthy areas, in some cases much more than double. He was writing about mid-20th century peacetime conditions in one of the wealthiest industrialised countries of the world. These few pages of Orwell's book underline how far social conditions and nutrition of most poorer people in Britain have improved over the last 50 years despite the disparity between the health and nutrition of rich and poor that still remains.

One practical consequence of the kind of effect described by Orwell will be to make it even more difficult to persuade the less affluent to make dietary changes that they perceive as reducing either the palatability or prestige of their diet. While diet-related disease is more prevalent in the poorer groups they also seem to be more resistant to nutritional and other health education advice. The decline in prevalence of breastfeeding with social class (White *et al.*, 1992) is a very clear example of this. This increases the onus upon those seeking to effect dietary change amongst all social groups to suggest changes that are simple, that are easy to permanently incorporate in usual culinary practices and that are not overly restrictive of highly palatable and high prestige foods. Change must not require the consumption of a diet that, although wholesome by current nutritional criteria, is perceived as dull and unpalatable and uses low prestige ingredients.

Changes must also be within a group's economic means if those changes are really expected to be implemented. Groom (1993) reviews a number of attempts to devise "healthy" diets that comply with current UK dietary guidelines and are also within the economic means of poorer families. A "least change" diet that involved no drastic changes in any of the food categories in the average UK diet cost 3% less than the current average food expenditure but 10% more than the amount spent by low income families. Less expensive healthy diets could be devised, but these involved greater changes, and she questions whether such diets would be acceptable and whether families without detailed nutrition knowledge would know which foods to select. If high fat, high sugar foods are replaced by starchy staples, then this may well involve reduced expenditure. However, to stay as close as possible to current eating patterns but to choose "healthier" alternatives such as leaner meat, wholemeal bread and fruit would increase food costs by 6–13%, which would not be possible for many low income families.

Effects of migration upon eating habits

Migrant groups are frequently used by epidemiologists in order to separate out the environmental and genetic influences upon patterns of mortality and morbidity (see Chapter 3). Migrants may also suffer from nutrition-related problems that may be much rarer both in their native homeland and amongst the indigenous population of their new homeland. For example, migrants to the UK from the Indian subcontinent have suffered from mini-epidemics of rickets, a condition that had been largely eliminated in the white population. It is therefore useful to try to establish and understand trends and patterns to the changes in dietary habits that inevitably occur after migration. Conflicts will inevitably arise between traditional influences and influences from the new culture, and these may adversely affect the dietary practices of migrants. What factors influence the speed of change? Why are the health records of migrant groups often worse than those of the indigenous population? Are there any measures that might facilitate the healthful assimilation of migrant groups into their new environment?

Why should change occur at all? Culture, including food habits, is a learned phenomenon rather than something that is innate or biologically determined. Culture is transmitted between generations by the process of socialisation. There is an inherent tendency of cultures to change over time and this process of change is almost inevitably greatly hastened by migration and exposure to the different cultural practices of the indigenous population. **Acculturation** is the term used to describe this acceleration of cultural change that occurs when different cultures interact. Both indigenous and migrant cultures are likely to be changed by their interaction, but migrants may feel the need to adopt aspects of the indigenous culture to facilitate their acceptance and assimilation into their new country. They will usually be in a minority and be dependent upon the goodwill of the indigenous population, they may therefore feel great pressure to conform in order to be accepted and to succeed in their new homeland.

Paradoxically, every culture also has a built-in resistance to change. Culture is mostly internalised, routine activities done unthinkingly in a particular way because that is the way they have always been done. After migration, however, there is repeated exposure to different cultural practices and familiarity may eventually lead to acceptance of initially strange and alien practices as normal. Dietary practices of the indigenous culture that are inconsistent with the values and beliefs of the migrant's culture may be the slowest to be adopted and also those most likely to cause social divisions within migrant communities or families. For example, migrants may be most reluctant to absorb dietary practices that would involve breaking of the food rules of their religion. The older, more conservative, migrants will probably be most resistant to such changes and those older folk may also be hostile to changes in the behaviour of younger, less ethnocentric members of their community or family. Dietary practices of migrants that are inconsistent with the values of the indigenous culture may also be a source of considerable friction between migrants and their fellow citizens. For example, Moslem and Jewish rules concerning the slaughter of animals sometimes provoke hostility in Britain from people concerned about animal welfare.

Bavly (1966) analysed changes over three generation in the diets of immigrants to Israel. She considered that several factors had a major accelerating effect upon the speed at which change occurred:

- marriage between different ethnic groups
- a home-maker working outside the home

- children receiving nutrition education at school
- children having school meals
- and, nutrition education via the media for immigrants of European origin.

These specific influences may be generalised to factors that increase interaction with the indigenous population and increase familiarity with, and understanding of, indigenous dietary practices. Conversely, any factors that tend to isolate the migrant from the indigenous population and culture may be expected to slow down acculturation, such as:

- an inability to read or speak the new language restricts interaction at the personal level and restricts access to the media
- cultural beliefs that discourage the homemaker from independent socialising outside the family
- religious beliefs and dietary rules that are at odds with the dietary practices of the indigenous majority
- living within a fairly self-contained immigrant area where shops are run by fellow migrants and where familiar foods and even native language media are available.

Many of these isolating influences would apply to many new immigrants from the Indian subcontinent to Britain.

Migration is often prompted by the attraction of improved economic opportunities in industrialised countries. Thus large scale migration is often accompanied by a complete change of social structure from a rural agrarian to a Western industrial type of society. In the rural agrarian community, society is likely to be based upon extended and close-knit family groupings with a constant flow of food between families and individuals. In Western industrialised societies this informal family and community support may no longer be available because people are organised into relatively isolated family groups, food is normally shared only with the immediate family and this sharing may help to define the family. These changes in social organisation may mean that in times of hardship, the missing informal neighbourhood and family support will have to be replaced by formal charitable or state welfare support. Accepting such "charity" may reduce the migrants' self esteem and perhaps engender hostility in the indigenous population. The impact of such changes may be ameliorated where movement is into an already well-established ethnic community.

Migrants from a rural food-orientated economy may suddenly be confronted with a cash-dominated economy. Family incomes of new immigrants are likely to be relatively low (inappropriate skills, language problems, discrimination, etc.). This combination of low income and lack of experience in cash budgeting may make immigrant people unable to cope adequately, even though their income may be technically adequate. An educational induction programme might reduce the impact of this potential problem. Food selection for migrants may be complicated by the unavailability of recognisable traditional foods; even where they are available, they may be relatively expensive because of their specialist nature. Food selection by immigrants may be particularly influenced by advertising pressures that encourage the excessive consumption of foods that are high in palatability and prestige but of relatively low nutritional value. Social and cultural pressures may tend to discourage migrant women from breastfeeding their infants.

Migration from a rural agrarian society in a developing country to a Western industrial society, will probably be associated with trends that are similar to the worldwide changes that accompany increasing affluence. The traditional starchy and predominantly vegetarian diet is likely to diversify, become more omnivorous, and sugars and fats will progressively replace some of the starch. The diseases of undernutrition will decline, but the dis-

eases of industrialisation will almost certainly become increasingly prevalent.

Wenham and Wolff (1970) surveyed the changes in the dietary habits of Japanese immigrants and their descendants to Hawaii. Japanese migrants began arriving in Hawaii at the end of the 19th century to become plantation workers in Hawaii. The typical Japanese diet at this time was a high carbohydrate, predominantly rice and plant-food diet. The major animal foods would have been fish and other seafood. Initially these migrants maintained their traditional diet; many regarded their stay in Hawaii as temporary and ate frugally in order to save for their return to Japan. After the annexation of Hawaii by the USA in 1898, these Japanese migrants started working outside of the plantations, and businesses specialising in the importation of traditional Japanese foods sprang up. Initially this change resulted in increased consumption of imported and high status Japanese foods. As these Japanese foods became cheaper, their status diminished and they came to be regarded as old-fashioned by many younger Japanese who preferred to eat American foods.

The traditional Japanese social structure with its strong family tradition, worship of ancestors and subordination of personal desires to the welfare of the family was replaced by a more fragmented society orientated by the notion of personal freedom. The traditional Buddhist constraints on meat consumption weakened as meat was plentiful in Hawaii.

Public education seems to have been a catalyst for change amongst the second generation as the schools encouraged newcomers to change their habits. There also seems little doubt that World War II accelerated the "Americanisation" of Japanese people in Hawaii. Wenham and Wolff describe a Japanese wedding in Hawaii before the war as being typically Japanese in character with no wedding cake, but by 1945 the food at such a wedding was likely to be much more cosmopolitan, with a Western wedding cake as the highlight.

Wenham and Wolff concluded that in 1970, the Japanese in Hawaii could be classified into three groups, namely:

- a traditional group of mainly older people who maintained a very Japanese cuisine
- a group that, although relatively acculturated, still consumed Japanese foods on some occasions
- an "Americanised" group that rejected Japanese heritage and the foods associated with it.

There may now exist a further category of Japanese-Americans who are moving back to traditional foods for health reasons as well as to re-affirm their ethnic identity (i.e. for reasons of self-actualisation).

Williams and Qureshi (1988) suggested a similar "four generation" concept that could be a useful way of explaining some of the variations in food choices within any particular ethnic minority group in the UK:

- *First generation A* – migrants who arrived as dependent relatives of migrant workers. They are usually retired and prefer to eat their native foods.
- *First generation B* – migrants who arrived as workers. They are usually aged 21–65 years and they accept both native and British foods.
- *Second generation* – young people aged 7–21 years who went to school in Britain and in many cases were born here. They prefer the new diet and may strongly resist attempts to force them to consume their native diet which is alien to them.
- *Third generation* – children who were born in Britain, who feel British but who have become interested in tracing their ethnic roots. They will accept both British and native foods.

The changes in the diet of the Japanese in Hawaii reviewed by Wenham and Wolff (1970) have been accompanied by a large increase in height of the typical Hawaiian Japanese and a lengthening of life expectancy. Deficiency diseases, in particular beriberi, have now been all but eliminated. On the debit side, the Hawaiian Japanese have very high rates of tooth decay and are four times more likely than the Japanese in Japan to have heart attacks.

Dietary taboos

The word taboo is derived from the Polynesian name for a system of religious prohibitions against the use of sacred things. It has come to mean any sacred prohibition and, with common usage, the religious connotation is no longer obligatory. One could define a dietary taboo as any avoidance that is maintained solely because failure to do so would generate disapproval, ostracism or punishment within one's own cultural group or because it would compromise one's own ethical standards. A food taboo should be distinguished from avoidances that are based upon sound empirical evidence of harm.

Many taboos are aimed at avoidance of flesh and these flesh taboos are often the most rigorously adhered to. It is said that the initial spark that ignited the Indian Mutiny against British rule in 1857 was the introduction of cartridges supposedly greased with animal fat. Hindu troops were unwilling to bite the ends off of these cartridges or, indeed, even to handle them. On May 6th 1857, 85 of 90 members of the 3rd native cavalry in Meerut refused direct orders to handle cartridges which, according to a contemporary account, they mistakenly believed to be contaminated with animal fat. They were subsequently sentenced to terms of imprisonment of between 6 and 10 years. These men would undoubtedly have been aware of the likely consequences of disobeying a direct military order, an awareness that would certainly underline the potential strength of such taboos.

The taboos of other cultures tend to be viewed as illogical restraints often imposed upon individuals by authoritarian religious leaders. This model leads to the belief that taboos should be discouraged. This is almost certainly a misreading of the situation in most cases. Most taboos need little external compulsion to ensure adherence; people feel secure when maintaining cultural standards that have been ingrained since childhood. There are nonetheless a few examples of essentially religious taboos being incorporated into the secular law and of severe penalties being imposed upon transgressors. In many Indian states the cow is legally protected, and there are severe penalties for alcohol consumption in some Moslem countries.

Most people of western European origin would not consider dietary taboos to have any significant influence upon their food selection, but no society is completely free of dietary prohibitions. It is not too long ago that Roman Catholics were required to abstain from meat on Fridays and some Christians still avoid meat on Good Friday. In the UK cannibalism is clearly prohibited but, equally, the consumption of animals like cats, dogs and horses would result in widespread hostility from and probably ostracism by other members of society. Most British people would not recognise these latter avoidances as taboos because ideologically they do not classify these creatures as potential food despite their being highly regarded as foods in some other countries. In France, for example, horsemeat is eaten, sometimes even meat from British horses!

In the UK, vegetarianism would seem to be an obvious candidate for an example of a dietary taboo that may have negative nutritional implications. Certainly many omnivores would like to think so, as the vegetarians' rejection of flesh is often perceived as a threat to highly desired and high prestige foods. There are some problems associated with a strictly vegetarian (vegan) diet (see Chapter 14), but it is also clear that a well-constructed vegetarian diet can be healthy. In the current climate of nutrition opinion, a well-constructed vegetarian diet may even be regarded as healthier than the typical omnivorous diet. Vegetarianism must be socially inconvenient where most of the population is omnivorous and where often only nominal provision is made for vegetarians by caterers. These inconveniences may, however, be more than compensated for by a comradeship, akin to religious fellowship, seemingly shared by many vegetarians which can lead to an enhancement of self-actualisation.

Perhaps, taboo has played some part in the dramatic decline in breastfeeding that occurred in Britain in the decades following World War II or perhaps it has played a part in thwarting current efforts to encourage breastfeeding. The inconvenience of breastfeeding and its "prestige" can only have been worsened by a very strong taboo against breastfeeding amongst strangers and in many cases even amongst friends and relatives. The arrival of a modern, scientifically developed and socially acceptable alternative provided women with an ideal opportunity to free themselves of the need to continue with this "inconvenient and embarrassing process". A decade ago a woman's magazine reported numerous examples of women arousing hostility from other customers in restaurants by publicly breastfeeding infants. Some restaurant managers had asked women to stop the feeding or even to leave the restaurant. Two recent surveys by the Royal College of Midwives (briefly summarised in Laurent, 1993) indicate this type of attitude still persists and is widespread. More than a third of the 700 restaurants surveyed either would not permit breastfeeding at the table or would ask women to stop if another customer complained. In the second survey, half a sample of 900 men disagreed with women breastfeeding "in any place they choose". They gave reasons for their objections like "it's unnecessary" "it's a form of exhibitionism" "it's disgusting behaviour". Clearly breastfeeding is seen by many men (and perhaps many women, too) as a distasteful or an embarrassing task that needs to be performed furtively. In Britain, images of bare female breasts are ubiquitous in popular newspapers, television, films and even on some beaches, and yet the sight of a woman breastfeeding her baby apparently still has the potential to shock and embarrass a high proportion of British adults.

The most widely familiar taboos – religious perhaps – generally cause few nutritional problems. Some taboos may apply only during certain phases of the life-cycle or during illness, however. Likewise some taboos may be restricted to certain groups of people. These kinds of taboos will also not usually give rise to adverse nutritional consequences unless they are imposed at times of rapid growth or when a body is under extreme physiological stress. An example of a taboo gone awry quoted by Fieldhouse (1986) is the varied food avoidances amongst the women of the southern Indian state of Tamilnadu, during lactation, during which time women are supposed to avoid: meat, eggs, rice, dhal, chillies, cow milk, sardines, fruits, potato, yam, cashew nuts and, onions. These avoidances compound with previous restrictions during pregnancy and the possibility of serious adverse nutritional consequences is clear. Additionally there is a widespread belief amongst various peoples that sick children should not be fed or should only be offered very restricted diets, thus potentially precipitating Protein Energy Malnutrition. There is also a widespread belief that many adult foods, especially meat and fish, are unsuitable for young children, leaving the starchy staple foods with their problems of low energy and nutrient density as the major permitted food at a time of relatively high physiological demand for both energy and nutrients.

If most dietary taboos are not usually associated with any major adverse nutritional consequences, then why should nutritionists and nutrition educators study them? The answer to this question is that taboos provide an insight into a culture, and some understanding of a culture is necessary if the general philosophy of giving advice that is culturally compatible is to be maintained. If advice is given that involves breaking an important dietary taboo then all of the advice may be ignored and, perhaps, the future credibility of the adviser destroyed. Maybe, even worse, if certain individuals are persuaded to conform to this advice, then this may provoke friction and divisions within a community or family.

If a taboo is nutritionally only marginally detrimental, neutral or perhaps even beneficial in its impact, then, no matter how bizarre or irrational it may seem, the cultural choice of the client should be respected – some of the practices of the adviser may seem equally bizarre to the client. If a taboo is manifestly harmful, then the aim of the adviser should be to eliminate the harmful impact with the minimum disruption to the cultural life of the client.

The conclusion that a taboo is harmful should be based upon a wide analysis of its impact. Fieldhouse (1986) uses the example of the Hindu sacred cow to make this point. There are nearly 200 million cows in India and yet their slaughter for food is generally forbidden even in times of famine – illogical? harmful? He points out that cows provide milk, their dead carcasses provide leather and are used as food by the lower castes. Cows provide the oxen traditionally vital for Indian agriculture; cow dung is also a major source of fuel and fertiliser in rural India. And much of the cow's food is scavenged and would be basically inedible to humans. The conclusion of adverseness is now less secure and the value of the taboo in preventing destruction of these valuable and well-adapted animals in adverse conditions is, at least, arguable.

How do taboos originate? As with much historical research, the sources of factual information are limited, and the scope for speculation is, in consequence, very great. Many theories as to their origins exist, each can give plausible explanations of some taboos and often these different theories can be used to give equally plausible explanations of the same taboo. Taboos are often derived from some religious commandment; be it in the religious book of the group, the oral mythology or the edict of some historical religious leader or teacher. Fieldhouse (1986) gives several examples of theories concerning the origins of taboos, such as:

1 *Aesthetic* – particular animals are rejected because of the perceived unpleasant lifestyle of the animal, e.g. some people consider the flesh of the mackerel as low prestige or inferior because they regard the mackerel as a scavenger. All meat may be rejected because of the perceived cruelty involved in rearing and slaughter.
2 *Health and sanitation* – the belief that there is, or was, some inherent logic underlying the exclusion of particular foods on health grounds. In effect, it is suggested that taboos originate from food avoidances based upon well-founded evidence of harm.

It has been suggested that Jewish prohibitions against shellfish consumption may have been prompted by the risk of poisoning by the toxin produced by the plankton species *Gonyaulux tamarensis* that the shellfish may have consumed (see Chapter 15).

3 *Ecology* – that there is some underlying environmental logic behind a particular prohibition. The exclusion of meat and fish at particular times to conserve stocks is an obvious example; the avoidance of meat by some present day vegetarians to prevent inefficient use of grain and thus to increase world food availability would be another.
4 *Religious distinction* – taboos serve to demonstrate the separateness of a religious group from non-believers and the self-restraint required to obey them may serve as a symbol of piety and obedience to the religious leaders.

The avoidance of pork by Jews is a very well-known taboo and Fieldhouse (1986) shows how each of the above explanations can been used to explain the origins of this particular taboo:

1 Jewish dietary law states that only animals that have cloven hooves and that chew the cud are clean and therefore edible – the pig is therefore unclean and inedible. The pig is widely viewed as a dirty and scavenging animal even by people who value its flesh.
2 Pork is a source of a parasitic worm that causes a disease, Trichinosis. Perhaps this is the origin of the Jewish taboo against pork, which is shared by other Middle Eastern peoples. Opponents of this theory argue that this is merely a later attempt at scientific rationalisation. The danger of Trichinosis is being used as one argument in a current campaign against horsemeat consumption in France; this is despite the fact that there have been only two outbreaks of the disease in France in the last 15 years, each outbreak due to a single, infected carcass.
3 It is suggested that supernatural prohibitions against the consumption of pork arose because the desert conditions of the Middle East were unsuitable for efficient pig rearing. It is suggested that taboos rarely involve abundant species that can be eaten with no threat to total food supplies.
4 Finally it is suggested that the pork taboo was originally part of a relatively lax and general prohibition against "imperfect" animals, including flightless birds and shellfish. Its symbolic importance was heightened when Syrian invaders forced Jews to eat pork as a visible sign of submission, and, thus,

once Jews regained their independ-
ence, strict pork avoidance came to
symbolise their Jewishness and their
opposition to pagan rule.

Endpiece

Cream has traditionally been a highly
prized, high prestige, luxury food in the
UK – a "high calorie treat". It is also, of
course, rich in saturated fat and cholesterol. In many health conscious people,
cream consumption now evokes feelings
of guilt or even fear – one UK advertising
campaign for cream used the catchphrase
"naughty but nice". I was once asked to
participate in an experiment that involved
consuming porridge (oatmeal) made with
cream. I did not volunteer because the
experiment involved repeated venepunc-
ture. Several of my colleagues at the time
assumed that I was really frightened of
eating the cream! Have we the origins of a
new dietary taboo loosely based upon
some notion of "health and sanitation"?
Will future generations of nutritionists
speculate upon the origins of the cream
taboo in some Western countries?

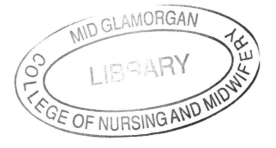
3 Methods of nutritional surveillance and research

Contents

Aim

The methods used in the scientific study of nutrition range from the high precision measurements of the analytical chemist through to the inevitably much less precise methods of the social scientist and behavioural psychologist. All approaches can be equally valid and rigorous and the complete range of approaches is necessary to study all of the various aspects of nutrition. The aim of this chapter is to give readers a sufficient insight into the methods of nutritional surveillance and research to enable them to read the literature critically. An understanding of the relative strengths and the limitations of the methods used is essential for any critical evaluation of the conclusions drawn from reported data. Some perception of the errors inherent in methods of measurement is necessary for realistic appraisal of the results that they produce.

Food analysis

Food tables

Food tables are an essential tool of both nutritional surveillance and research. Printed food tables contain lists of thousands of foods with the quantities of each nutrient in a standard amount (100 g) for each food. To translate food intakes into nutrient intakes with such printed tables is very tedious and time-consuming – the content of each nutrient in the consumed portion of each food has to be calculated from the tables and eventually the total consumption of each nutrient determined. Nowadays, the information contained within these printed tables is available on computer software, requiring the investigator merely to key in the foods and portion sizes and the computer will then automatically translate these into nutrient intakes. These programmes will also often calculate the nutrient intakes as proportions of the standard reference values appropriate for a subject whose size, age, sex, activity level and reproductive status has also been entered.

Both forms of these tables are the result of many hours of meticulous analytical work; to give the nutrient contents of a thousand foods requires more than thirty thousand individual determinations. The analytical methods used in the construction of food tables are briefly surveyed below. A number of general sources of error are inherent in the use of food tables, and these may produce errors and uncertainties that are orders of magnitude greater than the errors in analytical methods. Some of these flaws are listed below:

1 *Limited range of foods covered by tables* – Some of the software available for dietary analysis lists several thousand different food items including, in some cases, many menu items from the major restaurant chains. Despite this, there will inevitably be foods eaten that are not specifically listed in the tables – in such circumstances the operator either has to find alternative sources of information (such as nutritional information on the food label) or has to judge which is the nearest equivalent in the food tables. Continued innovation on the part of food manufacturers and increasing availability of foods from different parts of the world means that this will be an ongoing problem. Thus kiwi fruit, hoki (a fish from New Zealand) and Quorn (a mycoprotein meat substitute) were rare or unknown in Britain a few years ago but are now widely available and used – none of them is listed in the 1978 British food tables.

2 *Recipe variations* – Many dishes are extensive mixtures of foods, and it is often not practical in diet records or histories to obtain the precise mixture of ingredients used in the preparation of a particular dish. Even though the food tables may list this dish, the recipe used for the analysis in the tables may be quite different from the recipe used to prepare the food that was consumed. Thus, for example, beef and vegetable stew is something that will vary markedly in its composition from cook to cook. The ratio of vegetables to meat, the range and proportions of the vegetable mixture, the leanness of the meat, the amount of thickening agent (e.g. flour), and the proportion of water may all vary considerably. When estimating the nutrients in say, a slice of pie, then the proportions of crust and filling used by the analyst may be different from those that were actually eaten.

Different brands of the same commercially prepared foods will also vary, and the composition of any single brand may vary significantly from batch to batch. There are several brands of "baked beans canned in tomato sauce"; food tables can only give an average or typical composition. Some foods such as white flour may be supplemented with nutrients; this could be a source of considerable error if the supplementation in the analysed and eaten food is different, e.g. if American food tables are used to analyse British bread.

3 *Biological variation* – Just as different brands and recipes of prepared foods will vary in their composition, so different varieties of natural foods will vary in their composition – there may even be marked variation, particularly seasonal variation, within the same variety. Rump (buttock) steak from different cattle may have markedly different proportions of fat. The extent to which fat is removed during preparation and at the table will also vary greatly. As another example, the vitamin C content of apples may vary by up to 600% in different varieties. Once again, food tables can only indicate an average or a typical composition.

4 *Method and duration of storage* – The nutrient content of foods may change during storage. Milk left in strong sunlight may lose much of its riboflavin (vitamin B_2). The vitamin C content of maincrop potatoes after 8–9 months of storage will be only about a quarter of that when they were freshly dug. Foods upon which mould has grown may acquire dietetically significant amounts of vitamin B_{12}.

Energy content of foods

The processes of oxidative metabolism of foodstuffs are frequently equated to the oxidative processes of combustion or burning. This would suggest that the heat energy released during the combustion of a food should be a reliable indicator of its metabolic energy yield. In a **bomb calorimeter**, a small sample of food is placed in a sealed chamber which is pressurised with oxygen (to facilitate complete combustion) and the food then ignited electrically. The heat energy released during combustion of the food sample is then measured. This heat energy of combustion will significantly overestimate the energy that is metabolically available from most foods. The predictive value of the heat of combustion is worsened if the food is high in indigestible material or high in protein.

Some components of a food, such as dietary fibre, may burn and release heat energy but not be digested and absorbed, and this fraction of the energy of combustion will be lost in the faeces.

In the bomb calorimeter there is complete oxidation of protein to water, carbon dioxide and oxide of nitrogen, whereas in metabolic oxidation most of the nitrogen is excreted in the urine as urea. The metabolic energy yield from protein is only about 70% of the heat energy released during combustion, the other 30% is lost in the urine.

To determine the **metabolisable energy** from the heat energy released during combustion, it must be corrected for the energy lost in the faeces and for energy losses in urine as discussed above.

Nowadays, the usual way of determining the energy value of foods is to measure the available carbohydrate, fat, protein and alcohol content of the food and then to use standard conversion values for the metabolisable energy of each of these nutrients:

- 1 g of carbohydrate is assumed to yield 3.75 kilocalories (kcal) or 16 kilojoules (kJ)
- 1 g of protein 4 kcal (17 kJ)
- 1 g of fat 9 kcal (37 kJ)
- 1 g of alcohol 7 kcal (29 kJ).

Small variations in these conversion factors are of little significance, given the many other sources of error and uncertainty in estimating dietary energy intake. Non starch polysaccharide or dietary fibre has traditionally been assumed to contribute nothing to metabolisable energy, but recent studies suggest that it may yield up to 2 kcal per gram (via its fermentation by intestinal bacteria to volatile fatty acids and the subsequent absorption and metabolism of those acids).

Estimation of protein content

During the last century the German chemist, Liebig, noted that proteins from different sources all contained approximately 16% by weight of nitrogen. This observation remains the basis of estimating the protein content of foods; if the nitrogen content is determined and then multiplied by 6.25 (i.e. 100/16) then this will give an estimate of the protein content:

$$\text{wt. of protein} = \text{wt. of nitrogen} \times 6.25$$

This 6.25 figure is an approximation, and more precise values may be used for some foods. Some foods may contain non-protein nitrogen, but in most foods this non-protein nitrogen is largely amino acid and thus would not produce any dietetic error.

The chemical procedure used to determine the nitrogen content of foods is called the Kjeldahl method – the food is first digested by boiling it with concentrated sulphuric acid and a catalyst which converts the nitrogen into ammonium sulphate. Alkali is then added to the digest and liberated ammonia is distilled into acid; the amount of ammonia liberated is determined by titration.

Estimation of fat content

Fat is organic material that is insoluble in water but, unlike the other components of food, soluble in organic fat solvents such as petroleum spirit, ether and chloroform. Fat content may be simply measured by determining the amount of material that can be extracted from a sample of food by such solvents.

The proportions of the individual fatty acids contained within food fats are now considered to be of particular significance, this may be determined using **gas liquid chromatography (GLC)**. The fat is chemically broken down into its component fatty acids (hydrolysed) and these fatty acids converted to their methyl derivatives to make them volatile. The individual acids can then be separated by GLC because they will be pulled through a column of lipophilic (lipid attracting) material at different speeds by a flow of gas. The amount of the now-separated individual fatty acids emerging at the end of the column is determined by flame ionisation – the ions produced by the fatty acids in a flame generate a current that is proportional to the amount. Standardisation and calibration is by the use of known amounts of known fatty acid as standards; the time it takes for an unknown acid to pass through the column enables it to be identified, and the size of the current generated by flame ionisation indicates the quantity.

Estimation of carbohydrate content

Available carbohydrate in foods is made up of sugars and starches. Chemical methods are used to directly measure the amount of water soluble sugars in the food. Starch content is determined by measuring the amount of sugar released by hydrolysis with a starch-digesting enzyme system.

Dietary fibre is made up of a variable mixture of non-starch polysaccharides or indigestible carbohydrate plus the woody material lignin and resistant starch. Dietary fibre has traditionally been estimated by difference i.e. what remains when the weight of the other components has been subtracted. It is now usually measured by separate analysis of each of the component substances. Different methods of measuring dietary fibre yield sometimes quite different results, and this can be a source of considerable confusion and controversy (see Chapter 7).

Vitamin content of foods

Detailed descriptions of the individual analytical methods used to measure vitamins is beyond the scope of this book; only the general principles and problems can be overviewed. The vitamin must first be extracted from the food; some vitamins are water soluble and others fat soluble – the former would be extracted into water and the latter into an organic fat solvent. The extracted vitamin may then be assayed by one of a range of different types of methods, such as:

1 *Chemical analytical methods* – The vitamin is usually converted to a derivative that is coloured or fluorescent and the amount then determined by electronically comparing the colour or fluorescent intensity to that obtained using standards of known vitamin concentration.

2 *Gas-liquid chromatography*–The principle has already been outlined for determining the fatty acid composition of fat.

3 *Microbiological assay* – The extract containing the vitamin is added to a culture medium for a micro-organism that requires the vitamin for growth. Prior to addition of the extract, the culture medium contains all of the growth requirements for the organism except the vitamin. The extent of bacterial growth will, under these circumstances, indicate the amount of vitamin added. Bacterial growth is assessed by comparing the turbidity or cloudiness of the medium to other samples to which known amounts of the vitamin were added.

4 *Radio-immunoassay*–The vitamin-containing extract is added to known amounts of vitamin antibody and radioactive vitamin. The vitamin in the sample will compete with the radioactive vitamin for binding sites on the antibody. The amount of radioactivity in the vitamin-antibody fraction (which usually precipitates out of solution) will be inversely related to the amount of vitamin present in the extract. As with the other methods it would be calibrated using vitamin samples of known concentration.

Some general problems that may be encountered when foods are assayed for vitamin content:

- The vitamin may be present in the food in extremely low concentrations which means that extremely sensitive detection methods may be required. For example, milk contains only 0.3 µg of vitamin B_{12} per 100 g, i.e. a dilution of more than one in three hundred million.
- Some vitamins may have several different chemical forms or may be present in the form of a precursor. When the vitamin activity of foods is assessed then the activity contributed by the different chemical forms must be estimated and added together. Vitamin A activity in milk is partly due to vitamin A itself, retinol, and partly due to the plant-derived pigment carotene (see Chapter 10). The niacin (vitamin B3) derived from food may either come directly from vitamin in the food or indirectly by conversion of the amino acid tryptophan to niacin.
- The vitamin activity of certain chemical substances in food may be uncertain. Breast milk contains a water soluble substance with uncertain vitamin D activity. Folic acid (folacin) is present in several different forms in food; the extent to which these different forms are absorbed varies, making precise estimation of available folic acid in some foods problematical.

Mineral content of foods

The minerals present in foods are all assayed by the precise methods of analytical chemistry – it does not necessarily follow that the mineral content of a diet determined using food tables will be reliable. For example:

- Salt is frequently added to food during cooking and at the table. Standard food tables are therefore an unreliable means of estimating an individual's total salt intake.
- Pieces of bone in meat and fish may greatly increase the calcium content. With canned fish, the bones are softened and made more readily edible and cutting meat with a saw produces powdered bone that may stick to the meat and be eaten.
- Contact of foods with processing machines or with cooking utensils may significantly affect the content of metallic elements. Cooking or brewing in iron pots may enhance the iron content of foods very considerably, e.g. beer brewed in iron vessels has been a cause

of frequent toxic iron overload amongst the Bantu people of South Africa.

- Cooking food in hard tap water may significantly increase the content of calcium and other minerals.
- Contamination of food with small amounts of soil may affect mineral content.

Dietary standards and nutrient requirements (after Webb, 1994)

Origins of dietary standards

Just over 50 years ago the National Research Council in the USA established a committee, the brief of which was to produce a comprehensive set of dietary standards. These standards were intended to be used as a yardstick against which diets or food supplies could be assessed to determine their likely adequacy. The first printed version of these standards appeared in 1943 and they were called **Recommended Dietary Allowances (RDAs)**. These were the first official and comprehensive set of dietary standards. Many other governments and international agencies now regularly publish their own dietary standards, and the American RDAs have been revised and re-published nine times since 1943. The first edition of these American RDAs (NRC, 1943) covered just 6 pages and dealt with only 10 nutrients; the current British and American versions of these standards (COMA, 1991 and NRC, 1989a respectively) each cover more than 200 pages and deal with more than 30 nutrients.

The first British RDAs were published by the British Medical Association in 1950, and in 1969 a truly official set of UK standards was published by the Department of Health and Social Security (BMA, 1950; DHSS, 1969).

Definitions and explanations

For the purposes of setting dietary standards, the population is divided up into subgroups; children are divided up into bands according to their age and sex. Adults are subdivided according to their age and sex with separate standards for pregnant and lactating women. These standards are intended for use with healthy people, and they make no allowance for the effects of illness and injury upon nutrient needs.

The RDA in the USA is the suggested average daily intake of that nutrient for healthy people. It represents the best estimate of the requirement of those people in the population with a particularly high need for that nutrient. The RDA does not represent the minimum requirement when it is used to assess the diets of individuals. Rather, it should be thought of as lying within a "zone of safety"; the further intake is below the RDA, then the greater is the risk of deficiency; and the further above the RDA, then the greater is the risk of toxic effects.

Until 1991, the British standards were also termed RDAs. However, in the latest version (COMA, 1991) the general term **Dietary Reference Values (DRVs)** is used to cover a range of differently defined values. The word "recommended" has been specifically avoided as it was felt to wrongly imply that the RDA represented the minimum desirable intake for health. Instead of a single RDA three reference values are offered for protein, vitamins and minerals in these new British standards. The highest of these three values is called the **Reference Nutrient Intake (RNI)** – it is essentially equivalent to the old RDA as it also represents the estimated requirement of those people with the highest need for the nutrient. The other two DRVs offered for these nutrients are the **Estimated Average Requirement (EAR)** which is self explanatory and the **Lower Reference Nutrient Intake (LRNI)**. The LRNI is the best estimate of the needs of those individuals with a low need for the nutrient. The requirement of almost everyone should lie within the range covered by the LRNI and the RNI.

COMA (1991) assumed that the variation in nutrient requirements of individuals will follow a **normal distribution** (see Figure 3.1). Approximately half of the population should require more and half less than the Estimated Average Requirement. The **standard deviation** is a precisely defined statistical measure of the variation of individual values around the mean or average in a normal distribution. The RNI is set at a notional two of these standard deviations above the mean, and the LRNI at a notional two standard deviations below the mean (Figure 3.1). The characteristics of a normal distribution mean that the

requirements of all but 5% of the population should lie within the range covered by two standard deviations on either side of the mean. Thus the RNI and LRNI should theoretically satisfy the needs of 97.5% and 2.5% of the population respectively. The RNI should represent an amount sufficient, or more than sufficient, to satisfy the needs of practically all healthy people.

COMA (1991) suggested that this more complex system of standards would allow more meaningful interpretation of measured or predicted intakes that fall below the RNI (i.e. the old RDA). At the extremes, if an individual's habitual intake is below the LRNI then the diet is almost certainly not able to maintain adequacy as it has been defined for that nutrient. If intake is above the RNI then the individual is receiving an adequate

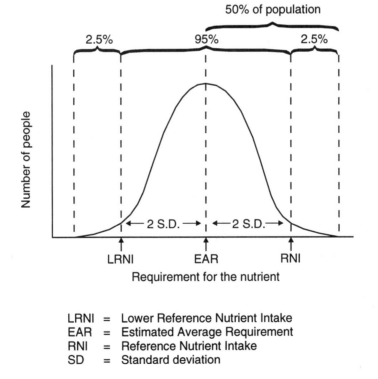

LRNI = Lower Reference Nutrient Intake
EAR = Estimated Average Requirement
RNI = Reference Nutrient Intake
SD = Standard deviation

Figure 3.1 A normal distribution of individual nutrient needs within a population with the theoretical positions of the UK Dietary Reference Values. Source: Webb, G. P. (1994) *Journal of Biological Education* 28(1), 102

supply. In between these two extremes the chances of adequacy fall, to a statistically predictable extent, as the intake approaches the LRNI, e.g. an individual consuming the EAR has a 50% chance of adequacy. Note that the iron requirements of women are an example where requirements for a nutrient are known not to be normally distributed; high iron losses in menstrual blood in some women skew or distort the distribution.

The RDAs for energy have traditionally been set at the best estimate of **average** requirement, rather than at the upper extremity of estimated requirement. This is true for the current energy RDA in the US. Whereas for most nutrients a modest surplus over requirement is not considered likely to be detrimental, this is not so with excessive energy intake that may lead to obesity. Consistent with this traditional practice, the latest UK standards give only an EAR for energy.

The COMA panel considered that, for eight nutrients, they did not have sufficient information to estimate the rather precisely defined set of values discussed above. In these cases, therefore, they merely suggested a **safe intake** – a level or range of intakes at which there is little risk of either deficiency or toxic effects. The NRC panel in the US also use this term.

The latest UK standards also, for the first time, set reference values for the various fat and carbohydrate fractions, including dietary fibre. These values are clearly directed towards reducing the diseases of industrialisation which breaks new ground for these standards because their traditional function has been solely to set standards of nutritional adequacy (see Chapter 4 for details of these fat and carbohydrate reference values).

The formal and precise statistical definitions detailed above, should not be allowed to obscure the fact that judgement plays a major part in the setting of these values. The three key elements in the setting of dietary standards all depend upon the judgement of the expert committee, namely:

- the criterion used to define adequacy
- the estimate of the average amount require to fulfil that criterion
- and, the estimated standard deviation of requirement.

Any particular reference value is the consensus view of one panel of experts based upon the information available to them in the prevailing social, political and economic climate. There may be genuine differences of opinion between different panels of experts and probably even between the experts within any given panel. Any particular panel's reference values are likely to be the result of compromises between the differing views of its individual members. Many other, not strictly scientific pressures, may also influence different committees to differing extents. Thus, the dairy industry might lobby for the calcium standard to be high, fruit growers lobby for a high vitamin C standard and meat and fish suppliers keen to keep the protein standard high. Where fruit is cheap and plentiful, a committee may be generous with vitamin C allowances because the cost of erring on the high side is perceived as minimal. However, where fruit is, for much of the year, an expensive imported luxury, then a panel may be more conservative in setting vitamin C standards.

There have been some very significant variations in these dietary standards over the years and there still are quite marked variations in the dietary standards used in different countries. Historical differences can be partly explained by the differences in scientific information available to different panels, but current international differences are largely due to variations in the way the same information has been interpreted by different panels of experts. Comparison of the current American RDAs and the British RNIs, which are essentially equivalent, reveals numerous differences, some of which are very substantial. In general, American RDAs are higher than UK RNIs; some examples are shown in Table 3:1. Note that, for example, the American RDA is around half as much again as the British RNI for vitamins A and C. In Chapter 8, the huge historical variations in protein standards for children are reviewed and discussed. In Chapter 12, the large differences in the current UK and US standards for pregnant women are highlighted and discussed.

Uses of dietary standards

A set of dietary standards enables nutritionists to predict the nutritional requirements of groups of people or of nations. Governments and food aid agencies can use them to identify the needs of populations, to decide whether available supplies are adequate for the population to be fed, and to identify nutrients the supply of which is deficient or only marginally adequate. They thus provide the means to make informed food policy decisions, for example decisions about:

- the amount and type of food aid that may be required
- the correct emphasis that should be applied when trying to influence agricultural producers, food processors or importers of food

- the determination of which foods might be beneficially subsidised or which need to be rationed with the size of any ration that should be allowed.

Similarly these standards can be used by institutional caterers (e.g. in prisons or schools), and those catering for the armed forces to assess the food requirements of the client population and also to check proposed menus for nutritional adequacy. Those devising therapeutic or reducing diets can check any proposed diets for adequacy using these standards.

These standards provide the means to assess nutritional adequacy after an intake survey. They are ideally used as a yardstick for assessing the adequacy of groups rather than individuals. They can nonetheless also be a useful tool for evaluating individual intakes provided it is recognised that the RDA or RNI is not a minimum requirement but a generous estimate of the requirement of those with a particularly high need. When assessing the nutritional adequacy of individuals, then it should be recognised that there will be very substantial fluctuations in the intakes of some nutrients from day to day. The habitual intake of the individual over a period of some days should, ideally, be the one that is compared to the standard.

Table 3.1 *Some current UK Reference Nutrient Intakes (RNIs) and American Recommended Dietary Allowances (RDAs) for an adult man. Values in parentheses are US values as a percentage of UK value Data sources: COMA (1991) and NRC (1989a)*

Nutrient	RDA (US)	RNI (UK)
Energy (kcal)	2900 (114)	2550* (* EAR)
(MJ)	12.14	10.60
Protein (grams)	63 (114)	55.5
Vitamin A (μg)	1000 (143)	700
Vitamin C (mg)	60 (150)	40
Riboflavin (mg)	1.7 (131)	1.3
Iron (mg)	10 (115)	8.7
Calcium (mg)	800 (114)	700

Most consumers will be exposed to these standards when they are used to make food labelling of nutrient content more intelligible. Absolute numerical amounts of nutrients will be meaningless to most consumers, but when expressed as a percentage of the RDA or EAR nutrient amounts become more meaningful. COMA (1991) suggested that the EAR was the most appropriate reference value to use for food labelling. In America, a Reference Daily Intake (RDI) is now used to indicate essential nutrient content on food labels; it is set at the higher of the two adult RDA values. These differing labelling standards may considerably widen the disparity between British and American values already seen in Table 3.1, e.g. the American RDI used for labelling of vitamin A content is 1000 μg/day (the RDA for an adult male), that recommended to be used in the UK is around half this value (the EAR for an adult male).

Methods used to determine requirements and set standards

Innaccurate standards

Setting dietary standards at erroneously low levels will negate their purpose. A yardstick of adequacy that does not meet the criterion of adequacy is of no use, and such a yardstick is probably worse than no standard at all because it will tend to induce a false sense of security and complacency. A serious underestimate of the standards for a nutrient could result in a nutrient deficiency being falsely ruled out as the cause of some pathology. Perhaps more probably, it could result in a suboptimally nourished group being reassured as to dietary adequacy.

Such arguments about the obvious hazards of setting standards too low means that there will be a strong temptation to err on the side of generosity, especially in affluent countries where the need to avoid waste of resources is less

acute. There are, however, potentially adverse consequences that may result if these standards are set too high:

- some nutrients (e.g. iron and some fat soluble vitamins) are toxic in excess; an unrealistically high standard might encourage sensitive individuals to consume hazardous amounts
- high standards may encourage the production or supply of unnecessary excesses which will result in wasteful use of sometimes scarce resources
- high standard values may create the illusion of widespread deficiency and result in unnecessary and wasteful measures to combat an illusory problem
- unreasonably high "target" values for particular nutrients may lead to distortion of the diet with deleterious effects on the intake of other nutrients
- if an unreasonably high standard results in the classification of large numbers of people as deficient but there are no other manifestations of deficiency, then this may discredit the standards and may, in the long run, undermine the credibility of nutrition education in general.

Some of the consequences of earlier exaggeration of human protein requirements are discussed in Chapter 8, and this may serve as a case-study to illustrate most of these points.

Defining requirement

The first problem that has to be confronted when devising a set of dietary standards is to decide upon the criteria that will be used to define adequacy. Ideally one would like to determine the intake that maximises growth, health and longevity, but these are not a readily measurable set of parameters. Overt deficiency of a nutrient will often produce a well-defined deficiency syndrome so that the minimum requirement will be an intake that prevents clinical signs of deficiency. Optimal intakes are assumed to be some way above this minimum requirement; subclinical indications of impairment or depletion of nutrient stores may occur long before overt clinical signs of deficiency. COMA (1991) decided that the EAR should allow for "a degree of storage of the nutrient to allow for periods of low intake or high demand without detriment to health".

This problem of defining an adequate intake is well illustrated by vitamin C. It is generally agreed that in adults, around 10 mg per day of this vitamin is sufficient to prevent the deficiency disease, scurvy. Below 30 mg/day negligible levels of the vitamin are detectable in plasma, at intakes of between 30 and 70 mg/day plasma vitamin levels rise steeply and they plateau at intakes of between 70 and 100 mg/day. COMA (1991) chose an adult RNI of 40 mg/day because, at this intake, most individuals would have measurable amounts of vitamin C in their plasma that is available for transfer to sites of depletion. NRC (1989a) chose an adult RDA of 60 mg/day, at which intake plasma concentrations would be approaching maximum. Yet some people advocate daily intakes of gram quantities of this vitamin in order to maximise resistance to infection. COMA (1991) list numerous suggested benefits of very high vitamin C intakes, but none of these influenced the ultimate RNI value. The underlying criterion in setting the RNI (and RDA in the US) is dietary adequacy, even though the additional requirement for adequate stores represents a large safety margin over that required for minimal adequacy, i.e. prevention of scurvy.

Deprivation studies

The most obvious and direct way of assessing the minimum requirement for a nutrient is to use a diet that is devoid of the nutrient and to see how much of the nutrient needs to be added to this experimental diet to prevent or cure the signs of deficiency. Experiments in Sheffield, England during World War II demonstrated

that volunteers started to dev
the deficiency disease scurvy
ple of months on a diet essent
of vitamin C. Intakes of around
were shown to prevent the deve_ ₚₘₑₙₜ of
scurvy and to cure the clinical signs
(COMA, 1991); this represents the minimum requirement for vitamin C, and COMA chose this as the LRNI for vitamin C.

Deprivation studies of this type may necessitate the consumption of very restricted diets for extended periods of time before clinical signs of deficiency develop in previously well-nourished adults. For example, it takes up to two years of depletion before previously well nourished adults develop even limited signs of vitamin A deficiency. This is because the livers of well-nourished adults contain large amounts of stored vitamin A. Such prolonged periods of deprivation may possibly have long term adverse consequences on the volunteers. Volunteers will, at the very least, be required to consume a very restricted and perhaps unpalatable diet for an extended period. Most people would consider it ethically unacceptable to deliberately subject vulnerable groups to this type of deprivation, e.g. children and pregnant or lactating women. This means that the extra requirements of these groups usually have to be inferred from less direct methods. As an alternative to controlled experiments it is possible to use epidemiological data relating average intakes of a nutrient to the presence or absence of clinical signs of deficiency in populations. For example, it has been observed that the deficiency disease beriberi occurs when the average intake of thiamin falls below 0.2 mg/1000 kcal, but when the average intake is above this level, beriberi does not occur (Passmore and Eastwood, 1986).

Radioactive tracer studies

If a known amount of radioactively labelled vitamin, or other nutrient, is administered to a volunteer, then assuming that this labelled vitamin disperses evenly in the body pool of that vitamin, the dilution of the radioactivity can be used to estimate the total size of that body pool. A sample of, say, plasma is taken, and the amount of vitamin and the amount of radioactivity in the sample is measured. The **specific activity** of vitamin in the sample (i.e. the radioactivity per unit weight of vitamin) can be used to calculate the total pool size, provided that the amount of radioactivity administered is known:

- administer 1 million units of radioactivity, the specific activity in the sample is measured as 1000 units of radioactivity per mg of vitamin
- therefore, radioactivity has been diluted in 1000 mg of vitamin, i.e. in a 1000 mg body pool of the vitamin.

If, after administration of a radioactive vitamin load, the body losses of radioactivity are monitored, this will enable the rate of vitamin loss or depletion to be determined.

Using this approach Baker *et al.* (1971) found that the average body pool of vitamin C in a group of healthy, well-nourished American men was around 1500 mg. On a vitamin C free diet, it was shown that this pool depleted at a rate of around 3% per day and that this **fractional catabolic rate** was independent of the pool size – i.e. 3% of whatever is in the body is lost no matter how much or how little is present in the body. When the body pool fell below 300 mg then symptoms of scurvy started to appear. The estimate of the replacement intake required to maintain the body pool above 300 mg and thus to prevent scurvy corresponds very well with the much earlier Sheffield depletion studies (i.e. 3% of 300 mg needs to be replaced daily – 9 mg/day c.f. 10 mg/day to prevent scurvy in the Sheffield study).

Balance studies

These methods rely upon the assumption that in healthy, well-nourished adults of stable body weight the body pool size of some nutrients remains constant. Healthy adults are, for example, in approximate balance for nitrogen (i.e. protein), calcium and sodium. Over a wide range of intakes and suitable measurement period, the intake is approximately equal to the output; variations in intake are compensated for by changes in the rate of absorption from the gut and/or changes in the rate of excretion. If say calcium intake is progressively reduced, then, initially, losses of calcium in urine and faeces will also decline and balance will be maintained. Eventually, however, a point will be reached when balance can no longer be maintained and output starts to exceed input. It would seem reasonable to propose that the minimum intake at which balance can be maintained represents the subject's minimum requirement for calcium. Such short term experiments do not exclude the very real possibility that long term adaptation to chronically low calcium intakes will occur.

COMA (1991) assumed that average daily losses of calcium via urine and skin in British adults were 160 mg/day. In order to replace this daily loss, they estimated that an intake of 525 mg/day would be required assuming that around 30% of dietary calcium is absorbed. They chose this as the adult EAR for calcium. They added or subtracted 30% to allow for individual variation and, therefore, came up with 700 mg/day and 400 mg/day as the RNI and LRNI respectively.

Factorial methods

Factorial calculations are essentially predictions of the requirements of particular groups or individuals taking into account a number of measured variables (or factors) and making a number of apparently logical assumptions. For example, during growth or pregnancy certain nutrients will be retained and accumulate in the growing body or pregnant woman. Knowing the rate at which these nutrients accumulate during pregnancy or growth, one can then make predictions of the amount required, for example

estimated requirement for pregnancy
equals
amount to achieve balance (from value for non-pregnant woman)
plus
daily accumulation rate of nutrient during pregnancy
multiplied by
factor to allow for assumed efficiency of absorption and assimilation.

COMA (1991) predicted the increase in Estimated Average Requirement for energy of women during lactation thus:

average energy content of daily milk production
multiplied by
1.25, i.e. an assumed 80% efficiency of conversion of dietary energy to milk energy
minus
an allowance for the contribution from the extra maternal fat stores laid down during pregnancy.

No matter how logical they may seem, such values are theoretical predictions and they may not represent actual physiological need. Physiological adaptations may occur which will reduce the predicted requirement, e.g. the efficiency of calcium absorption from the gut increases during pregnancy (see Chapter 12).

Measurement of blood or tissue levels

COMA (1991) defined some reference values according to the intake required to maintain a particular circulating level or tissue level of the nutrient. Thus the LRNI for vitamin C is set at the intake that prevents scurvy (10 mg/day in adults) but

the RNI is set at a level which maintains a measurable amount of vitamin C in plasma in most adults (40 mg/day); the EAR (25 mg/day) is set half way between the LRNI and the RNI.

The reference values for vitamin A in the UK are based upon the intake that is estimated as necessary to maintain a liver concentration of 20 μg vitamin A per gram of liver. In order to estimate the intake of vitamin required to maintain the target liver concentration, the panel had to perform quite an elaborate factorial calculation (summarised in Figure 3.2).

First they had to predict the size of the body pool required to achieve this liver concentration. To do this they had to make assumptions about what proportion of the body is liver and also assumptions about how the total body pool of vitamin A partitions between liver and extra hepatic tissues. The fractional catabolic rate of vitamin A has been measured at 0.5% of the body pool lost per, day and so an amount equivalent to 0.5% of this estimated pool would have to be replaced each day. Finally assumptions had to be made about the efficiency with which ingested vitamin A is stored in the liver in order to convert this replacement requirement into an intake requirement.

Biochemical markers

COMA (1991) used the intake required to "maintain a given degree of enzyme saturation" as another criterion for determining reference values. An example of this is the use of the erythrocyte glutathione reductase activation test to assess and define nutritional status for the B vitamin riboflavin.

Glutathione reductase is an enzyme present in red blood cells the activity of which is dependent upon the presence of a cofactor that is derived from riboflavin; the enzyme cannot function in the absence of the cofactor. In riboflavin deficiency the activity of this enzyme is low because of a reduced availability of the cofactor; in red blood cells taken from

Target liver concentration – 20 µg/g

↓

Estimate body pool size required to give this liver concentration. Assume liver represents 3% of total body weight and contains 90% of body vitamin A.

↓

Estimate daily replacement amount required to keep body pool at this level. Assume fractional catabolic rate of 0.5%, i.e. 0.5% of pool is lost each day.

↓

Estimate dietary intake required to achieve this replacement. Assume efficiency of absorption and storage of vitamin A is 50%.

↓

EAR of 496 µg/day for 74 kg male.

↓

Assume 21% coefficient of variation to give RNI and LRNI of 700 and 300 µg/day respectively.

Figure 3.2 *An illustration of the calculations and assumptions required to estimate the vitamin A intake required to maintain a designated liver concentration and thus to set the Dietary Reference Values for vitamin A (after COMA, 1991)*

well-nourished subjects, the activity of this enzyme will be higher because it is not limited by the availability of the cofactor. To perform the activation test, the activity of glutathione reductase is measured in two samples of red cells from the subject – one has had excess riboflavin added the other has not had riboflavin added. The ratio of these two activities – the **glutathione reductase activation coefficient (EGRAC)** – is a measure of the extent to which enzyme activity has been limited by riboflavin availability in the unsupplemented sample, representing a measure of the subject's dietary riboflavin status. The RNI is set at the intake which maintains the EGRAC at 1.3 or less in almost all people. Similar enzyme activation tests are used to assess status for other vitamins, e.g. activation of the enzyme transketolase in red cells is used to determine thiamin status – a thiamin-derived cofactor is necessary for transketolase to function.

Biological markers

Blood haemoglobin concentration has been widely used in the past as a measure of nutritional status for iron. It is now regarded as an insensitive and unreliable indicator of iron status because, for example: haemoglobin levels change in response to a number of physiological factors such as training, altitude and pregnancy; and, iron stores may be depleted without any change in blood haemoglobin concentration (see Chapter 11 and "biochemical assessment" in this chapter for further discussion of iron status assessment).

Vitamin K status is frequently assessed by functional tests of prothrombin levels in blood. Prothrombin is one of several clotting factors the synthesis of which in the liver depends upon vitamin K as an essential cofactor. Thus in vitamin K deficiency prothrombin levels fall and blood clotting is impaired. In order to measure the **prothrombin time,** excess calcium and tissue thromboplastin are added to fresh plasma that has been previously depleted of calcium to prevent clotting. The time taken for the plasma to clot under these conditions is dependent upon the amount of prothrombin present, and thus upon the vitamin K status of the donor. Anti-coagulant drugs, like warfarin, work by blocking the effect of vitamin K – prothrombin time is thus a useful way of monitoring vitamin K status and thus of regulating drug dosage during anti-coagulant therapy.

Animal experiments

Animal experiments are likely to be of very limited value in quantifying the nutrient needs of human beings; they may even encourage widely erroneous estimates to be made. It is extremely difficult to allow for species differences in nutrient requirements and to scale between species as different in size as rats and people. The examples below illustrate some of the difficulties of predicting human nutrient needs from those of laboratory animals.

Most rapidly growing young animals need a relatively high proportion of their dietary energy as protein, but human babies grow relatively slowly and thus are likely to need proportionally less dietary protein. Rat milk has around 25% of its energy as protein compared to only about 6% in human milk. Predicting the protein needs of human children from those of young rats is likely to exaggerate the needs of children.

Pauling (1972) has used the measured rate of vitamin C synthesis in the rat (which does not require dietary vitamin C) to support his highly controversial view that gram quantities of the vitamin are required for optimal human health. He has scaled up the rats' rate of production on a simple weight-to-weight basis and come up with estimates that rats of human size would make 2–4 g/day of the vitamin – he has suggested that this indicates human requirements. This procedure seems extremely dubious on several grounds, not least of which is the decision to scale on a simple weight-to-weight basis. Vitamin needs may be more related to metabolic needs than simple body weight. If one scales according to relative metabolic rate, then one might predict that the human size rat would only make around a quarter of the amount predicted by body weight scaling.

The expected nutritional burdens of pregnancy and lactation are also relatively much greater in small laboratory animals than in women – laboratory animals have relatively larger litters, short gestations and rapidly growing infants when compared to human beings. Extrapolating from laboratory animals is thus likely to exaggerate any extra nutritional requirements of pregnant and lactating women (see Chapter 12).

Despite these reservations about the use of animal experiments to quantify human nutrient needs, they have, nonetheless, played a vital role in the identification of the essential nutrients and their physiological and biochemical functions. Several of those awarded Nobel prizes for work on vitamins used animals in their work. The need for essential fatty acids was, for example, identified in the rat 40 years before unequivocal confirmation of the need for human beings.

Animal experiments may also be very useful in providing in depth information on the pathological changes that accompany prolonged deficiency and in determining whether prolonged marginal adequacy is likely to have any long term detrimental effects.

Assessment of nutritional status

Clinical assessment

Nutrient deficiencies ultimately lead to clinically recognisable deficiency diseases. Identification of the clinical signs of these deficiency diseases usually requires little or no specialised equipment, is cheap, simple and quick, enabling assessment surveys to be conducted rapidly and cheaply even in the most inaccessible places. Even non-medical personnel can be trained to conduct clinical surveys of nutritional status by recording the presence or absence of various clinical signs from checklists of clinical signs that are likely to be associated with nutrient deficiencies. Passmore and Eastwood (1986) list around 50 clinical signs that are likely to indicate a nutritional deficiency, e.g. loss of hair pigment and easy pluckability; spongy and bleeding gums; flaking and depigmentation of the skin; oedema; enlargement of the liver; loss of sensation; mottled tooth enamel; excessively smooth or red tongue; redness and cracking at the corners of the mouth; drying of the cornea and white foamy spots on the cornea; mental confusion or apathy.

Those conducting any type of nutritional survey must take steps to actively ensure that those assessed are representative of the whole population under investigation. Those most badly affected by deficiency diseases may well be those least accessible to the survey team – the weak, the frail, the elderly, pregnant and lactating women and babies are the least likely to be out and about. Sampling people in the street, or those mobile enough to attend a centre may well overestimate the nutritional status of the population.

The clinical signs of deficiency usually become recognisable only after severe and/or prolonged deficiency, and thus they are relatively insensitive indicators of nutritional status. It is generally assumed that suboptimal intakes of nutrients and subclinical impairment of physiological functioning occur long before any deficiency disease becomes clinically apparent. In surveys in affluent countries, very few cases of clinical deficiency would be found and thus very limited information about the nutrient status of the population would be forthcoming, except that there are no deficiencies severe enough or long standing enough to induce overt clinical deficiency. Clinical signs are therefore not useful as early indicators of nutritional problems that can warn of the need to implement preventative measures.

Clinical signs tend to be qualitative and subjective. Any attempt to grade or quantify clinical signs is likely to depend upon subjective judgements on the part of the operator. For example, grading the severity of goitre (swelling of the thyroid gland due to iodine deficiency) depends upon the judgement of the assessor about the degree of thyroid enlargement; different clinicians may produce considerably different gradings for the same population.

Clinical signs are not very specific indicators of nutrient deficiencies. Some symptoms are common to several deficiency diseases and also to non-nutritional causes. Some form of dermatitis is, for example, common to several deficiency diseases and may also be induced by a variety of non-nutritional causes; oedema may be a symptom of beriberi, Protein Energy Malnutrition, heart failure, kidney disease, etc.

Anthropometric assessment

Uses of anthropometric assessment

Anthropometric assessment means physical measurements of body weight and dimensions. Body composition may be estimated from anthropometric measurements. These physical measurements have a variety of uses:

1 They allow assessment of nutritional status. They can be used to detect undernutrition or obesity in adults and to indicate whether the growth of children is satisfactory.
2 They allow for more useful comparisons of metabolic rate between individuals or groups. Adipose tissue has a low metabolic rate, and so expressing metabolic rate per unit of lean body mass is more meaningful than simply expressing it per unit total weight.
3 Certain drug dosages may be calculated per unit of lean body weight.
4 Changes in body weight may be due to gain or loss of water, lean tissue or fat. Longitudinal measurements of body composition may help to decide the composition of any weight change. Most of the measures currently available for assessing body composition are relatively insensitive and thus could only be reliably used for this purpose if the weight change were substantial.

Anthropometric assessment in children

Anthropometric measurements are cumulative indicators of the nutritional status and general health of children. Low values for height or length provide evidence of the chronic effects of malnutrition; weight for height is a more acute measure and indicates current nutritional status. These simple measures require little equipment or professional training, thus reliable results may be readily and cheaply produced by non-specialists. Interpretation of these results requires that they be compared with standards; the need for reliable standards is a recurrent problem when interpreting anthropometric measurements. The standards of height and weight for children at various ages tend to be derived from children in affluent countries – poor children in developing countries may not correspond well with such standards. These differences between rich and poor are largely a reflection of chronic adapta-

tion to undernutrition by the poor, which may make interpretation of results and deciding upon appropriate responses difficult. An anthropometric survey of children in rural Bangladesh is likely to show that their average heights and weights are some way below those of typical American children of the same age, but they may be typical of children living in rural Bangladesh and thus they are not specifically "at risk". This point is well illustrated by considering some of the changes that have occurred in the anthropometric characteristics of affluent populations during this century. Britons are on average several inches taller than they were at the start of the century – those in the higher socioeconomic groups have always been taller than those in the lower groups, but this gap has narrowed considerably during this century. Sexual maturation occurs earlier now than at the start of the century; girls start menstruating 2–3 years earlier than they did on average at the start of the century, and boys reach their adult stature at 19 years of age rather than their mid-20s. Standards of height and weight of British children have thus changed very significantly during the course of this century.

Body size is not only dependent upon environmental factors, like diet, but it is also genetically determined. Some races of people may be genetically smaller than others – this might make the use of non-local standards problematical. This will obviously create difficulties in assessing the nutritional status of an individual child from single anthropometric measurements – is a child short because it is genetically small or because it is chronically malnourished? Growth curves are more useful ways of monitoring the nutritional status of individual children – provided the child remains on its predicted growth curve, whether the absolute values are low or high is in most cases unimportant. If a child on a high growth curve dips significantly below that curve, then this may indicate a nutrition or health problem, even though it may be average for its age. A child who remains on a low growth curve will be assessed as growing satisfactorily even though it may be well below average size for its age.

Centiles are frequently used when discussing or interpreting anthropometric measures in children. If the growth curves of a population are plotted, then one can produce growth curves that are typical of each per cent (or centile) of the population, i.e. the largest 1% through to the smallest 1%. If, for example, point measurements on a group indicate an average height for age that is substantially below the 50th centile, this would suggest impaired growth in the sample group. If a point measurement on an individual shows a value at the extremes of the range, e.g. below the 3rd centile, then this indicates

a probability that growth has been unsatisfactory. Figure 3.3 illustrates this by showing World Health Organisation standards of height for age in girls, the 3rd, 10th, 50th, 90th and 97th centiles are given; if a girl has a height for age below the 3rd centile, then there is a less than 3% probability that she has been growing satisfactorily.

The body mass index

In adults, low weight for height may indicate inadequate nutrition, whereas high weight for height may indicate

Figure 3.3 WHO standards of height (length) for age in girls aged up to five years. The 97th, 90th, 50th, 10th and 3rd centiles are shown. Source: Passmore, R. and Eastwood, M. A. (1986) *Human nutrition and dietetics.* 8th edition. Edinburgh: Churchill Livingstone. p.519

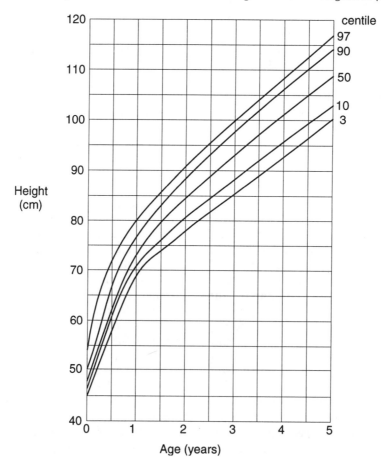

overweight or obesity. If the recent nutritional adequacy of an individual (e.g. a hospital patient) is being assessed, then recent weight change may be a more sensitive indicator than absolute weight for height.

Weight for height tables listing acceptable weight ranges for given heights have traditionally been used as anthropometric standards to assess the nutritional status and fatness of adults.

In recent years, the **body mass index (BMI)** has been very widely used. This measure has been shown empirically to be the best simple and quantitative anthropometric indicator of body composition and thus of nutritional status.

$$BMI = \frac{Body\ weight\ (kg)}{Height^2\ (m^2)}$$

The normal range for the BMI is set at 20–25 kg/m^2, any value significantly below this range is taken to indicate underweight, while values above this range would be considered to indicate varying degrees of overweight or obesity, e.g.:

less than 20 kg/m^2	underweight
20 – 25	normal
25 – 30	overweight
30 – 40	obesity
40+	severe obesity

When the BMI is being used to assess degree of obesity, then it is assumed that variations in weight for a given height are primarily due to variations in adiposity. This assumption generally holds reasonably well, but there are some groups for whom it clearly does not hold. People with very well developed musculature (e.g. body builders) will be heavy but have very low fat content – their BMI may falsely indicate obesity. In elderly women, loss of lean tissue and bone mass may mean that BMI remains within the normal range even though more direct measures of fatness may indicate excess adiposity.

Skinfold calipers

The most widely used direct measure of fatness in people is measurement of skinfold thickness using skinfold calipers. These spring loaded calipers exert a constant pressure on a fold of skin; the thickness of the skinfold is indicated on a meter. The thickness of the skinfold will be largely dependent upon the amount of fat stored subcutaneously in the region of the skinfold. Skinfold thicknesses are measured at several sites, and the assumption is made that the amount of fat stored subcutaneously at these sites (as measured by the skinfold thickness) will be representative of the total amount of body fat. Typically, skinfold thickness is determined at four sites: over the triceps muscle; over the biceps; in the subscapular region; and, in the supra iliac region. The total of these four skinfolds is then translated into an estimate of percentage body fat using a calibration table or formula. Figure 3.4 shows the relationship between the sum of these four skinfolds and the percentage body fat (estimated by body density) in 17–29 year old men and women. The single triceps skinfold thickness is sometimes used in nutritional surveys – it has the obvious advantage, in such circumstances, that it can be measured quickly and without the need for subjects to undress. There are racial differences in the way that fat is distributed between the various storage sites, and so using calibration tables derived from subjects from a different racial group may be an additional source of uncertainty.

Estimation of fatness from body density

The calibration of the skinfold method of determining fatness has been obtained by using body density as a reference method. The density of fat (0.9 kg/l) is less than that of lean tissue (1.1 kg/l), and so measurement of whole body density

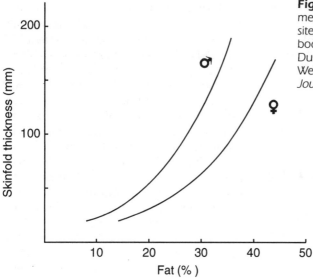

Figure 3.4 Relationship between caliper measurements of skinfold thickness at four sites and body fat content estimated from body density in young adults. Data of Durnin and Wormersley (1974). Source: Webb, G.P. and Jackobson, M.E. (1980) *Journal of Biological Education* 14(4), 321.

enables one to estimate the proportion of fat in the body.

$$\text{Density} = \frac{\text{Mass}}{\text{Volume}}$$

Mass may be determined by simple weighing. Volume is measured by comparing the weight of the body in air and its weight when fully immersed in water. The difference between these two values is the weight of water displaced by the body (Archimedes principle) and knowing the density of water (1 kg/l); then one can calculate the volume of water displaced, i.e. the volume of the body. The principle is very simple, but the technical procedures required to obtain accurate and valid values are quite elaborate, e.g. subjects wear a weighted belt to ensure that they are fully immersed and correction has to be made for this; corrections will need to be made for the residual air in the lungs during the immersion, which will greatly distort density measurements. This method requires sentient and co-operative subjects; it is not suitable for routine use, but has traditionally been used as the reference method against which other methods are calibrated and validated.

Body water content as a predictor of body fat content

Measurement of body water content should enable good estimates of body fatness to be made. The body is envisaged as consisting of two compartments – lean tissue with a constant proportion of water (around 73%) and water-free fat. Thus some measure of body water enables proportions of lean and fat to be estimated. In order to estimate body water content in a living person or animal, then one needs some chemical substance that is not toxic, that will readily and evenly disperse in all of the body water and that is readily measurable. Water that is labelled with the deuterium isotope of hydrogen (heavy water) or the radioactive isotope of hydrogen (tritiated water) seems to fulfil these criteria.

After allowing time for dispersal, the concentration of the chemical in a sample of body fluid is measured; knowing the amount of the substance introduced into the body, one can then estimate the amount of diluting fluid (i.e. the body water):

- administer 100 units of chemical
- allow time for dispersal in body water

- measure concentration in body water sample, let us say 2 units per litre
- volume of body water estimated at 50 litres i.e. 50 kg
- estimate lean body mass assuming this 50 kg of water represents 73% of lean tissue, i.e. 50 × 100/73
- total weight – lean weight = weight of body fat.

This method should yield reliable and valid measures of body water and thus good estimates of body fat. Garrow (1993) has reviewed methods of measuring human body composition, including some methods involving use of modern high technology apparatus.

Estimating fatness in animals

The fat content of dead animals can be measured directly by extracting the fat with a suitable solvent (e.g. chloroform). Animal experimenters thus have the option of using this precise analytical method at the end of their experiment. This analytical method also provides an absolute standard against which other methods of estimating fatness can be calibrated and validated. In humans, of course, any method of estimating fatness can only be validated and calibrated against another estimate.

Experimental animals can be used to show that there is an almost perfect negative correlation between the percentage of body water and the percentage of body fat (see Figure 3.5). This validates the use of body water measurements to predict body fatness. In the mice used for Figure 3.5, when body water was expressed as a percentage of the fat-free weight, then all values were within the range 74–76%; this validates the earlier assumption that the body is made up of lean tissue with a constant proportion of water plus water-free fat. Other methods, similar to those described for people, are also available to estimate the fatness of animals: weight/length indices; density; and, in animals that store fat subcutaneously, like pigs, skinfold thickness. Rodents do not store much of their fat subcutaneously but dissection and weighing of one fat storage organ may be used to predict total fat content in dead animals (Webb and Jakobson, 1980).

Mid-arm circumference measures

In immobile adults who cannot be weighed (e.g. unconscious hospital patients) **mid arm circumference** of the upper arm can be a useful anthropometric indicator

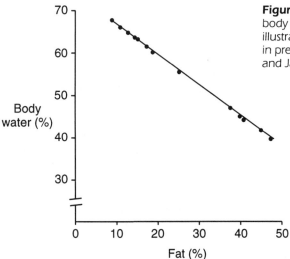

Figure 3.5 The relationship between percentage body fat and percentage body water in mice. To illustrate the value of body water measurements in predicting body fat content. Data from Webb and Jakobson (1980)

of nutritional status. A single measurement needs standards for interpretation, but longitudinal changes in this measure are a reasonably sensitive indicator of changes in body weight. Mid arm circumference has been widely used as a simple and rapid means of assessing nutritional status in children. A piece of previously calibrated and colour coded tape can be used. If the circumference lies within the green region, then this can be taken to indicate normality, in the yellow region, mild malnutrition, and in the red region, frank malnutrition (Passmore and Eastwood, 1986).

Mid-arm muscle circumference (MAMC) has been widely used as a simple measure of lean body mass. The circumference of the mid arm is measured with a tape and the triceps skinfold measured with calipers. Then:

$$\text{MAMC} = \text{mid-arm circumference} - (\pi \times \text{triceps skinfold})$$

Changes in MAMC are taken to indicate changes in lean body mass, and, once again, may be a useful longitudinal measure of nutritional status in hospital patients.

Biochemical assessment

Biochemical measures of nutrient status yield objective and quantitative measures and are the most sensitive indicators of nutritional status. A number of these biochemical measures of nutrient status were discussed in the section dealing with the methods used to assess nutrient requirements, e.g. measures of blood and tissue levels of nutrients or metabolites; measuring nutrient excretion rates; enzyme saturation tests; and, functional biochemical tests such as prothrombin time.

Biochemical measurements need laboratory facilities, and they are relatively expensive and time consuming. Interpretation of the values obtained will depend upon the limits of normality that have been set and these will often be a matter of judgement. For example, blood haemo-globin concentration can be measured with considerable precision, but deciding upon the level that should be taken to indicate anaemia will be a matter of judgement. Thus translating surveys of haemoglobin measurements into assessments of the prevalence of anaemia will depend very much on the limits of normality that are used. A figure of 12 g of haemoglobin per 100 ml of blood has traditionally been regarded as the level below which there is a progressively increasing risk of anaemia. If this value is taken as the lower limit of normality then the prevalence of iron deficiency anaemia in menstruating women is high even in industrialised countries (10–20%). However, clinical symptoms of anaemia may only become apparent with haemoglobin levels substantially below 10 g per 100 ml of blood (see Chapter 11).

Measurements made upon urine samples have the obvious advantage of requiring no invasive procedures and of giving relatively large samples, thus avoiding the need for special micro-analytical techniques. They can be useful if excretion rate of an intact nutrient or readily identifiable derivative can be related to nutritional status. Rates of urine flow, and thus the concentration of solutes in urine samples, are very variable and greatly influenced by, for example: recent fluid consumption, physical activity, and consumption of substances that have diuretic or antidiuretic activity (e.g. caffeine or nicotine). Twenty-four hour samples may give more meaningful results; their collection will be impractical in many survey situations and, even where they are feasible, checks will be required to ensure that the samples are complete in non-captive subjects. Thus, for example, it is generally agreed that the best method of assessing salt intake is to measure sodium excretion in a 24-hour urine sample (see Chapter 11). In order to ensure that the 24-hour sample is complete, subjects may be asked to take doses of a marker substance (para amino benzoic acid) with their meals –

only where there is practically complete recovery of the marker in the urine sample will the sample be accepted as complete.

Urinary levels of the B vitamins have traditionally been used as measures of nutritional status for these vitamins. The values are often expressed as amount of nutrient or nutrient derivative per gram of creatinine in the urine sample. It is assumed that the excretion of creatinine is approximately constant, thus giving a more meaningful value than the amount of nutrient per unit volume of urine because the latter is so dependent upon the rate of urine flow.

Blood samples give much greater scope for assessing nutrient status – plasma or blood cell concentrations of nutrients and enzyme reactivation tests using red blood cell enzymes are extensively used as specific measures of nutritional status. Plasma albumin concentration drops in Protein Energy Malnutrition, and albumin concentration is widely used as a sensitive and general biochemical indicator of nutritional status. Blood tests require facilities and personnel for taking samples; analysis of the samples often requires special microanalytical techniques because of the limited volumes taken for analysis.

Table 3.2 gives a summary of the relative advantages and disadvantages of using clinical signs, anthropometric measurements and biochemical measurements in the assessment of nutritional status.

Measurement of food and nutrient intake

Measures of food intake have a variety of purposes, e.g. they can be used to:

1 assess the adequacy of the diets of populations, groups or individuals and to identify problem nutrients
2 relate dietary factors in populations or individuals to disease incidence or risk markers like serum cholesterol concentration
3 monitor the effects of socioeconomic factors upon diet

Table 3.2 Some advantages and disadvatages of using clinical, anthropometric and biochemical methods of nutritional assessment

Advantages	Disadvantages
Clinical	
Quick	Insensitive, not useful for early warning
Simple	Not specific
Cheap	Qualitative
No specialist equipment needed	Subjective
Specialist personnel not required	
Anthropometric	
Quantitative	Need reliable standards
Objective	Previous obesity makes current weight-for-
Specialist personnel not required	height an insensitive indicator of current status
Quick	Genetic variation makes current height-for-age
Simple	an insensitive measure in children
Simple equipment	
Biochemical	
Quantitative	Laboratory facilities needed
Objective	Time consuming
Sensitive	Expensive
Trained personnel needed	
Difficult to set standards of normality	

4 monitor changes in the diets of populations, groups or individuals over time and thus, for example, to monitor the effectiveness of nutrition education programmes.

Almost all of these methods use food tables to translate food intakes into nutrient intakes and so all of the errors, uncertainties and limitations previously discussed for food tables use will also apply to these methods.

Population or group methods

1 *Food balance sheets* – These are used to estimate the average *per capita* food and nutrient consumption of nations (see Figure 3.6 for summary). Food balance sheets usually yield no information about distribution within the population – they will not show up, for example, regional differences in nutrient intakes, socio-economic influences upon nutrient intakes or age and sex differences in nutrient intakes. Domestic food production must first be estimated – any food imports are added to this total and any exports subtracted. Food balance sheets must also be corrected for any change in food stocks within the country during the period. This estimate of food available for consumption must then be corrected for wastage and for food not consumed by humans, e.g. animal fodder and pet foods (see Figure 3.6). Such methods allow crude estimates of population adequacy and allow crude comparisons of actual intakes with nutrition education guidelines to be made. They also enable international comparisons to be

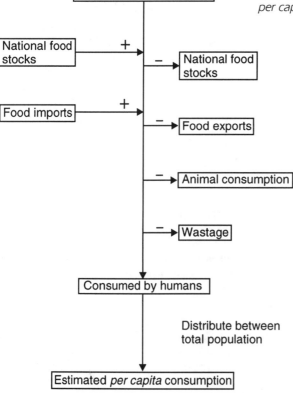

Figure 3.6 Schematic diagram to illustrate how food balance sheets can be used to estimate *per capita* food consumption in a country

made, e.g. one could relate average *per capita* sugar consumption to rates of dental caries in different populations.

Home produced food will be one potential source of error in these estimates. Wastage will be difficult to estimate accurately and is likely to depend upon the affluence of the population – the rich are likely to waste more than the poor. Within the EC, construction of national food balance sheets is likely to be complicated by the introduction of the single market with the consequent reduction in checks upon imports and exports between member nations.

2 *Household surveys* – The National Food Survey (NFS) of the United Kingdom is an example of a national household survey that has now been undertaken annually for over 50 years (e.g. MAFF, 1993). Each participant of this nationally representative survey of around 7500 households is asked to record in a log book all food entering the household for human consumption during a 14-day period. The log is checked by a trained interviewer at the end of the survey period. Home grown food is included in the log, but detailed information about food eaten outside the home is not collected, only the number of external meals taken by each family member, is recorded. Up until 1992 no information was collected about alcoholic drinks, soft drinks (soda) or confectionery (candies) as these are often purchased by individual family members although those purchased for home consumption are now recorded. Information is also recorded concerning the composition of the family, its socio-economic status and the region of the country in which it makes its home. No attempt is made to record distribution within the family although assumptions about wastage and distribution are made in order to estimate individual intakes of food and nutrients. Expenditure during the 14-day survey period may overestimate usual rates of purchasing, especially in lower socio-economic groups.

The NFS is not a complete record of food purchases because outside meals and foods purchased and consumed directly by family members other than the record keeper go unrecorded. Neither does the NFS attempt to record what food is actually eaten during the record period. Nevertheless, despite its limitations, the National Food Survey provides an invaluable record of the changing dietary habits of the British population over half a century; it gives indications about regional and socio-economic influences upon food selection (see MAFF, 1991 for a review of 50 years of the NFS). Many other countries conduct similar expenditure surveys, but rarely are these other surveys as regular or long-lasting as the British National Food Survey.

Individual methods

Individual methods of assessing food intake may either involve prospective recording of food as it is eaten or may assess intake retrospectively by the use of interviews or questionnaires. These methods, almost inevitably, rely to a large extent upon the honesty of the subjects.

Retrospective methods

Twenty-four hour recall is very frequently used to retrospectively assess the food and nutrient intakes of subjects. An interviewer asks subjects to recount the types and amounts of all food and drink consumed during the previous day. This recalled list is then translated into estimates of energy and nutrient intakes by the use of food tables. The method is frequently used in large scale epidemiological surveys where large numbers of subjects need to be dealt with quickly and cheaply and where precision in assessing the intake of any individual is not essential. The method requires relatively little commitment from the subject and thus co-operation rates tend to be good. As the assessment is retrospective the subjects do not alter their intakes in response to monitoring.

Some of the limitations and sources of error in this method:

- *Memory errors* – subjects are likely to forget some of the items that have been consumed. This method tends to significantly underestimate total calorie intake and seems to particularly underestimate, for example, alcohol intake.
- *Quantification* – it is difficult to quantify portions in retrospect. It may be particularly difficult for the very young and the very old to conceptualise amounts. Food models are sometimes used to aid this quantification process.
- *Intake may not be representative of usual intake* – the day chosen for the record may not be typical of the subjects' usual daily intake. Week-end and weekday intakes may be very different for some subjects – subjects' appetites may be affected by illness or stress –subjects' usual intake may be exaggerated by some social occasion or event. Even where subjects are of regular habits and no factors have distorted that day's intake, the intake of many nutrients tends to fluctuate quite markedly from day to day and thus one day's intake cannot be taken to represent the subjects' habitual intake.
- *Interviewer bias* – an interview-based survey is liable to bias. The interviewer may encourage subjects to remember particular dietary items more than others and thus may obtain a distorted picture of the real diet. If the interviewer indicates approval or disapproval of certain foods or drinks this may also encourage distorted recall.

It might seem logical to extend the recall period if one wishes to get a more representative picture of a subject's usual dietary pattern, but one would, of course, expect memory errors to increase exponentially as the recall period is extended. In order to try to get more of a representative picture of dietary pattern detailed **dietary histories** may be taken by interview or self-administered **food frequency questionnaires** can be used. The investigators may be interested in the intakes of particular nutrients, and thus the frequency of consumption of the types of foods that contain these nutrients may give a useful indication of the usual intake of that nutrient, e.g. assessing the frequency, types and amounts of fruits and vegetables consumed would be a useful guide to discovering approximate vitamin C or carotene intakes.

Prospective methods

The **weighed inventory** requires that the subjects weigh and record all items of food and drink consumed over a pre-determined period. The operator must then translate this food inventory into nutrient intakes with food tables. Household measures (e.g. cup, spoon, slice, etc.) can be recorded; this means that subjects do not have to weigh everything without sacrificing accuracy unduly. Such methods have the advantage of being direct, accurate, current and of variable length, enabling more representative assessments of average intakes to be made.

Some disadvantages of these methods:

- Subjects may still forget to record some items consumed, especially snack items.
- They are labour intensive for both subject and operator – considerable motivation and skill on the part of the subject is required for accurate and complete recording. Participation rates may therefore be low, and this may make the population sampled unrepresentative of that being surveyed. Recording usually requires numerate and literate subjects; in order to get records from subjects who do not have these skills, a variety of methods have been tried, e.g. subjects have been issued with cameras to photograph

their food and drink; subjects have been given balances that have a tape recorder incorporated so that the subject's oral description of the weighed food can be recorded.

• Prospective methods may be invalidated if subjects modify their behaviour in response to monitoring, by attempting to impress the operator, in order to simplify the recording process, or simply because their awareness of their food and drink intake has been heightened by the recording process.

Measurement of energy expenditure and metabolic rate

Metabolic rate is the rate at which energy is expended by the body. Energy expenditure may be rather crudely and indirectly assessed from measurements of energy intake. As energy can neither be created nor destroyed, then energy expenditure over any given period must be equal to the intake plus or minus any change in body energy stores.

Energy expenditure = energy intake ±
                     change in
                     body energy

If expenditure is measured in this way then the errors in measuring intake and changes in body energy will be compounded. The methods of measuring changes in body energy are insensitive, making this method unreliable for measurement of expenditure over short periods. Tens of thousands of calories may be added to or lost from body energy without being quantifiable by the available methods of measuring body composition. This error is minimised with a long sample period, but using a lot of time also means that subjects might lose motivation

All of the energy expended by the body is ultimately lost as heat, and it is theoretically possible to measure this directly in a

whole body calorimeter, i.e. a chamber surrounded by a water jacket in which the heat released by the subject in the chamber is measured by a rise in temperature in the surrounding water. It is usual, however, to predict energy expenditure from measures of oxygen consumption and/or carbon dioxide evolution. Foodstuffs are metabolically oxidised to carbon dioxide, water and, in the case of protein, nitrogenous waste products like urea; this oxidation process consumes atmospheric oxygen. The chemical equations for the oxidation of the various foodstuffs can be used to predict the **energy equivalent of oxygen** – the amount of energy released when a litre of oxygen is used to metabolically oxidise food.

The equation for the oxidation of glucose is:

$$C_6H_{12}O_6 + 6O_2 = 6CO_2 + 6H_2O$$

$$\frac{180\ g}{glucose} + \frac{6 \times 22.41}{oxygen} = \frac{6 \times 22.41}{carbon\ dioxide} + \frac{6 \times 18\ g}{water}$$

and, therefore, oxidation of 180 g of glucose yields around 665 kcal. Thus one litre of oxygen yields approximately 4.95 kcal when it is being used to metabolise glucose, i.e. 665 divided by (6 × 22.4). Similar calculations can be performed using the other substrates, and such calculations yield energy equivalents for oxygen that are not very different from that for glucose; if a mixture of substrates is being oxidised, then a figure of 4.86 kcal per litre of oxygen can be used as the approximate energy equivalent of oxygen. If more precise estimation is required then the ratio of carbon dioxide evolution to oxygen consumption, the **respiratory quotient (RQ)**, gives an indication of the balance of substrates being metabolised. The RQ is 1.0 if carbohydrate is being oxidised but only 0.71 if fat is being oxidised – tables listing the energy equivalent of oxygen at various RQs are available.

The simplest way of measuring oxygen consumption (and carbon dioxide evolution) is to use a **Douglas bag**. This is a large plastic bag fitted with a two way valve so that the subject who breathes through a mouthpiece attached to the valve, sucks in air from the atmosphere and then blows it out into the bag. All of the expired air can be collected over a period of time and then the volume and composition of this expired air can be measured. Knowing the composition of the inspired atmospheric air means that the subject's oxygen consumption and carbon dioxide evolution can be calculated. Note that the collection period is limited to a few minutes even if the capacity of the bag is large (100 litres).

The **static spirometer** is essentially a metal bell that is filled with oxygen and is suspended with its open end under water. The subject breathes through a tube connected to the oxygen-containing chamber of the bell. The bell rises and falls as the volume of gas inside the bell changes, and thus it will fall and rise with subject's inspiration and expiration. If the system contains a carbon dioxide absorber, then the bell will gradually sink as the subject uses up the oxygen in the bell. This change in volume of oxygen inside the bell can be recorded on a calibrated chart, and thus the rate of oxygen consumption can be determined. This is a standard undergraduate practical exercise – it is limited to short term (i.e. a few minutes) of measurements of resting oxygen consumption or very short periods of consumption with static exercise, e.g. on an exercise bicycle.

Portable respirometers have been developed that can be strapped onto the back and thus used and worn whilst performing everyday domestic, leisure or employment tasks. These respirometers such as the **Max Planck respirometer**, monitor the volume of gas expired by the wearer and divert a small proportion of the expired gas to a collection bag for later analysis. They are once again only suitable for relatively short term recording, but they can be used to quantify the energy costs of a variety of tasks.

If subjects keep a detailed record of their 5 minute by 5 minute activities over a day (**activity diary**), then total energy expenditure can be roughly estimated using the measured energy costs of the various activities.

A number of research units have **respiration chambers** that allow relatively long term measurement of energy expenditure of subjects performing any routine tasks that may be done within the chamber. The respiration chamber is essentially a small room which has a controlled and measured flow of air through it. Oxygen consumption and carbon dioxide production by the subject can be measured by the difference in the composition of air as it enters and leaves the chamber. These pieces of equipment are, in practice, complex and expensive and thus restricted to a relatively few well-funded research units. They can be used to monitor long term energy expenditure of subjects who can live in the chamber for several days and perform everyday tasks, thus simulating normal daily activity.

Over the last few years, the **doubly-labelled-water method** has been widely used to determine the long term energy expenditure of free-living subjects going about their normal daily activities. If people are given a dose of doubly-labelled-water ($^2H_2^{18}O$), i.e. water containing the heavy isotopes of hydrogen (^2H) and oxygen (^{18}O), then the subjects lose the labelled oxygen more rapidly than the labelled hydrogen because the hydrogen is lost only as water whereas the oxygen is lost as both water and carbon dioxide (this is due to the action of the enzyme carbonic anhydrase that promotes the exchange of oxygen between water and carbon dioxide). The difference between the rate of loss of labelled hydrogen and labelled oxygen is a measure of the rate of carbon dioxide evolution and thus it can be used to estimate long term rates of carbon dioxide evolution representing long term energy expenditure.

Comparisons of total energy expenditure measurements by respiration chamber and by doubly-labelled-water method suggest that, under strictly controlled conditions, this less expensive method accurately measures energy expenditure. Much work is currently being undertaken to determine how the reliability and validity of this method is altered under different circumstances, e.g. high water consumption. This method offers, for the first time, the realistic prospect of an acceptably accurate means of estimating the long term energy expenditure of free-living people, it has thus, not surprisingly, generated much scientific interest, been the subject of numerous scientific symposia and enabled large numbers of scientific publications (see for example, Nutrition Society, 1988).

Comparisons of metabolic rates between individuals

Absolute metabolic rates obviously tend to increase with increasing body size – large animals have higher absolute metabolic rates than small ones – fully grown adults have larger absolute metabolic rates than small children. However, relative metabolic rate (i.e. per unit body mass) declines with increasing body size – small animals have larger relative metabolic rates than large ones – small children have higher relative metabolic rates than adults. The equation:

metabolic rate = constant (k) × weight $^{3/4}$

is found to approximately predict the metabolic rates of mammals of different sizes both within and between species.

Human metabolic rates have traditionally been expressed per unit of body surface area, e.g. kcal/hour/m^2. Even in human adults, if metabolic rates are expressed per unit of body weight, then large variations between individuals are found, particularly between fat and thin individuals. Adipose tissue has a much

lower metabolic rate than lean tiss' increasing adipose tissue mass tively much less effect in increasing whole body metabolic rate than increasing lean tissue mass. Increasing adipose tissue mass also has relatively little effect in increasing body surface area, and so expressing metabolic rate per unit surface area tends to reduce the individual variation in metabolic rate and has been a useful way of comparing metabolic rates in different individuals. Nomograms are available that enable surface area to be predicted from measurements of height and weight.

Nowadays, it is considered that the best way of comparing and expressing metabolic rates of people is to express it per unit weight of lean tissue, e.g. kcal/hour/kg lean tissue. When expressed in this way, the metabolic rates of men and women are not different, whereas, when expressed per unit surface area, then the metabolic rates of women are about 10% less than those of men – this is an artefact due to the much higher body fat content of women.

Methods used to establish links between diet and disease

Human observational studies – epidemiology

Cross cultural comparisons

The first indication that diet or some other environmental factor is implicated in the aetiology of a particular disease often comes from cross cultural associations between some average population measure of the dietary variable and population mortality or morbidity rates from the disease in question. Some examples:

● a positive association between the average saturated fat intakes of populations and their mortality rates from coronary heart disease point towards high saturated fat intakes as an aetiological factor in coronary heart disease

- a positive association between *per capita* sugar consumption in different countries and the average number of decayed, missing and filled teeth in young people implicates sugar in the aetiology of dental caries
- a positive association between *per capita* salt consumption and blood pressure in various adult populations implicates high salt intake in the aetiology of hypertension
- a negative association between *per capita* fibre consumption and bowel cancer mortality in various populations has been used to implicate the fibre-depletion of Western diets in the aetiology of bowel cancer.

Information about the diets of populations are derived from the methods discussed earlier in this chapter – often food balance sheets or household expenditure surveys are the basis for international dietary comparisons. The many sources of error and uncertainty in making population estimates of dietary intakes have been discussed earlier – acceptably accurate and representative measures of dietary intake are clearly a prerequisite for making useful cross population comparisons of this type.

Information about rates of mortality from specific diseases is usually obtained through some analysis of information recorded on death certificates. There have now been efforts made to standardise death certificates internationally and to standardise the nomenclature and diagnostic criteria for the various causes of death. There will, however, still be differences between individual physicians, and this variation is likely to be even greater between those in different regions or nations.

There may be straightforward errors of diagnosis, different diagnostic criteria or terminology may be used at different times or in different centres,

even the accuracy of the age recording on death certificates may vary. When autopsies have been used to confirm the accuracy of previously recorded causes of death then they show that errors in diagnosing the causes of death in individual patients may be frequent (Barker and Rose, 1990). Both false positives (i.e. people falsely diagnosed as dying of the disease) and false negatives (i.e. people dying of the disease but not recognised as such) tend to occur, but these also tend to cancel out when population mortality is calculated. Even though the number of individual errors of diagnosis may be quite large, provided false negatives and false positives occur at similar rates, then the estimate of population mortality from diseases may still be acceptably accurate. Any factor which leads to systematic over or under recording of deaths from any cause may seriously distort population comparisons, e.g. any attempt to play down the prevalence of AIDS in order to protect the tourist industry or to exaggerate death rates from diseases of poverty to attract more international aid.

The simplest measure of mortality is the **crude death rate** for the specified cause:

$$\frac{\text{Number of deaths}}{\text{(by cause) in one year}} \times 1000$$
$$\frac{}{\begin{array}{c}\text{Number of people}\\\text{in the population}\end{array}}$$

This crude figure is of limited usefulness as mortality from many causes is age-dependant and because the age structure of different populations may vary considerably. Higher birth rates and shorter life expectancies mean, for example, that populations in developing countries tend to be much younger than those in Western industrialised countries. A more useful measure for comparisons would be the **age–specific death rate**, e.g.:

$$\frac{\text{Annual number of deaths}}{\text{in males aged 45–54 years}} \times 1000$$
$$\text{Number of men in this age}$$
$$\text{group in the population}$$

To make more complete comparisons, the **standard mortality ratio (SMR)** is a useful and widely used measure. In order to calculate the SMR, it is necessary to use as a standard or reference population, a population where all of the various age-specific mortality rates for the cause under investigation have been established. Then for each age band of the test population, one must calculate how many deaths would be expected or predicted given:

1 the number of persons of that age in the test population

and

2 assuming the same age-specific death rate as in the reference population. e.g. Number of males aged 45–49 years in the test population × death rate from the cause for males aged 45–49 years in the reference population = number of predicted deaths in 45–49 year old males in the test population.

This calculation is made for each age group in the population and the total number of predicted deaths in the test population is calculated. The total number of actual deaths in the test population is then expressed as a percentage or ratio of the predicted number of deaths from that cause in that test population.

$$\text{SMR} = \frac{\text{Actual number of deaths}}{\text{Predicted number of deaths}}$$

The SMR is not only used for international comparisons, but it is also used to make regional comparisons within a given country; in this case, the national population will probably be used as a reference population. For example, comparisons of the SMRs for gastric cancer in different regions of Britain in the early 1980s showed that the SMR was over 1.15 in Wales but less than 0.85 in parts of East Anglia (Barker and Rose, 1990). People in Wales have a greater risk of dying (115%) of this disease than the national population, whereas those in East Anglia have less than 85% of the risk of the whole population. Differences in diet, lifestyle and environment can now also be compared within the regions of Britain to see if any particular variable is associated with this variation in gastric cancer mortality, which may in turn give important clues about the aetiology of gastric cancer.

Accurate and representative measures of morbidity are likely to be more difficult to obtain than mortality data. Investigators will almost certainly have to rely upon less rigorous and uniform methods of collecting data than death certificates. Sources of information about disease frequency include: notification or registration of particular diseases; analysis of reasons for hospital admission or general practitioner consultation; social security data on reasons for absences from work; or extrapolation from relatively small scale and possibly unrepresentative survey samples. Similarly, if a symptomless risk marker, like serum cholesterol level or blood pressure, is being related to diet, then investigators will probably have to rely upon data obtained from several surveys conducted in the various countries by different investigators who will have been using different protocols.

Incidence and **prevalence** are terms used to indicate disease frequency. Incidence is the number of new cases of the disease occurring within a specified time period. Prevalence is the number of cases of the disease existing at a any particular point in time – it is dependent both upon the incidence and the duration of the disease. A chronic disease will have a much greater prevalence than an acute one of similar incidence. The chronic diseases of industrialisation, almost by definition therefore, have high prevalence and not only do they cause reduced quality of life for large numbers of people, but also exert a considerable drain on health and social care budgets.

There are large variations between nations in mortality and morbidity rates from the diet-related diseases of industrialisation. It is, therefore, common to see cross population associations between a dietary variable and one of these diseases used to implicate that particular dietary factor in the aetiology of the disease such as the sugar/caries, fat/heart disease, salt/hypertension and fibre-depletion/bowel cancer examples given earlier. Such associations do not, however, necessarily mean that there is a cause and effect relationship between that particular dietary factor and the disease. As populations become more affluent, then numerous changes in diet, lifestyle and environmental conditions tend to occur together. With increasing affluence and industrialisation may come:

- increased fat and saturated fat consumption
- less consumption of starches and fibre
- increased use of simple sugars, salt and perhaps alcohol and tobacco
- reduced physical activity
- increased consumption of animal protein
- reduced incidence of nutritional deficiencies
- increased levels of overweight and obesity
- improved medical care
- numerous other nutritional, social and environmental changes.

Accompanying these trends for change in diet and lifestyle there will be general trends in patterns of mortality and morbidity; life expectancy will increase, mortality from infectious diseases will decline, but there will be increased prevalence of and mortality from the various diseases of industrialisation. Cross cultural studies tend to focus upon individual associations between one of these lifestyle or dietary changes and one of the diseases of industrialisation. Thus the association

between saturated fat intake and coronary heart disease mortality is used to support the proposition that high saturated fat intake causes heart disease, and the negative association between fibre intake and bowel cancer used to support the proposition that low fibre intakes cause bowel cancer. As high fat diets tend to be low in fibre and vice versa, it would certainly be possible to produce equally convincing correlations between fibre intake and coronary heart disease (negatively correlated) and between saturated fat intake and bowel cancer. Epidemiological association does not necessarily mean that there is a cause and effect relationship between the two variables; the association may be coincidental and dependent upon a relationship between both tested variables and a third unconsidered or **confounding variable**.

Barker and Rose (1990) list six characteristics which would make it more likely that a demonstrated association was causal, namely that the association is:

1 *Strong* – The stronger the association the less the likelihood that it is due to some unforeseen confounding factor.
2 *Graded or dose dependent* – There is usually a graded effect of true causes rather than a threshold effect.
3 *Independent* – The relationship remains even after correction for potentially confounding variables.
4 *Consistent* – The relationship is found in studies using different investigative approaches.
5 *Reversible* – If reduced exposure to the suspected cause leads to reduced incidence of the disease, this increases the likelihood of it being a true cause.
6 *Plausible* – There is a believable mechanism to explain the causality of the association and that this mechanism can be supported by laboratory studies. A plausible mechanism unsupported by corroborating laboratory studies probably adds little weight to the argument – it is quite possible to devise plausible

mechanisms for most observations, often equally plausible mechanisms for opposing findings. The most plausible and intellectually satisfying mechanism may not be the one that ultimately proves to be correct.

The problem of confounding variables pervades all types of epidemiological investigation, and epidemiologists use various means and statistical devices to correct for variables they suspect to be confounding. There is, however, no statistical magic wand that is able to identify and perfectly correct for all confounding variables; the quality of this correction is likely to vary considerably from study to study.

If, as claimed by McCormick and Skrabanek (1988) there really are 250 risk markers for coronary heart disease, then the task of identifying any one of them as independent of all of the others is a formidable one. As another particular example, many authors have reported an apparent preventative effect of moderate doses of alcohol on coronary heart disease (e.g. Rimm *et al.*, 1991) but how many will have considered or corrected for level of physical activity as a potential confounding variable? A recent representative survey in England reported a strong positive association between alcohol consumption and level of physical activity (White *et al.*, 1993).

The classic paper of Gleibermann (1973) on the relationship between the average salt intake and blood pressure of adult populations illustrates several of these problems of cross cultural studies. She gleaned from the literature estimates of the salt intakes and blood pressures of middle-aged persons in 27 populations from various parts of the world. The data for the male populations has been used to construct a simple scatter diagram (Figure 3.7), and the correlation coefficient and regression line have also been calculated; there is a highly significant, positive and apparently linear relation-

ship between the average salt intake and the mean blood pressure of these populations, consistent with the hypothesis that high salt intake is causally linked to the development of hypertension.

The two variables in Figure 3.7 have been measured by numerous different investigators – the methods, conditions of measurement and quality of measurement are therefore not consistent across the groups. As has already been noted earlier in the chapter, salt intake is a particularly problematical measurement. The methods used to determine salt intakes in these 27 populations are variable, and in some cases unspecified; they range from the high precision 24-hour sodium excretion method to "educated guesses" made by Gleibermann herself. Recorded blood pressure may be very much influenced by the method used and the care taken by the measurer to standardise the conditions – e.g. blood pressure may be raised if measured in anxious subjects.

Although the correlation shown on Figure 3.7 is highly statistically significant, there is a considerable scatter of points around the line of best fit. The correlation coefficient (r) is 0.61, suggesting that only about 37% (r^2) of the variation in population blood pressures is accounted for by variation in their salt intake. It is possible that this association is due to some confounding variable or variables, e.g. the populations with the lowest blood pressures and lowest salt intakes would also tend to be active, have low levels of obesity, have relatively low alcohol intakes, have high potassium intakes, etc. All of these factors are thought to favour lower blood pressure.

The range of salt intakes shown in Figure 3.7 is huge, from around 1 g/day to well over 25 g/day. The US and UK average salt intakes fall some way below the middle of this range. If one takes the linear relationship at face value, then one could predict that specified falls in a population's average salt intake would be

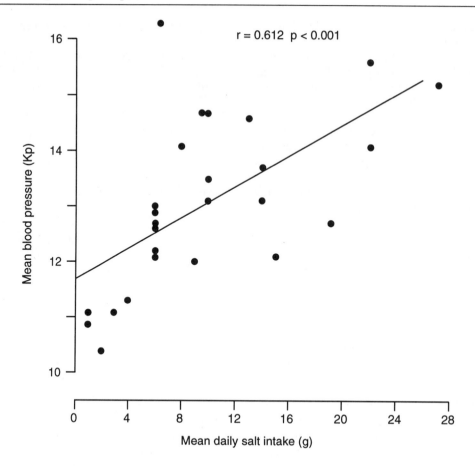

Figure 3.7 *A simple scatter diagram showing the relationship between the estimated salt intake and the mean blood pressure in 27 male populations. Data of Gleibermann (1973). Source: Webb, G.P. (1992a)* Journal of Biological Education *26(4), 264*

associated with specified falls in average blood pressure. One could then go on to make predictions about the expected benefits for that population (reductions in the prevalence of hypertension and hypertension-related diseases). It would be hard to demonstrate conclusively that this association was linear over the whole range and, of course, that is what one is assuming when predicting that small or moderate reductions in salt intakes of the populations around the centre of the range will have predictable effects on average blood pressure.

There have been numerous studies conducted in Western industrialised countries that have measured blood pressure and salt intakes in large samples of individuals living in particular towns or regions. In these studies no association is generally found between individual salt intake and individual blood pressure. Such disparity between cross cultural and within population studies are common in epidemiology and also tend to be found, for example, when dietary saturated fat intake and serum cholesterol are related and probably also if calorie intake and levels of adiposity are related. Taking the results of both approaches at face value, one would be led to conclude that whilst average salt intake may be an important determinant of average population blood pressure, individual differences in salt intake are not a major factor in producing the differences in blood pressure within a single population. This may initially seem like a contradiction because, of course, the influence of salt on population blood pressure would have to be a summation of its effects on the blood pressure of individuals. However, numerous other factors may also affect an individual's blood pressure, such as:

- individual genetic variation
- levels of activity and obesity
- alcohol consumption
- variation in genetic susceptibility to the hypertensive effects of salt.

These other influences on blood pressure may mask any effect of salt on individual blood pressure, e.g. some people may have high blood pressure because they are overweight, inactive and consume large amounts of alcohol yet their salt consumption may be low; others may have low blood pressure despite high salt intake because they are fit, abstemious, and relatively salt-insensitive. Significant numbers of such people would, of course, make it difficult to find a statistically significant association between salt intake and blood pressure, especially as most people within any given population will be concentrated around the mean value and the total range of salt intake may be relatively narrow. This problem is discussed further in the section dealing with short term human experiments later in this chapter.

Studies on migrants

One possible explanation of the differences between the morbidity and mortality patterns of different nations is that they are due to genetic differences between the populations. Studies on migrants are a useful means of distinguishing between environmental and genetic influences on disease frequency. People who migrate are immediately exposed to the new environmental conditions, and they also tend to acculturate, i.e. progressively adopt aspects of the dietary habits of the indigenous pop ever, unless widespread occurs, migrants retain th acteristics of their country oɪ Migrant populations generally also tenu to progressively acquire the morbidity and mortality characteristics of their new homeland (Barker and Rose, 1990). These trends indicate that despite there being variations in genetic susceptibility to different diseases both within and between populations, environmental factors have a predominant influence upon disease rates in populations. The differences in the mortality and morbidity patterns in different nations are predominantly due to differences in environment, lifestyle and diet rather than to the genetic differences between populations.

Mortality rates from gastric cancer and stroke are much higher in Japan than in the USA. Mortality from coronary heart disease and bowel cancer are much higher in the USA than in Japan. In Japanese migrants to the USA and their descendants, mortality rates for these four diseases move over time towards those typical of other Americans. This would indicate that these differences in mortality rates in the two countries are due to environmental factors and thus that they are potentially alterable by intervention.

Anomalous populations

When cross cultural correlations are made between dietary variables and mortality/ morbidity rates for specific diseases, then there are often anomalous populations that deviate very significantly from the general trend. These anomalous populations may provide useful information that can lead to modification of existing theories or to additional areas of investigation. Observations that Greenland eskimos had low rates of heart disease despite a diet high in fats of animal origin were important in focusing attention upon the potential dietary and therapeutic benefits of fish oils (Bang *et al.*, 1980).

In the UK, the Asian population has higher rates of coronary heart disease than the white population. This is despite their apparently lower exposure to many of the traditional risk markers for coronary heart disease (Mckeigue *et al.*, 1985), e.g. they have lower serum cholesterol levels, smoke less, drink less alcohol, consume less saturated fat and cholesterol and many are lactovegetarian. This Asian population also has low rates of bowel cancer and yet high rates of bowel cancer and coronary heart disease tend to go together. Studies on this Asian population may help to clarify the relative importance and interaction of risk factors for coronary heart disease; it may also be useful in differentiating risk factors for coronary heart disease from those for bowel cancer.

Special groups

These are groups, the people from which by reason of, for example, their religion or occupation have dietary habits or lifestyles that deviate markedly from the majority of the population that shares their particular environment. Such groups are often the subject of intensive study by epidemiologists because many of the confounding variables of other cross cultural studies will not exist between these groups and the rest of their own population. Seventh Day Adventists in the USA have been the subject of numerous investigations relating diet and lifestyle to disease. This religious group abstain from alcohol and tobacco and around half of them are ovolactovegetarian – they also have lower rates of coronary heart disease and many types of cancers (including bowel cancer) than the American population as a whole.

Despite the use of such groups because of better matching than in most cross cultural studies, there may still be numerous differences in the diet and lifestyle of these groups compared to say, the average American. Picking out one dietary or other lifestyle difference between such groups and the rest of population may still produce false assumptions about cause and effect. A religion may "impose" numerous lifestyle and dietary constraints upon its adherents; religious groups may be socially, intellectually or even genetically unrepresentative of the population as a whole, and of course the people's religious faith may provide emotional comfort that lessens the impact of stresses upon mental and physical health. A recent report claims, for example, that being religious may in itself protect against the development of bowel cancer (Kune *et al.*, 1993). See Chapter 13 for discussion of vegetarianism and health.

Time trends

Populations diets and lifestyles tend to change with the passage of time, these changes may be particularly rapid and pronounced if there has been rapid economic development and industrialisation. Epidemiologists may look for associations between the changes in a population diet and its mortality and morbidity rates for particular diseases.

In America and Western Europe salt consumption has declined during this century as the dominance of salting as a means of preserving food has been reduced by the increasing use of refrigeration and alternative methods of preservation. This decline in salt consumption in these countries has been associated with reduced mortality rates for stroke and gastric cancer (note that high blood pressure is a risk factor for stroke). These observations have been used to support the proposition that salt is an aetiological influence for both of these diseases (Joossens and Geboers, 1981). Figure 3.8 shows a very strong correlation between average death rates from stroke and gastric cancer in twelve industrialised countries between 1955 and 1972. This is consistent with the hypothesis that a change in exposure to a common aetiological influence was responsible for the decline in mortality from both diseases i.e. reduced intake of dietary salt. The apparent, relative acceleration in the decline of stroke mortality after 1972 is attributed to the population impact of anti-hypertensive drugs, which would be expected to reduce mortality from stroke but not gastric cancer.

The Japanese are frequently used by those investigating links between diet and disease as an example of a nation that, though affluent and industrialised, has a diet very different from the typical American and Western European diet. The Japanese diet has much less meat and dairy produce but much more vegetable matter and seafood. Since World War II, however, the Japanese diet has undergone considerable "westernisation". For example, since 1950 total fat intake has trebled; the ratio of animal to vegetable fat has doubled; and American-style fast food outlets have mushroomed. Mortality patterns of the Japanese have also changed over this time scale. Two thirds of deaths in Japan are now due to cardiovascular diseases, cancer and diabetes, whereas in 1950 only one third were due to these causes. Deaths from cancer have increased two and a half times since 1950 as have deaths from heart disease.

These changes in Japanese mortality patterns are consistent with most current

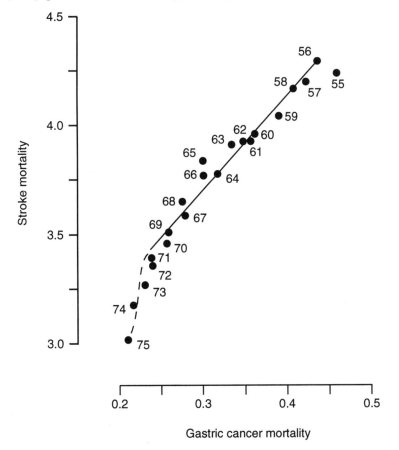

Figure 3.8 Time trends in mortality rates from gastric cancer and stroke over 20 years. Each point represents average death rates from these diseases in 12 industrialised countries for that year, e.g. 55 represents rates in 1955

Source: Webb, G.P. (1992a) *Journal of Biological Education* 26(4), 266. Simplified from Joossens, J.Y. and Geboers, J. (1981) *Proceedings of the Nutrition Society* 40, 40

views on the specific roles of diet in the aetiology of particular diseases of industrialisation. Note, however that Japanese boys are 20% taller than they were in 1950 and total life expectancy of the Japanese has also shown very big increases over the same time scale, making them now probably the most long-lived population in the world. Fujita (1993) has reviewed these changes from a Japanese perspective. He concludes that these post war dietary changes "have greatly improved the nutritional status of the Japanese people". He further concludes that the rise in crude mortality rates from the diseases of industrialisation is "mainly due to increases in the actual numbers of elderly people, rather than to westernizing effects in dietary habits". Of course, this does not mean that the current Japanese diet is optimal, and it certainly does not mean that further "westernisation" of the Japanese diet will lead to further benefits. The example does illustrate the potential hazards of focusing too narrowly upon individual causes of mortality or morbidity.

Cohort studies

In a **cohort study**, a sample of people, or cohort, is selected from either within the same population or, less commonly, from several populations. Details of the individual diets, lifestyle and other characteristics of all members of the cohort are then recorded and their subsequent health and mortality monitored for a period of years or even decades. The investigators then look for associations between the measured characteristics and the subsequent risks of mortality or morbidity. They look for dietary, lifestyle or other characteristics that are predictive of increased risk of a particular disease. To use a simple non health example, a university could record the entry qualifications of its new students and see if these predict the eventual level of achievement of students at the end of their course – is there a significant association between

level of entry qualification and final level of attainment?

Cohort studies usually require large sample groups and long follow-up times in order to get enough cases of a disease for meaningful statistical analysis, e.g. a sample of 100 000 middle-aged northern Europeans would be required in order to get 150 cases of colon cancer within a 5 year follow-up period. Cohort studies inevitably require major commitments of time, effort and money. They have, in the past, been considered impractical for all but the most common of diseases because for less common diseases impossibly long follow-up times or impossibly large sample groups are required in order to get enough cases for statistical analysis. In recent decades, however, several vast cohort studies have been instigated; there is currently underway a European cohort study looking at the relationship between diet and disease that is using a cohort of 500 000 people from nine European countries (see Coghlan, 1991). Such a study is not limited to investigating any one diet-disease relationship, it can potentially be used to provide data on dozens of such relationships. For example, data from the American Nurses Study has been used to investigate several relationships between environmental factors and diseases, some of which are discussed in this book and listed in the references:

- obesity/coronary heart disease (Manson *et al.,* 1990)
- vitamin E/coronary heart disease (Stampfer *et al.,* 1993)
- meat, fat, fibre/colon or breast cancer (Willett *et al.,* 1990)
- *trans* fatty acids/coronary heart disease (Willett *et al.,* 1993).

Many problems of such studies are common to other areas of epidemiology, for example: the accuracy of the end point diagnosis; the reliability, range and validity of the original measurements; the problem of confounding variables.

Morris *et al.*, (1980) asked 18 000 middle-aged British civil servants to complete a questionnaire on a Monday morning detailing, amongst other things, a 5 minute by 5 minute record of how they spent the previous Friday and Saturday. They found that over the next eight years, those who had reported engaging in vigorous leisure time activity, had only around half of the incidence of coronary heart disease of their colleagues who reported having participated in no such vigorous activity (even allowing for differences in smoking of the two groups).

This is consistent with the hypothesis that exercise reduces the risk of coronary heart disease but of course does not necessarily prove that the differences between these groups is caused by differences in exercise levels – perhaps, for example, those best equipped for vigorous physical activity and thus more inclined to participate are also less prone to coronary heart disease; perhaps a reluctance to participate in vigorous leisure time activity is an early indication of existing but undiagnosed coronary heart disease.

When cohort studies are used to assess the relationships between exposure to an environmental factor and disease then the term **relative risk** is widely used:

$$\text{Relative risk} = \frac{\text{Incidence in exposed group}}{\text{Incidence in unexposed group}}$$

In the example of Morris *et al.* (1980) the relative risk of coronary heart disease in the inactive smokers was compared to that of the active non smokers:

$$\frac{\text{Incidence in inactive smokers}}{\text{Incidence in active non smokers}}$$

In many dietary studies, the population is divided up into fifths or **quintiles** according to their level of consumption of a particular nutrient i.e. the fifth with the lowest consumption (or exposure) through to the fifth with the highest consumption. The relative risk in each quintile can then be expressed in relation to that of the lowest quintile:

$$\text{Relative risk} = \frac{\begin{array}{c}\text{Incidence of disease in}\\\text{any other quintile}\end{array}}{\text{Incidence in lowest quintile}}$$

Figure 3.9 shows the relative risk of developing colon cancer in differing quintiles of a cohort of almost 90 000 American nurses divided according to their consumption of animal fat (Willett *et al.*, 1990). The results indicate that there is a progressive increase in risk of colon cancer associated with increased animal fat consumption; the effect was statistically significant.

Positive results from an apparently rigorous cohort study are usually given particular weight when conclusions are made about relationships between lifestyle factors and disease.

Case-control studies

In **case–control studies,** investigators try to identify differences in the diet, lifestyle or other characteristics of matched groups of disease sufferers and controls. Often such studies are retrospective and involve matching a group of those suffering from or dying of a particular disease with a group that can act as a control and then trying to retrospectively identify differences in the past diets, behaviours or occupations of the two groups that might account for the presence of the disease in the case group. Returning to our example of predicting final degree results from entry qualifications; using a case-control type of approach one might try to identify the entry characteristics of students who have attained first class degrees. One could take a group of students attaining first class degrees (cases) and match them with some obtaining lower grades (controls)

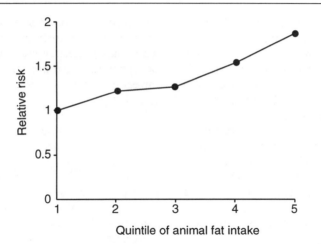

Figure 3.9 Relative risk of colon cancer according to quintile of animal fat intake. A cohort of almost 90 000 American nurses was followed for six years and there were 150 recorded cases. Source: simplified from Willett, W.C. *et al* (1990) *New England Journal of Medicine* 323, 1669.

and see if the entry characteristics of the two groups were different.

Matching of cases and controls is clearly a critical factor in such investigations; because the sample sizes are usually small, testing and correction for the effects of confounding variables cannot be undertaken in the final analysis of the results. One would wish to match only for confounding variables, i.e. those that are independently linked to both the suspected cause and the disease under investigation. Matching for factors that are linked to the cause but not independently to the disease will actually tend to obscure any relationship between the suspected cause and the disease. In addition to the problem of control selection, it may be extremely difficult to obtain reliable information about past behaviour, especially past dietary practices. Present behaviour may be an unreliable guide to past behaviour because the disease or awareness of it may modify current behaviour; differences between controls and cases may be as a result of the disease rather than its cause. Some diseases, like cancer, are thought to be initiated many years before overt clinical symptoms appear – this may make it desirable to compare the behaviours of people from case and control groups from years back.

Cramer *et al.* (1989) set out to test the hypothesis that high dietary galactose consumption (from lactose or milk sugar) was implicated in the aetiology of ovarian cancer. Approximately equal numbers of sufferers and non sufferers from the disease were asked to fill in a food frequency questionnaire, focusing upon the dietary patterns in the previous five years but asking the "cases" to ignore changes in food preferences since their diagnosis of cancer. Lactose consumption was not significantly different in the cases and controls, neither were there any significant differences when several other specific dairy foods were considered separately. However, eating yoghurt at least once a month was associated with significantly increased relative risk of ovarian cancer. The implication is that yoghurt consumption is causally linked to the development of ovarian cancer but there are many other explanations for these results.

Yoghurt is a food with a "healthy image" and ovarian cancer is sometimes called the silent cancer because the disease has often progressed to an advanced stage before its clinical recognition – perhaps minor subclinical effects of the disease persuaded the cases to include more healthy foods in their diets prior to the onset of clinically overt symptoms. The sufferers also differed from the controls in several other respects – the sufferers were more likely: to be Jewish; to be college-educated; to have never been married; to have never had children; and, never to have used oral contraceptives. It is not unreasonable to suggest that women with such characteristics might also be more likely to eat yoghurt, i.e. that the differences in yoghurt consumption are due to some other characteristic of women who develop ovarian cancer, rather than yoghurt consumption being directly, causally, linked to the development of ovarian cancer.

Case-control studies may be prospective. Clinical records or stored samples may be used to yield information that is more reliable or at least less subject to bias than asking questions about past behaviour. On occasion, such information may be recorded or stored with the specific intention of referring back to it when cases have become apparent. Wald *et al* (1980) investigated the possibility of a link between vitamin A status and risk of cancer. Serum samples were collected and frozen from 16 000 men over a three year period. 86 men from this large sample subsequently developed cancer and were matched with 172 men who did not develop cancer. They were matched for age, smoking habits and time at which the samples were collected. The serum retinol (vitamin A) concentrations were then measured in the stored samples from both groups of men. Serum retinol concentrations were found to be lower in the cases than in the controls; consistent with the hypothesis that poor dietary vitamin A status increases cancer risk. However, the time between sample collection and clinical diagnosis was short (i.e. 1 to 4 years) – it is again possible that an existing undiagnosed cancerous condition may have resulted in reduced serum retinol

concentration, i.e. that the difference in serum retinol concentrations is due to rather than the cause of the cancers. It is also generally agreed that serum retinol concentration is an insensitive measure of dietary status for vitamin A; serum retinol concentrations normally only start to fall when body pools of the vitamin are seriously depleted.

In cohort studies, then relative risk could be calculated directly, but in case-control studies an indirect measure of relative risk, the **odds ratio,** has to be used. This is defined as the odds of exposure to the suspected cause amongst the cases divided by the odds of exposure amongst the controls.

$$\text{Odds ratio} = \frac{\text{Odds of case exposure}}{\text{Odds of control exposure}}$$

In most case-control studies this is calculated using the equation:

$$\text{Odds ratio} = \frac{\text{No. exposed cases} \times \text{No. unexposed controls}}{\text{No. unexposed cases} \times \text{No. exposed controls}}$$

If the experiment has been designed using matched pairs of cases and controls then:

$$\text{Odds ratio} = \frac{\text{No. pairs with case exposed but control unexposed}}{\text{No. pairs with case unexposed but control exposed}}$$

As with relative risk in cohort studies, the odds ratio can be calculated at each of several different levels of exposure as was seen in Figure 3.9.

Case-control studies of some type account for many of the putative links between diet or lifestyle and disease that fleetingly attract the attention of the health correspondents of the media. This type of study is clearly an important tool for the epidemiologist seeking to identify causes of many diseases but clearly also many of these studies are open to several interpretations and often they do no more than point to the possibility of a causative link that is worthy of further investigation.

Experiments of nature

Observations made upon victims of some congenital or acquired disorder may provide useful evidence about the relationships between diet and disease. The observation that people with familial hypercholesteraemia (a genetic tendency to very high plasma cholesterol concentration) are very prone to premature coronary heart disease supports the idea that serum cholesterol levels and coronary heart disease risk are positively associated. The work of Brown and Goldstein (1984) indicates that high plasma cholesterol is a primary consequence of the genetic defect, and this supports the proposition that the association is causal.

Animal experiments (after Webb, 1990 and 1992b)

Animal experiments afford the opportunity to perform high precision, well-controlled and, if necessary, long term experiments to directly test hypotheses. Technical, ethical or financial considerations would often make it difficult or impossible to undertake such experiments using human subjects. The **reliability** of well designed and competently executed animal experiments should be high, i.e. the experimenter can have confidence that a difference between, say, an experimental group and a control group is due to the treatment being tested and results should be repeatable if the experimental circumstances are replicated.

Epidemiological studies rely upon investigators attempting to demonstrate correlations or associations between naturalistic observations. These are not truly experiments because the investigator does not impose any constraint or intervention upon the subjects to test an hypothesis.

These observational human studies cannot be properly controlled; confounding variables may result in a false assumption that two associated variables are causally linked and, conversely, other influences upon the dependent variable (the disease) may obscure a causative association.

The problem with animal experiments is their questionable **validity**; the extent to which hypotheses supported by animal experiments may be applied to people. Strictly speaking, animal experiments can only be used to generate hypotheses about humans. The new hypothesis should then be tested by direct experiment with humans, or, if that is not possible, then the extent to which human observations are consistent with the animal-generated hypothesis can be assessed. In practice, however, results from animal experiments may be extrapolated to people with little experimental confirmation in people and sometimes with little consideration of biological factors which may make such projections unsafe. It is a measure of the robustness of animal experimentation that often, despite such lack of rigour, essentially correct conclusions about humans are drawn.

There is abundant evidence for those willing to be convinced, that animal experiments have played a key role in progressing our knowledge of human biology, and, therefore, also a key role in generating the practical medical, surgical and nutritional benefits that have resulted from the application of that knowledge. Only around 20% of the Nobel prize-winners in Physiology and Medicine have used human subjects for their research, and only around 10% have not made use of some non-human species. These Nobel prizes represent a yardstick to assess the contribution of animal experiments, because they acknowledge landmark achievements in advancing physiological and medical knowledge; almost all prize-winners have made use of non-human species in their research.

There is also clear evidence that animal experiments have sometimes mislead researchers. Dietary cholesterol was once widely regarded as the dominant influence upon serum cholesterol concentration. Frantz and Moore (1969) in a review of "the sterol hypothesis of atherogenesis" concluded that, although saturated fat was an important influence upon serum cholesterol, its effect was probably to potentiate the effects of dietary cholesterol. Most current nutrition education advice suggests that dietary cholesterol is normally a relatively minor, perhaps even insignificant, influence upon serum cholesterol concentration. According to Frantz and Moore, experiments with herbivorous, laboratory rabbits were the major evidence directly supporting the now apparently exaggerated influence of dietary cholesterol upon blood cholesterol concentration. In Chapter 8 it is argued that experiments with laboratory rats were an important factor in exaggerating the protein requirements of children and thus in falsely indicating a huge deficit in world protein supplies.

Animal experiments are a vital research tool in human nutrition and the other biomedical sciences. In the past, they have made major contributions to advancing understanding of human biology and will continue to be vital for the foreseeable future. Animal experiments also have a considerable potential to mislead the human nutritionist, especially if results generated in experiments with small laboratory animals are extrapolated to people with little consideration of the factors that might invalidate such projections and with little attempt to corroborate the animal-generated hypothesis with studies in people.

Some particular factors that need to be considered when projecting from nutrition experiments with animals to people:

1 *Species differences in nutrient requirements* – There may be both qualitative and quantitative differences in the nutritional requirements of different species. Most mammals, unlike primates and guinea-pigs, make their own vitamin C and therefore do not require a dietary supply.

All mammals require an exogenous source of protein but equally, the requirements of children and other young primates are relatively low because of their slow growth rate – the milk of most mammals has 20–25% of the energy as protein whereas in humans and chimpanzees this figure is only around 6% (see Chapter 8).

2 *Species differences in feeding pattern and diet character* – Experiments that involve exposing animals to a type of diet or a mode of feeding that is totally different from their natural behaviour might not predict the response of people, especially if the experimental diet or feeding pattern is much more akin to the natural one in humans.

Rabbits are herbivores and would not normally encounter cholesterol in their diets because cholesterol is found in foods of animal origin. This might be expected to leave them metabolically ill-equipped to handle large dietary loads of cholesterol. They certainly seem to be much more sensitive to the atherogenic effects of cholesterol than many other laboratory species. One might expect omnivorous and carnivorous species to be better adapted to handling dietary loads of cholesterol and thus less susceptible to its atherogenic effects. The assumption that the rabbit's response to dietary cholesterol would predict the human response seems, with the benefit of hindsight, like a very unsafe assumption.

This partly explains the much higher emphasis in past years put upon dietary cholesterol as a major influence upon serum cholesterol and atherogenesis. Some animals spend long periods of time nibbling or grazing whereas other species consume large amounts of food rapidly in short duration and during relatively infrequent meals. The idea that nibbling regimes might be useful in the treatment of human obesity were largely based upon experiments that monitored the effect of meal feeding upon naturally nibbling species, like rats and mice.

3 *Controlled experimental conditions versus real life* – Animal experiments are usually performed under highly controlled conditions – experimental and control groups are matched and treated identically except for imposed differences in the experimental variables. Strictly speaking one is then only able to assume that the test treatment produces the results obtained under the specified conditions of the experiment. In practice, one tends to assume that essentially similar effects would result from the treatment even if some of the background conditions were changed (e.g. in free-living, genetically diverse, wild animals of the same species). Changes in background conditions might sometimes substantially alter the response of even the experimental species to the experimental treatment, i.e. controlled experiments with laboratory animals might sometimes not even predict the response of free-living wild animals of the same species, let alone the response of human beings.

Animal experiments play a key role in the toxicological testing of food additives. Such tests often involve exposing experimental animals to huge doses of single additives over their whole life-span under laboratory conditions – if additives show no adverse effects under these test conditions it is then assumed that they are generally non-toxic to that species in those doses. Under different conditions, however, the additive might have harmful effects – there might be interactions between the additive and some other factor – the additive might become harmful, e.g. in the presence of other additives, drugs or chemicals; with particular dietary inadequacies; with exposure to cigarette smoke or alcohol; or if animals with differing genotypes are exposed. There is, for example, a well known interaction between certain anti-depressant drugs (mono amine oxidase inhibitors) and certain foods containing tyramine (e.g. cheese); the tyramine causes a dangerous rise in blood pressure in people taking these drugs. There are several other well known interactions between drugs and diet.

4 *Differences in species' sizes* – One of the major advantages of using most laboratory animals is their small size, which greatly reduces the cost of experiments. More than 90% of all animals used for experiments in the UK are rodents or rabbits. This small size also leaves experimenters with the difficulty of how to allow for differences in size when projecting results from animal experiments to humans. It is usual to scale dosages and requirements according to body weight but this is more because of convention and convenience than because there is convincing evidence of its validity. Earlier in the chapter, four fold differences were obtained when projecting the rat's rate of vitamin C synthesis to human size depending upon whether relative body weight or relative metabolic rate was used as the basis for the scaling.

Let us assume that one might wish to model in a mouse experiment, the sugar consumption of two human populations – one consuming around 40 kg per person per year and one consuming around half this amount. These amounts represent somewhere near 20% and 10% of total calorie intake respectively for the human populations. If one scales this human consumption according to relative body weight to set the experimental consumption in the mice then sugar would only represent only around 2.5% and 1.3% of total calories in the two groups of mice.

As discussed earlier in this chapter, the relative metabolic rate (i.e. energy expenditure per unit weight) declines with increasing body size in mammals. Small animals like rats and mice have much more rapid metabolic rates than larger species like man. This accounts for the large differences produced when the scaling is by relative body weight or relative metabolic rate in the two examples above.

Rodents are widely used in studies upon energy balance that are directed towards increasing understanding of human energy balance regulation. The size difference in relative metabolic rate is just one of several factors that greatly complicates the human nutritionist's interpretation of energy balance studies conducted with small mammals. It is sometimes difficult to project to humans, even qualitatively, the results from energy balance studies on rodents.

The relative energy costs of locomotion (i.e. energy required to move a specific mass a specific distance) declines with increasing body size, there is also the added complication that, in humans, bipedal locomotion seems to double the energy cost of walking compared to that of a similarly sized quadruped. This will make it difficult to assess the importance of activity level to overall human energy expenditure from small animal studies.

Small animals rely upon heat generation as their principal physiological response to cold, whereas large animals and people rely much more upon heat conservation to maintain body temperature in the cold. When mice are used, the situation may be still further complicated because mice have been shown to become torpid when fasted, i.e. they allow substantial and prolonged falls in body temperature in order to conserve energy. Most investigators, in the past, have assumed that mice are invariably homeothermic.

Such factors would clearly make it difficult to predict the effects of environmental temperature upon human energy needs from experiments with mice. They may also complicate more fundamental decisions about the relative importance of variations in energy intake or expenditure to overall energy balance and thus to the development of obesity.

Human experimental studies

These have been divided up into three categories for ease of discussion but these divisions are rather arbitrary. The overall design strategy is similar in the three types of study the differences are to do with the scale and duration of the study, the nature of the experimental constraints and whether or not the subject is expected to gain therapeutic benefit from the experimental treatment.

Short term experiments

Most of the hypotheses relating diet to diseases of industrialisation suggest that chronic exposure to the dietary risk factor leads eventually to increased risk of the development of clinical disease. Clearly such hypotheses are not directly testable in short term experiments. However, these diet-disease hypotheses often involve hypothetical chains of apparently reversible steps between exposure to the initial dietary risk factor and clinical disease; the diet-heart hypothesis, for example, envisages changes in plasma cholesterol resulting from high intake of dietary saturated fats leading to lipid deposition in artery walls, atherosclerosis and ultimately increased risk of coronary heart disease. It may be possible to test individual steps in such an hypothesis in short term experiments without exposing the experimental subjects to any significant long term risks. Keys *et al.* (1959) were able to demonstrate in short term experiments that changing the ratio of polyunsaturated to saturated fats in the diet had predictable effects upon serum cholesterol concentration. Subjects switched from diets high in saturates/low in polyunsaturates to low saturate/high polyunsaturate diets (i.e. from low to high P:S ratio); all showed some decline in plasma cholesterol concentration even though the degree of responsiveness varied and the total fat content of the two diets was the same (see Figure 3.10). It must be borne in mind that such short term experiments may not necessarily predict the long term response – subjects may adapt to any change in the longer term. Also, support for one element of an hypothesis does not confirm the whole hypothesis – thus even if high polyunsaturate/low saturate diets reduce serum cholesterol in the short term, it does not necessarily follow that this will lead to improved health and longevity or even necessarily to reduced risk of coronary heart disease.

Further consideration of the data in Figure 3.10 may help to explain how saturated fat intake could be a major determinant of average population serum cholesterol despite the fact that within populations there appears to be no significant association between serum cholesterol concentration and saturated fat intake. Clearly this dietary change in P:S ratio has had a cholesterol lowering effect in these individuals; the appropriate statistical test (a paired "t" test) would show that this effect was highly statistically significant. This dietary change appears to have shifted the whole distribution of individual serum cholesterol concentrations downwards; given a large enough sample one would expect this would significantly reduce average serum cholesterol of the sample population. Yet, the range of cholesterol concentrations of subjects consuming a matched diet, say diet A, is huge and the average reduction in serum

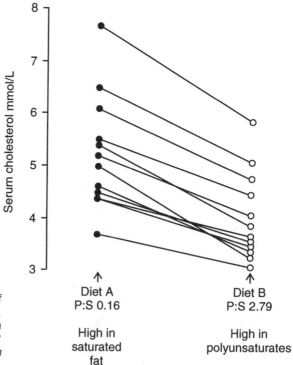

Figure 3.10 Effects of different types of dietary fat on serum cholesterol in 12 men. Total fat in the two diets was matched. Data of Keys *et al.* (1959). Source: Webb, G.P. (1992a) *Journal of Biological Education* 26(4), 266. After NACNE (1983)

cholesterol resulting from the dietary change to diet B is relatively small in comparison. The difference between the two means is less than a third of the difference between the highest and lowest values on diet A. This is despite the fact that the magnitude of this experimental dietary change is enormous – probably towards the extreme ends of the range of practical feasibility with regard to P:S ratio. Although the ratio of polyunsaturated to saturated fat clearly affects individual serum cholesterol levels, and therefore average population levels, it is not the primary factor determining where any individual lies within the population range of serum cholesterol concentrations.

Clinical trials

Clinical trials are usually used to test the effectiveness of a treatment on the course or severity of a disease or symptom. The aim of such trials is to isolate and quantify the effect of the treatment under test. It is, therefore necessary to eliminate, minimise or allow for other influences on the disease progression or severity, e.g.:

1 There may be variation in disease progression/severity that is unrelated to the intervention – this requires that there be a matched control group or control period. There may be considerable variation in the initial disease severity and this could be a source of bias if the control and experimental groups are not initially well-matched. Bias can be overcome by randomly assigning subjects to experimental or control groups; with large samples, this makes it likely that groups will be initially well matched. In some studies, particularly small scale studies, there may need to be more formal matching for disease severity.
2 A **placebo** effect of treatment may occur; a psychologically based improvement that results from an expectation that treatment will yield benefits. If the outcome measure involves any subjective grading of symptom severity, this placebo effect is likely to be particularly important. Ideally the control subjects would be offered a dummy treatment which they cannot distinguish from the real treatment – a placebo.
3 There may be unconscious bias on the part of the operator who measures outcomes and who administers the real and dummy treatments. Ideally the experimenter should also be unaware of which patients are receiving real and dummy treatments until after the data collection has been completed. This is particularly important if the outcome measure involves any subjective judgement to be made by the experimenter.

When dealing with clinical trials of dietary interventions, there may be particular problems that may make it impossible to achieve the design aims listed above, e.g.:

● a dietary intervention aimed at varying intake of a particular nutrient will usually involve consequential changes in the intakes of other nutrients
● if intervention is a special diet, then it may be difficult or impossible to allow for the placebo effect and to eliminate operator bias
● if the intervention is a special diet then there are likely to be variations in the degree of compliance and it may be difficult or impossible to objectively assess the level of compliance.

One ideal model of a clinical trial is the double-blind, random-crossover trial. Patients are given indistinguishable real or dummy treatments during two consecutive trial periods and some measure of treatment success made at the end of both treatment periods. Patients would be randomly assigned to receive either real or dummy treatment first. Neither patient nor experimenter knows whether real or dummy treatment is being given at any particular time. It may even be possible to ensure uniform compliance by administering treatment (e.g. a tablet) in the presence of the experimenter. Below is an example to illustrate this type of experimental design.

Macgregor *et al.* (1982) prescribed patients with mild to moderate hypertension a diet designed to be low in sodium. All subjects were required to remain on this experimental diet throughout the 10 week experimental period. After a two week adjustment period, the subjects then received either slow release sodium tablets or placebos during two consecutive monthly periods. The sodium tablets raised salt intake and negated the effects of the low salt diet. The real and dummy tablets were identical and were administered using the double-blind, random-crossover model (see Figure 3.11 for a summary of the experimental protocol). Blood pressure was found to be significantly lower at the end of the placebo period compared to the salt-supplementation period. This supports the hypothesis that moderate salt restriction can have at least some short term effect of lowering blood pressure in this category of patient.

In Chapter 12, a large double-blind clinical trial is described which was set up to test whether folate supplements given

Figure 3.11 A plan of the experimental protocol of Macgregor *et al.* (1982) to illustrate a double blind random crossover trial

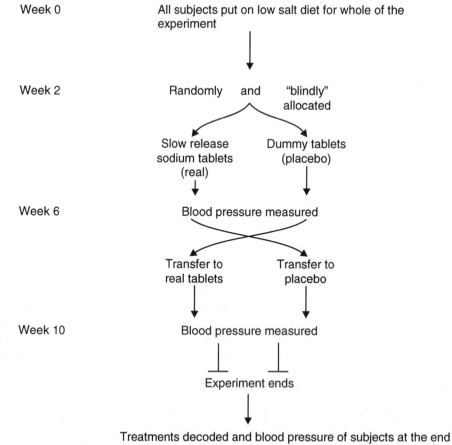

Week 0   All subjects put on low salt diet for whole of the experiment

Week 2   Randomly   and   "blindly" allocated

Slow release sodium tablets (real)   Dummy tablets (placebo)

Week 6   Blood pressure measured

Transfer to real tablets   Transfer to placebo

Week 10   Blood pressure measured

Experiment ends

Treatments decoded and blood pressure of subjects at the end of the "real" and placebo treatment periods compared.

to high risk pregnant women reduced the risk of babies being born with neural tube defects. Almost 2000 women, from 7 countries and 33 centres, who were at high risk of having babies with neural tube defects (because of a previously affected pregnancy) were randomly assigned to receive one of four treatments: folate supplements; other vitamin supplements; both of these; or, neither of these. There were many less affected babies in the two folic acid supplemented groups compared to the two groups not receiving folic acid supplements (MRC, 1991).

Intervention trials

These are essentially long term, population level experiments. The design aim, as in other experiments, is to make the intended variable or variables the only difference between matched control and experimental groups. The scale and duration of most intervention trials, and perhaps also the nature of the intervention itself, may make it impossible to impose the level of rigour in design that can be accomplished with small scale, short term experiments or clinical trials.

Some of the problems that may be encountered when designing intervention trials:

1 *Selection of subjects* – In some intervention trials, a "high risk" group may be used as subjects. Even if an intervention is convincingly shown to benefit such high risk subjects, this does not necessarily mean that the intervention will yield net benefit to the population as a whole.

When such high risk subjects are used, then there may be an ethical dilemma about how to treat the control group. If they are made aware of their high risk status, then control groups may significantly alter their behaviour during the course of the experiment.

2 *Multiple intervention* – Most of the diseases of industrialisation are assumed to have a multifactorial aetiology.

Multiple risk factor interventions may be used to maximise the likely benefits of intervention; in some cases the experimental aspects of the trial may be given low priority because the primary purpose is to promote health within a population rather than to test the efficacy of the intervention. Using such multiple interventions may make it impossible to quantify the contribution of any particular intervention to the overall benefits (or harm) demonstrated for the experimental group. Factorial design of experiments can aid in this respect but may not be practical in many trials. Note that the previously discussed clinical trial of folate supplementation in pregnant women is an example of a factorial design – with such a design it is possible to statistically test the effects of both of the interventions and also to test for any possible interaction between the two interventions.

3 *Measure of outcome* – An intervention trial may be designed to test the effect of the intervention upon a particular disease risk marker or upon morbidity or mortality from a particular disease. Even if the intervention produces the expected beneficial effect in such cases, the ultimate holistic test of the benefit of the intervention is whether such narrow benefits result in a reduction in total morbidity or mortality. Statistically significant reductions in these holistic measures may require impossibly large subject groups and long durations of study.

Passmore and Eastwood (1986) summarise studies on the effects of water fluoridation upon the dental health of UK children; these come closer to an "ideal" design than most intervention trials. In 1956, three experimental areas of the UK started to fluoridate their water supply whilst three neighbouring areas were used as controls. Prevalence of caries in the teeth of the children in the control and experimental areas was similar prior to fluoridation but by 1961 the experimental areas had shown a considerable relative improvement. One of the experimental areas later discontinued fluoridation and within five years, caries prevalence had risen back up to the level in the control areas. This trial provides very convincing evidence of the benefit of fluoridation to the dental health of children. The controversy that has prevented widespread fluoridation of water supplies in the UK revolve around its long term safety rather than its efficacy in preventing dental caries. Absolute, long term safety is, of course, much more difficult to demonstrate convincingly.

In The Multiple Risk Factor Intervention Trial (1982), a third of a million American men were screened to identify 13,000 who were classified as at "high risk" of coronary heart disease. These high risk men were then randomly assigned to experimental and control groups. The experimental group received intensive dietary counselling aimed at both normalisation of serum cholesterol concentration and body weight, they received aggressive treatment for hypertension and intensive counselling to help them reduce tobacco usage.

The control group received no counselling but they, and their personal physicians, were advised of their high risk status and the results of annual physical examinations were sent to their physicians; they were classified as "usual care". The experimental intervention was apparently very successful in modifying behaviour and in producing measurable reductions in the objective risk markers (e.g. serum cholesterol concentration), but the study failed to show any beneficial effects of intervention, i.e. there was no difference in either total mortality or even coronary heart disease mortality between the two groups after seven years of follow-up.

This failure has been partly explained by the behaviour of the control group, who also appeared to modify their behaviour once they, and their physicians became aware of their high risk status. It has also been suggested that harmful effects of the antihypertensive therapy may have cancelled out and obscured the beneficial effects of other aspects of the intervention.

Both of these trials could be described as primary intervention trials – they aimed to prevent the onset of disease in asymptomatic subjects. Rarely have such trials produced significant reductions in total mortality when dietary interventions have been used. Other trials are described as secondary intervention trials because they use subjects who have already experienced a disease event (e.g. have already had a myocardial infarction). These are an extreme example of a high risk group and one would need to be particularly cautious about assuming that any benefit demonstrated in such a group would have net beneficial effects on the population as a whole. Burr *et al.* (1991) tested the effects of three dietary interventions upon total two year mortality in 2000 men who had recovered from a myocardial infarction. The three dietary interventions were advice to: increase cereal fibre consumption; reduce total fat intake; and, to eat fatty fish or take fish oil capsules twice weekly. Subjects were randomly allocated to receive or not to receive advice on each of these three interventions and the allocations were made independently of allocations for the other two interventions. Thus there were eight possible combinations of interventions or non-interventions, including a group who received no intervention at all. The fish oil intervention almost uniquely, for a dietary intervention, did produce a significant reduction in total all cause mortality. One suggestion as to why this trial alone has produced a statistically significant fall in total mortality is because there appeared to be almost no tendency for non-fish advised men to increase their fish consumption. At the time, the potential therapeutic effects of fish oils were not widely known in the UK. In many other intervention trials, control subjects have also tended to modify their behaviour in the direction of that counselled for the intervention group.

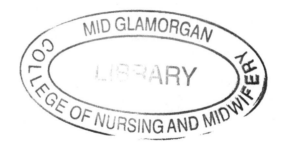

4 Dietary guidelines and recommendations

Contents

Overview

Over the past decade or so there have been dozens of reports emanating from governmental and other expert committees in industrialised countries that have suggested dietary changes and guidelines. The general aim of all of these reports is to offer advice that, if followed, would be expected to reduce the morbidity and mortality from the diseases of industrialisation. Some of these reports have focused upon one aspect of diet and health such as diet and coronary heart disease or diet and cancer prevention. Other reports have offered more general dietary guidelines that attempt to synthesise current ideas on the relationship between diet and individual diseases and to construct sets of general guidelines that might be expected to maximise health and longevity. Inevitably these reports vary somewhat in the scope of their recommendations, the precise quantitative targets and the priority attached to the various recommendations. Nevertheless, in general qualitative terms, there is a striking level

of agreement and consistency between almost all of these reports; examples of fundamental disagreement are rare. This certainly adds a cumulative weight to these recommendations and guidelines; nevertheless, even apparent consensus support amongst experts for a particular intervention does not guarantee that in the longer term it will continue to be regarded as useful or even safe (see Chapter 1).

As an illustration of this current consensus amongst "expert committees", Hamilton *et al.* (1991) give a summary of the recommendations in five reports published in the US between 1987 and 1990; they vary from those aimed specifically at reducing one disease, like cancer, to more general recommendations for "reducing chronic disease risk". These five reports are unanimous in recommending: varied food choices; maintenance of ideal body weight; a diet rich in starch and fibre; severe limitations on the consumption of fat; and, limits on the consumption of alcohol. Four of the five also recommend limiting cholesterol and salt intake and three recommend limiting sugar intake.

In the UK, the report of the National Advisory Committee on Nutrition Education (NACNE, 1983) has had, and continues to have, a great influence on nutrition education. This committee, for the first time in the UK, attempted to offer a comprehensive set of quantitative dietary targets for the UK population. This NACNE committee envisaged a 15 year time scale for implementing its long term goals (i.e. by around the end of the century) but suggested that around a third of the changes could be achieved by the end of the 1980s. The 1980s have now passed with relatively little progress made on achieving several of the key goals of the NACNE committee; its short term target for total dietary fat appeared in a recent report by the Department of Health on "The Health of the Nation" as a target for the year 2005! (DH, 1992). In the USA, the National Research Council report of 1989 (NRC, 1989b) also attempted to make a comprehensive set of dietary recommendations for health promotion. Other important and influential reports that have made recommendations for diet and health, in the UK, include the 1984 and 1991 reports of the Committee on Medical Aspects of Food Policy on "Diet and cardiovascular disease" and "Dietary Reference Values" (COMA, 1984 and 1991 respectively); Hamilton *et al.* (1991) give a comprehensive list of such reports aimed at Americans and Canadians.

The individual recommendations of these various expert committees are summarised and briefly discussed below, with particular emphasis on those of NACNE (1983) and the NRC (1989b). NACNE (1983) gave their recommendations in the form of goals for average population intakes of nutrients. They thought this was the most appropriate way of using largely epidemiological data. NACNE envisaged nutrition education seeking to shift the whole population distribution of the nutrient intakes upwards or downwards rather than aiming to truncate the distribution by concentrating on those with intakes at the extremities of the range. NRC (1989b) on the other hand, gave their recommendations in the form of individual minimum or maximum intakes. Where the two sets of recommendations apparently correspond, this difference in approach means that the NRC targets do in fact require greater change than those of NACNE. This is illustrated in Figure 4.1 by reference to the apparently common 30% target for proportion of total calories from fat. If individuals are all to meet this target as recommended by NRC, then the average population intake must be some way below 30% because of individual variation in fat intakes.

Guidelines for specific nutrients

Body weight and activity

Most dietary guidelines, including those in the NRC and NACNE reports, emphasise the importance of maintaining an ideal body weight by matching energy intake to expenditure. In Britain in 1987, almost a third of adults were considered to be overweight, and it was estimated that 8% of men and 12% of women were obese,, i.e. body mass index greater than 30 (Gregory *et al.*, 1990). A survey in 1991 indicated that incidence of obesity has risen sharply in recent years and may be as high as 13% among men and 15% amongst women (White *et al.*, 1993). This latter survey also found that 53% of men and 44% of women had a Body Mass Index of more than 25 and thus were either overweight or obese. Using different criteria, the incidence of being overweight in the US is estimated at 26% of all persons aged 20–74 years but with much higher incidence in particular ethnic groups, e.g. 44% in black American women (DHHS, 1992). The prevalence

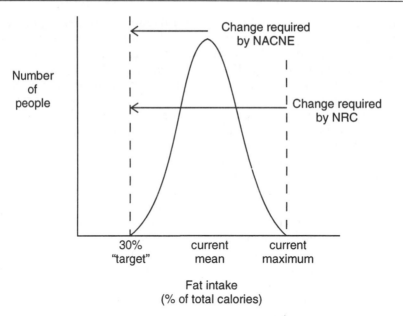

Figure 4.1 The theoretical changes in the current normal distribution of population intakes required to meet the receommended intakes of NACNE (1983) and NRC (1989b). NACNE recommended a new population average of 30% of calories from fat whereas NRC recommended 30% as an individual target

of being overweight and obesity together with the health and other consequences of obesity are discussed at length in Chapter 6.

Both NACNE and NRC highlight the importance of increased physical activity in the maintenance of an ideal body weight. NACNE specifically recommended maintenance of the then current energy intake but with increased levels of physical activity to balance expenditure to intake. Both the US and UK populations have become increasingly sedentary in recent decades. As a consequence of this increasingly sedentary lifestyle, average energy intakes have shown quite substantial recent falls in both countries (e.g. Chesher, 1990). Over the same period, the average body mass index has increased in both countries and being overweight and obesity have become more prevalent. A recent survey of activity and

physical fitness of British adults has confirmed the low level of physical activity of the population; around three-quarters of those surveyed reported taking less physical exercise than is considered necessary to produce any health benefits. Very low levels of aerobic fitness were also found; one third of middle-aged men and half of middle-aged women were "unfit" for continuous walking on the level at normal walking pace (DH, 1992).

Dietary fat

Both NRC and NACNE recommended reducing total fat intake to 30% of calories and reducing the saturated fat to 10% of total calories. NACNE suggested that to reduce total fat to 34% of total calories (i.e. total including alcohol) and saturated fat to 15% of total calories by the end of the 1980s were modest targets (from assumed baselines of 38% and 18% of calories respectively in 1980). Since 1983, average UK saturated fat intakes have dropped substantially in absolute terms but only modestly when corrected for the decline in total energy intake. This small decline in the proportion of calories derived from saturated fat reflects the switch from animal-based cooking and spreading fats to vegetable oils and margarines. There has also been a substantial decline in absolute fat intakes in the UK over the last decade but this is almost entirely accounted for by a decline in total food intake. There has been no significant progress in generally reducing the proportion of calories derived from fat, which has remained practically unchanged since the 1960s (MAFF, 1993). Other expert committees, including COMA (1984) and (1991), have taken a figure of 35% of food calories (i.e. excluding alcohol) derived from fat because even this is likely to prove very difficult to achieve in the foreseeable future. Gregory *et al.* (1990) found that in a nationally representative survey of British adults only 12% of men and 15% of women met even this 35% target. Only 6% of men and 8% of women met the two targets of no more than 35% of energy from fat and 15% from saturated fat.

NACNE suggested that the intakes of polyunsaturates should be allowed to rise modestly to facilitate the large reduction in saturated fat intake that they proposed; from 4% of calories in 1980 to 5% at the end of the 1980s and ultimately to 6%; they did not advocate a wholesale switch from saturated to polyunsaturated fats. NRC (1989b) recommended that intakes of polyunsaturates be maintained at the then current level in the US (7% of average calorie intake) with an individual maximum of 10% of calories. NRC did suggest that some increase in omega-3 polyunsaturates from fish would be acceptable although they came out against the use of concentrated fish oil supplements. Both NRC and NACNE expressed concern about the long term safety of diets with very high levels of polyunsaturates. More recently in the UK, COMA (1991) have re-inforced this message by suggesting a population average of 6% of calories from polyunsaturates with an individual maximum of 10%.

Current intakes of polyunsaturates represent very close to 6% of total calories in the UK and the ratio of polyunsaturated to saturated fatty acids in the UK diet (the P:S ratio) has risen from 0.24 at the time of NACNE to currently over 0.4.

NRC suggested that cholesterol intake should be limited to 300 mg per day whereas NACNE and other UK committees have, in recent years, tended to avoid making any specific cholesterol recommendations; it should be noted that implementing the NACNE and NRC recommendations on saturated fat would inevitably lead to a substantial decline in cholesterol intakes because many sources of saturated fat are also rich in cholesterol.

Dietary sugar

NACNE (1983) recommended a very substantial reduction in the consumption of simple sugars, this was one of the most contentious aspects of the report. They estimated *per capita* sucrose consumption in 1983 at 38 kg per year (14% of calories) and recommended a reduction to 34 kg per year by the end of the 1980s with a long term target of 20 kg per year (7% of calories). NACNE further recommended that no more than half of this sucrose should come from between meal snacks and soft drinks and that there should be a corresponding reduction in intakes of other sugars. In the latest UK dietary reference values it is suggested that **non-milk extrinsic sugars** should make up, on average, 10% of total calories and this same figure has also been widely advocated in the US. (The category non-milk extrinsic sugars excludes milk sugar and simple sugars naturally present in fruits and vegetables but includes all added sugars and is not restricted to sucrose). Simple sugars make up well over 20% of dietary energy in the US and yet NRC (1989b) did not make specific recommendations to substantially cut sugar intakes although they did counsel against any further increase.

Complex carbohydrates

Both NRC and NACNE recommended that any calories removed from the diet by reduced intakes of fats and sugars should be replaced by starches. NRC suggest calories from carbohydrate should be increased to at least 55% of the total but without increasing sugar intakes. The long term goal of NACNE is also 55% of calories as carbohydrate but with the additional requirement that consumption of sugars should be all but halved to around 10% of total calories. NACNE specifically recommended substantial increases in fibre (non starch polysaccharide) consumption; a 25% increase during the 1980s with a further 25% increase in the long term (from an assumed base-line of 20 g per day in 1980). These changes would be brought about by increased consumption of potatoes and cereals and, as specifically recommended by both committees, increased consumption of fruits and vegetables (five servings per day advocated by NRC). NRC did not make specific fibre recommendations but the recommended increases in consumption of fruits, vegetables and cereals would lead to substantial increases in consumption of dietary fibre.

Precise measures of fibre intakes are difficult and confused by differences in methodology and definition. COMA (1991) estimated that intakes of non-starch polysaccharide in the UK were in the range 11–13 g per day and they set a desirable population average of 18 g per day; non-starch polysaccharide would exclude some of the substances traditionally encompassed by the term fibre, notably, the non-carbohydrate substance, lignin and resistant starch. This, together with differences in analytical methods, accounts for the apparent numerical discrepancy between these values and the assumed base-line figure of 20 g/day used by NACNE. It is estimated that on any given day, half of the US population consume less than 10 g of fibre and the American Dietetic Association has suggested an optimal intake in the range 20–35 g/day (see Hamilton *et al.*, 1991).

Alcohol

NACNE recommended that, on average, alcohol should decline from 6% of calories in 1980 to 5% and ultimately to 4%. They suggested that the aim should be to truncate the distribution of alcohol intake rather than advocating that everyone should drink less, i.e. to moderate the intakes of those considered to be drinking excessively. NRC (1989b) recommended Americans to limit individual consumption to around 25 g of alcohol per day (around 14 units per week). Current recommendations in both countries seem to have settled on a safe intake for men of around 21 units per week and 14 units per week for women. One unit of alcohol is a half pint of beer, a glass of wine or a small pub measure of spirits (25 ml). NRC specifically recommend that pregnant women should avoid alcohol.

According to Gregory *et al.* (1990) 21% of British women and 47% of men obtained 5% or more of their dietary energy from alcohol and 7% of women and 28% of men more than 10% of their energy from this source. In DHHS (1992) annual *per capita* alcohol intake in the US is estimated at 2.54 US gallons in persons over 14 years. This represents about 7.5% of total energy assuming an intake of 2500 kcal (10.5 MJ) per day. American Indian men and black men are singled out as two groups whose health is particularly badly affected by alcohol-related problems.

Salt

NRC (1989b) recommended that salt intake should be limited to 6 g per day. NACNE (1983) suggested that during the 1980s salt intake should be cut by 1 g per day with a longer term reduction of 3 g per day. The NACNE committee assumed a baseline intake of about 12 g per day but current estimates (e.g. James *et al.,* 1986) suggest that this may have been a significant overestimate and the true figure might be as low as 9 g per day. If this later estimate of UK intake is combined with the long term NACNE recommendation, then this produces the same target figure as the NRC. The World Health Organisation have suggested 5 g per day as a target average for population salt intakes.

Protein

Both committees considered current protein intakes to be satisfactory and recommended that they be maintained. NRC suggested an upper limit to protein intake of twice the RDA and NACNE suggested that within the overall unchanged protein intake, a greater proportion should be of vegetable origin.

Other nutrients

NACNE acknowledged the importance of meeting the dietary standard for calcium intake and they recognised the importance of milk in achieving this standard. They suggested that the wider availability of lower fat milk (especially milk delivered to the doorstep) would facilitate maintenance of calcium intakes despite the recommended cuts in fat intake. Lower fat milks have indeed become more available in the UK and account for a markedly increased proportion of total milk sales. Nonetheless *per capita* calcium intakes in the UK did fall by around 12% in the period 1979–1989 which can be accounted for by a 12% fall in total energy intake over that same period (Chesher, 1990).

NRC (1989b) were also concerned that calcium and iron intakes should be maintained despite cuts in saturated fat consumption. They felt these dual objectives could be achieved if low fat dairy products, fish, lean meat and poultry were substituted for fatty meats, full fat dairy products and other fried and fatty foods.

NRC specifically recommended an optimal intake of fluoride especially in children whose teeth are developing. NACNE also suggested that health educators should continue to encourage the use of fluoride.

Expected benefits from the implementation of these guidelines

Several of these recommended changes would be expected to contribute to a decline in average blood pressure of the population. They should therefore reduce the incidence of hypertension and ultimately produce a fall in morbidity and mortality from those diseases for which hypertension is a risk factor, i.e. coronary heart disease, strokes and renal disease. The salt recommendations have been largely included because of the assumed causal link between high salt intake and the incidence of hypertension. Being overweight, inactive or consuming a lot of alcohol have well-established tendencies to raise blood pressure; losing weight, increasing exercise and moderating alcohol intakes can lead to marked reductions in an individual's blood pressure. The increased consumption of fruits and vegetables would also tend to increase potassium intakes, and this may also have a protective effect.

Reductions in total fat consumption, and saturated fat in particular, are expected to lead to reduced levels of plasma cholesterol. Plasma cholesterol is an established risk factor for coronary heart disease and other diseases of the vascular system associated with atherosclerotic changes in arteries, e.g. occlusive strokes. These changes are expected to lead to substantial reductions in mortality from coronary heart disease and these aetiologically related conditions. Increased fruit and vegetable fibre may also contribute to reducing serum cholesterol concentration and higher intakes of anti-oxidant vitamins (carotene, C and E) may also contribute to preventing atherosclerotic damage to blood vessels.

The shift away from fats and sugars and their replacement with foods high in complex carbohydrates will inevitable produce a bulkier diet. In order to obtain a given number of calories, people will need to consume a considerably higher volume of food and this is expected to assist in maintenance of energy balance and thus in maintenance of an ideal body weight. In general, reducing the proportion of calories derived from sugars, fats and alcohol should tend to increase the nutrient density of the diet (amount of nutrients per calorie) and thus should assist in producing nutrient-rich diets. However, any reduction in overall consumption of dairy foods is likely to reduce calcium intakes, and reducing consumption of meat may reduce dietary iron and also reduce its availability.

It is expected that these changes will contribute to a reduced incidence of several cancers: reduced fat intake (bowel cancers?); increased fibre intake (bowel cancer?); moderation of alcohol intake (cancers of the mouth, throat, oesophagus, liver, bowel and perhaps other sites); decreased salt intake (gastric cancer?); increased consumption of fruit and vegetables and their associated antioxidant vitamins may have a general protective effect.

Substantial reduction in sugar intake (especially between-meal sugar) coupled with ensuring adequate intake of fluoride is expected to lead to major improvements in dental health.

The increases in fibre intake are expected to reduce the risk of constipation and a number of disorders of the bowel (e.g. haemorrhoids and diverticulosis) in addition to any benefits they may have in reducing risk of bowel cancer and in lowering serum cholesterol concentration.

The role of dietary calcium in the prevention of osteoporosis is still very controversial but inactivity is well-established as a risk factor and high alcohol consumption has also been linked to this disease.

The maturity-onset form of diabetes accounts for about three-quarters of the cases of this disease. The acute symptoms of this form of diabetes are unpleasant even if rarely life threatening. Apart from the acute symptoms, diabetes of both types is strongly associated with a range of disabling and fatal long term complications including: blindness due to retinopathy or cataract; coronary heart disease; renal disease; and, gangrene. Inactivity and obesity are strongly implicated in the aetiology of maturity-onset diabetes.

The social and health dangers of excessive alcohol consumption are well known and widely accepted. Liver disease, increased accident risk, hypertension and increased cancer risk are well-established effects of high alcohol consumption. What constitutes excessive intake is a more contentious issue. Many studies have reported higher mortality in complete abstainers as compared to those consuming moderate amounts of alcohol; high intakes are associated with sharply increasing mortality rates, the so-called J-curve of mortality. It has been argued, that this J-curve of mortality is an artefact due to the inclusion of reformed alcoholics in the abstainers group, but recent evidence supports the idea that the protective association between moderate alcohol consumption and, in particular, coronary heart disease remains even after correcting for this effect (e.g. Rimm *et al.*, 1991). Neither NACNE nor NRC went so far as to recommend alcohol consumption but a substantial body of evidence now suggests some benefits may be associated with moderate alcohol intakes. Even if moderate amounts of alcohol are beneficial, however, any attempt to actively promote alcohol on health grounds runs a very high risk of encouraging excessive consumption by existing and new drinkers; the difference between a beneficial and a damaging dose may be quite small, and alcohol is addictive and reduces self-restraint. At the time of writing it seems quite possible that during the lifetime of this edition there may be some relaxation in the alcohol guideline limits given earlier. Average intakes of up to 75% higher than those given earlier may cause few problems in most people provided that the consumption is spread relatively evenly throughout the week and provided that alcohol is avoided at times when its adverse effects on judgement and co-ordination may precipitate accidental injury, e.g. prior to driving a car or operating machinery.

A number of the putative health benefits of individual dietary changes are still controversial but most of them are mutually consistent and point towards the same general trend, i.e. moderately reducing intakes of fatty and sugary foods and replacing them with foods higher in complex carbohydrates and increasing consumption of fruits and vegetables. Thus for example increased consumption of fruits and vegetables will tend to:

- increase fibre intakes
- make the diet more bulky
- increase the proportion of calories derived from carbohydrate and thus reduce the proportion from fat
- increase intakes of carotene and other anti-oxidant vitamins
- and, increase potassium intakes.

A relatively high proportion of nutritionists might be sceptical about the putative health benefits of any one of these compositional changes. Despite this, almost all would probably support recommendations to increase consumption of fruits and vegetables – the cumulative evidence supporting this food change is overwhelming.

Table 4.1 shows how the "ideal diet" as suggested by the NACNE recommendations compares with the typical current British diet. The "ideal diet" would also be consistent with the recommendations of NRC (1989b) and the general consensus of US dietary recommendations.

Conclusions

Although many nutritionists would argue about specific diet/disease issues, few would disagree with the proposition that significant health benefits would be likely to accrue if Americans and Britons were leaner, more active, consumed alcohol moderately, ate less fat, sugar and salt but more fruit, vegetables and cereals.

Some of the targets given in the "ideal" diet (Table 4.1) do, however, look rather unrealistic. No matter how great the likely benefits, it is difficult to foresee that within a reasonable time-span the British population as a whole will meet the sugar, fat and perhaps the salt recommendations although they are clearly achievable by highly-motivated individuals who have a sound knowledge of food and nutrition. It seems particularly improbable that the fat

Table 4.1 Current estimates of the average UK adult diet composition compared with the "ideal" of NACNE (1983). Values are % of total energy unless otherwise stated. Data source: Gregory et al. (1990)

Nutrient	Current	Ideal
Fat	38	30
Saturated fat	16	10
Protein	14	11
Total carbohydrate	42	55
Sugars	18	10
Alcohol	6	4
Salt (g/day)	9	6
Fibre (g/day)*	20	30

*Precise numerical values for fibre depend upon definition and method of estimation; using current estimations of non starch polysaccharide, then current and ideal values of 12 and 18 g/day could be substituted.

and sugar recommendations of NACNE will be implemented concurrently by the bulk of the population. To implement both of these recommendations whilst keeping total calorie intake constant and using only acceptable amounts of alcohol would involve approximately doubling current starch intakes. McColl (1988) suggests that in a free-living affluent population there is an inverse relationship between sugar and fat consumption; people who get a low proportion of their calories from fat tend to get a high proportion from sugar and vice versa - the so-called **"sugar-fat seesaw"**. Survey data quoted by McColl suggests that people who consumed less than 35% of their calories as fat derived, on average, more than 25% of their calories from sugars.

This sugar-fat seesaw might, in practice, tend to make the sugar and fat recommendations of NACNE almost mutually exclusive. In the light of this discussion, the NRC recommendation to Americans merely not to increase sugar intakes could be interpreted as a logical and pragmatic decision to make fat reduction their nutrition education priority.

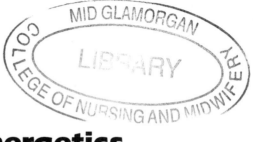

5 Cellular energetics

Contents

Aim

This very brief and greatly simplified outline of the energy conversions within the cell is not intended to be an introduction to the study of biochemistry. Only the minimum of factual biochemistry to allow illustration of the broad principles and concepts has been included. The purpose is to give the reader with no biochemical background enough perception of the biochemical processes of the cell so as to facilitate an understanding of nutrition. It is hoped that certain nutritionally important observations will be clarified by this discussion, such as:

- fat cannot be converted to glucose, but glucose is readily converted to fat
- the human brain cannot use fatty acids as substrates, but during starvation the brain obtains more than half of its energy from the metabolism of ketone bodies that are derived from fatty acids

- many vitamins are essential as precursors of the coenzymes that allow enzyme-mediated reactions to occur
- amino acids can serve as energy sources and can be used to generate glucose during fasting.

Introduction and overview

The catabolism (breakdown) of carbohydrates, fats and proteins within cells releases chemical energy. This energy is used to drive all of the energy requiring processes of the cell, e.g. synthetic processes, muscle contraction, transport of materials across cell membranes, nerve conduction. **Adenosine triphosphate, ATP** plays a pivotal role as a short term energy store within the cell. The chemical energy released during the catabolic metabolism of foodstuffs is "captured" as high energy ATP, and then the breakdown of ATP is used to drive the other energy requiring processes. Each cell produces its own ATP; it is not transported between cells.

Although they will not be listed or discussed in the following outline, it should be noted and borne in mind that every cellular reaction is catalysed (speeded up) by a specific **enzyme**. The reactions would not occur to any significant extent in the absence of the specific enzyme – it is the enzymes within the cell that determine what reactions can occur within the cell and thus determine the nature of the cell. Enzymes are proteins and the genetic code (contained within the DNA molecule) codes for the proteins of the cell. It is the proteins an organism produces that determines its characteristics. Genetic diseases are the result of an error in one of the proteins produced by that individual. Many enzymes require non-protein moieties known as **coenzymes** or cofactors in order to function. Several of these coenzymes are derivatives of vitamins, and it is their roles as precursors of coenzymes that accounts for the essentiality of several vitamins. Cofactors that are bound strongly to the enzyme and become an integral part of the enzyme structure are termed **prosthetic groups**.

Nature and functioning of ATP

Adenosine triphosphate is comprised of a purine base (adenine), a pentose sugar (ribose) and three phosphate groups. The hydrolysis of ATP to adenosine diphosphate (ADP), by removal of one of the phosphate groups, is a highly **exergonic reaction**, i.e. a considerable amount of chemical energy is released during the reaction. This energy would be released as heat if the ATP hydrolysis were conducted in a test tube. Similarly, the hydrolysis of ADP to adenosine monophosphate (AMP) is highly exergonic. Conversely, the conversions of AMP to ADP to ATP are highly **endergonic reactions**, they

absorb large amounts of energy; if these reactions were conducted in a test tube then one would expect to need to provide heat energy to make the thermodynamics of the reactions favourable.

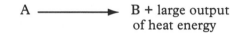

ATP: Adenine — Ribose — P — P — P
ADP: Adenine — Ribose — P — P
AMP: Adenine — Ribose — P
    P = phosphate

Within the cell, highly exergonic reactions in the catabolism of foodstuffs are coupled to ATP synthesis. The combined reaction remains slightly exergonic but much of the chemical energy of the exergonic, catabolic reaction is stored as ATP rather than being released into the cellular fluids as heat.

As an example take the hypothetical exergonic catabolic reaction:

A ⟶ B + large output of heat energy

in the cell:

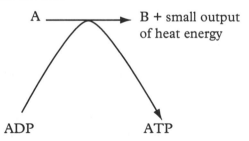

Other reactions within the cell are endergonic (energy consuming), and one would expect that if these reactions were being carried out in a test tube that one would have to provide heat to make them thermodynamically favourable and allow them to occur. Within the cell, however, such an endergonic reaction can be coupled to ATP hydrolysis to make the combined reaction exergonic and thus thermodynamically favourable at body temperature.

As an example take the hypothetical endergonic reaction:

$$X + \text{heat energy} \longrightarrow Y$$

in the cell:

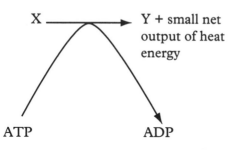

X ⟶ Y + small net output of heat energy

ATP   ADP

Substrate level phosphorylation

In catabolic pathways, some highly exergonic steps are directly linked to ATP formation (substrate level phosphorylation) as illustrated by the theoretical A → B reaction above e.g. in the glycolytic pathway one reaction involves the conversion of diphosphoglyceric acid to monophosphoglyceric acid, and this reaction is directly coupled to ATP synthesis:

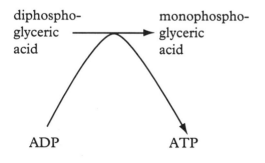

diphospho-glyceric acid ⟶ monophospho-glyceric acid

ADP   ATP

Oxidative phosphorylation

Much of the energy release in the catabolic pathways of metabolism occurs as a result of oxidation. Many oxidative steps involve the removal of hydrogen atoms from substrate molecules and their acceptance by hydrogen acceptor molecules such as **nicotinamide adenine dinucleotide (NAD)**.

As an example take the hypothetical oxidative reaction:

$$KH_2 + NAD \quad K + NADH_2$$

In this reaction, KH_2 has been oxidised to K and NAD has been reduced to $NADH_2$. As an example, in the Krebs cycle (discussed below) malic acid is oxidised to oxaloacetic acid by the removal of hydrogen and this reaction is coupled to the reduction of NAD by hydrogen addition:

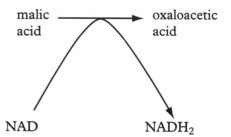

malic acid ⟶ oxaloacetic acid

NAD $NADH_2$

NAD is derived from the vitamin nicotinic acid or niacin; its role as a precursor of NAD and the phosphorylated derivative NADP explains the need for this vitamin. Re-oxidation of these reduced hydrogen acceptors in the **mitochondria** of cells results in the production of large quantities of ATP (three molecules of ATP per molecule of $NADH_2$ re-oxidised):

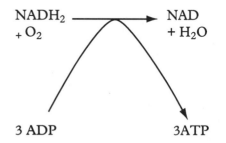

$NADH_2$ + O_2 ⟶ NAD + H_2O

3 ADP   3ATP

The details of this process of **oxidative phosphorylation** are beyond the scope of this text.

Oxidative phosphorylation normally yields the vast bulk of the energy released in catabolic metabolism – cells which do not have mitochondria (e.g. red blood cells) or which have insufficient oxygen supply (e.g. a muscle working beyond the capacity of the blood system to supply oxygen) have to rely upon the anaerobic metabolism of glucose to supply their energy needs. One molecule of glucose when metabolised anaerobically to lactic acid gives a net yield of only two molecules of ATP whereas when metabolised aerobically to carbon dioxide and water it yields 38 ATP molecules.

Metabolism of carbohydrate

Dietary carbohydrates are digested to their component monosaccharides before being absorbed. Digestion of starch yields glucose; digestion of disaccharides yields glucose plus other monosaccharides, fructose from sucrose (cane or beet sugar) and galactose from lactose (milk sugar).

The glycolytic sequence

This sequence is summarised in Figure 5.1, which is on the next page. The first three steps in this sequence involve activation of the glucose molecule by the addition of phosphate groups and a molecular rearrangement (**isomerisation**) of glucose phosphate to fructose phosphate. There is consumption of two ATP molecules during these activating steps. The fructose diphosphate thus produced is much more reactive (unstable) than glucose, and the six carbon (6C) molecule can be enzymically split into two, three carbon (3C) molecules. The other major dietary monosaccharides, fructose and galactose, also feed into the early stages of the glycolytic sequence as does glucose phosphate derived from the breakdown of body glycogen stores.

During the steps that convert glyceraldehyde phosphate into pyruvic acid, there is production of two molecules of reduced NAD and four molecules of ATP (giving a net yield of 2 ATP at the substrate level). Under aerobic conditions, the reduced NAD will be re-oxidised in the mitochondria using molecular oxygen and will yield a further six molecules of ATP – oxidative phosphorylation. Under anaerobic conditions then this reduced NAD must be re-oxidised by some other means, otherwise the very small quantities of oxidised NAD within the cell would be quickly exhausted and the whole process halted. In mammalian cells this NAD is regenerated under anaerobic conditions by the reduction of pyruvic acid to lactic acid:

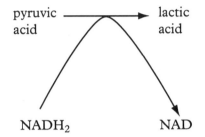

Lactic acid is the end product of anaerobic metabolism in mammalian cells, and anaerobic energy production is only possible from carbohydrate substrate. Red blood cells do not have mitochondria, and thus they metabolise glucose only as far as pyruvic acid or lactic acid. During heavy exercise, when the oxygen supply to a muscle may be limiting, muscles will generate some ATP anaerobically and produce lactic acid as a by-product – accumulation of lactic acid is one factor responsible for the fatigue of exercising muscles. Note also that in thiamin deficiency (beriberi) there is effectively a partial block in the metabolism of carbohydrate beyond pyruvic acid because the conversion of pyruvic acid to acetyl coenzyme A requires a coenzyme, thiamin

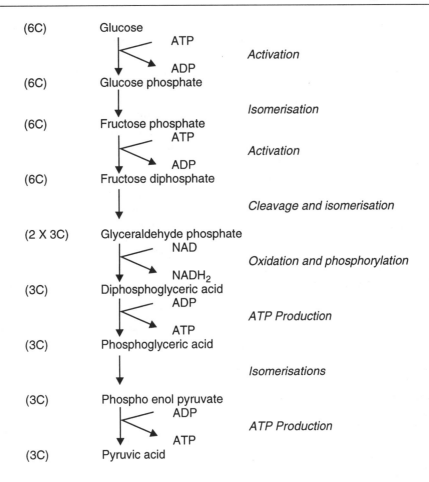

Figure 5.1 Outline of the glycolytic sequence (C) = Number of carbon atoms

pyrophosphate, that is derived from thiamin. Lactic acid and pyruvic acid therefore also accumulate in victims of beriberi because of this metabolic block.

The lactic acid produced by anaerobic metabolism is used for the re-synthesis of glucose in the liver (Cori cycle). This re-synthesis of glucose is effectively a reversal of glycolysis, and thus it is possible to synthesise glucose from any intermediate of the glycolytic sequence although the process does consume ATP.

Metabolism of pyruvic acid

Under aerobic conditions pyruvic acid will normally be converted to acetyl coenzyme A (activated acetate):

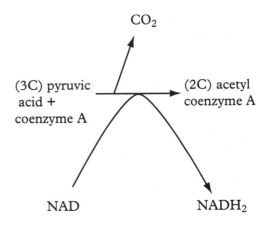

Coenzyme A is a large moiety that is derived from the B vitamin, pantothenic acid; addition of coenzyme A increases the reactivity of acetate and it is released in the next reaction and recycled.

This step cannot be reversed in mammalian cells, and thus glucose cannot be synthesised from acetyl coenzyme A.

The acetyl coenzyme A (2C) then enters a sequence known as the **Krebs cycle** (see Figure 5.2), it combines with oxaloacetic acid (4C) to give citric acid (6C). This citric acid then goes through a sequence of eight reactions which ultimately results, once again, in the production of oxaloacetic acid – hence this process is called a cycle. During two of the reactions, a molecule of carbon dioxide is produced, and in four of them a molecule of reduced coenzyme (e.g. $NADH_2$) is produced; in only one reaction is there direct substrate level ATP production. Each starting molecule of glucose yields two molecules of acetyl coenzyme A, and thus each molecule of glucose metabolised under aerobic conditions results in two "turns" of the Krebs cycle.

After undergoing all the reactions of the glycolytic sequence and Krebs cycle, all of the six carbon atoms of the original glucose molecule will thus have been evolved as carbon dioxide. When the reduced coenzyme is re-oxidised in the mitochondria this will result in the production of water. Thus overall, the glucose has been metabolised to carbon dioxide and water.

Figure 5.2 Outline of the Krebs cycle. Note that one reaction uses flavin adenine dinucleotide (FAD) rather than NAD. FAD is a derivative of the B vitamin, riboflavin. (C) = Number of carbon atoms

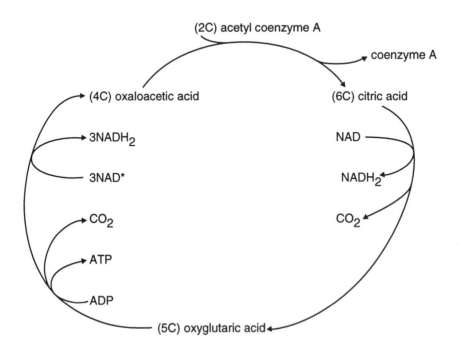

Metabolism of fats

Dietary fat, or the fat stored in adipose tissue, is largely triglyceride, and it yields for metabolism one molecule of glycerol and three fatty acid molecules. The 3C glycerol is converted to glyceraldehyde phosphate and enters the glycolytic sequence – it can thus be used directly as a source of energy or it can be used to generate glucose (by reversal of glycolysis). Fatty acids are metabolised to multiple units of acetyl coenzyme A, in a pathway known as the **beta-oxidation pathway**. A 16-carbon fatty acid (e.g. palmitic acid) would thus yield eight, 2C units of acetyl coenzyme A (summarised in Figure 5.3).

Note that, as the reconversion of acetyl coenzyme A back to pyruvic acid is not possible, fatty acids cannot be used to generate glucose. Brain cells, for example, do not have the enzymes necessary

for beta-oxidation and therefore they cannot directly use fatty acids as an energy source. Under conditions of good carbohydrate supply (i.e. regular eating of carbohydrate containing food) such cells use glucose as their substrate but they are not, as was previously thought, totally dependant upon carbohydrate as a substrate; during fasting, they can utilise certain ketones or **ketone bodies** that are made from acetyl coenzyme A. This means that during starvation the brain can indirectly utilise fatty acids that have been converted to these ketones in the liver (discussed more fully under metabolic adaptation to starvation in Chapter 6).

Fatty acids are synthesised by a process that is essentially a reversal of beta-oxidation, e.g. to synthesise 16C palmitic acid, eight units of 2C acetate (as acetyl coenzyme A) are progressively assembled. Thus fatty acids can be synthesised from carbohydrates via acetyl coenzyme A. Breakdown of fatty acids to acetyl coenzyme A is an oxidative process (hence

Figure 5.3 Outline of fat metabolism (C) = Number of carbon atoms

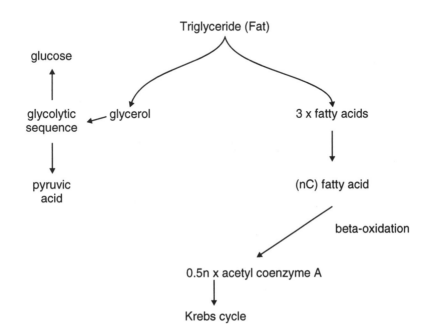

beta-oxidation), thus the synthesis of fatty acids from acetyl coenzyme A is a reductive process. The reduced form of the phosphorylated derivative of NAD, $NADPH_2$, is used as the source of reducing power in this pathway – $NADPH_2$ is generated in the **pentose phosphate pathway**.

Metabolism of protein

Protein digestion yields amino acids and surplus amino acids are used as an energy source. The nitrogen containing amino group is removed to leave a moiety, the keto acid, that can be converted to pyruvic acid, acetyl coenzyme A or one of the intermediates of the Krebs cycle. The amino group can be converted to the waste product urea or it can be transferred to another keto acid and thus produce another amino acid through a process called **transamination**.

It is possible to make glucose from protein. If the amino acid (e.g. alanine) yields pyruvic acid, then glucose synthesis merely involves the effective reversal of glycolysis. If the amino acid (e.g. glutamic acid) yields a Krebs cycle intermediate, then this intermediate will be converted to oxaloacetic acid which can then be converted to the phospho enol pyruvate of the glycolytic sequence:

Note that acetyl coenzyme A (and thus fatty acids) cannot be used to synthesise glucose via this route because the two atoms of the acetate that enter the Krebs cycle have been lost as carbon dioxide by the time oxaloacetic acid has been regenerated. Utilisation of existing Krebs cycle intermediates to synthesise glucose is theoretically possible, but they would be so rapidly depleted that their contribution to glucose supply would be insignificant. The metabolic routes for the metabolism of the different foodstuffs are summarised in Figure 5.4, which is on the next page.

During starvation or carbohydrate deprivation, the only routes available for the maintenance of carbohydrate supplies are by manufacture from amino acids or the glycerol component of fat. This process of generation of glucose from amino acids (**gluconeogenesis**) occurs in the liver, but it is energy expensive and will of course lead to depletion of the protein in muscle and vital organs. Note, however, that the need for gluconeogenesis is limited during starvation or carbohydrate deprivation by the use of ketone bodies as an alternative to carbohydrate substrate by, for example, nervous tissue.

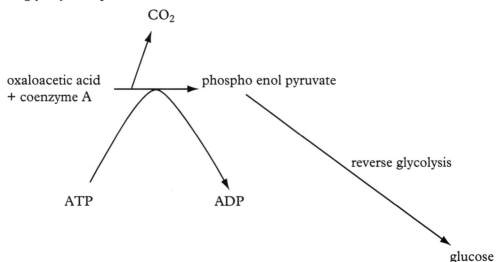

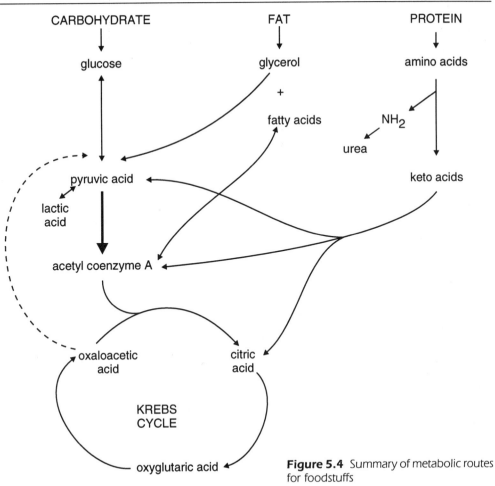

Figure 5.4 Summary of metabolic routes for foodstuffs

The pentose phosphate pathway

This pathway generates reducing power in the form of $NADPH_2$ (necessary, for example, in fatty acids biosynthesis) and also generates the pentose sugar, ribose phosphate, essential for nucleotide (e.g. ATP) biosynthesis and nucleic acid (RNA and DNA) synthesis. The first part of this pathway involves the conversion of glucose phosphate to ribose phosphate.

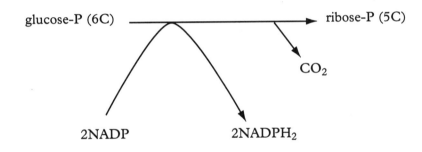

If the demand for $NADPH_2$ and ribose phosphate is balanced, then these two will represent end products of the pathway. If, however, the demand for $NADPH_2$, say for active lipid synthesis, exceeds the demand for ribose phosphate then the excess ribose is converted, by a complex series of reactions, to 3 carbon glyceraldehyde phosphate and 6 carbon fructose phosphate.

Overall reaction:

$$3 \times \text{ribose-P} (3 \times 5C) \longrightarrow$$

glyceraldehyde-P (3C) +
2 X fructose-P (2 X 6C)

The enzymes used in this series of reactions are called transketolase and transaldolase. Transketolase requires thiamin pyrophosphate, derived from the B vitamin thiamin, as a coenzyme. The glyceraldehyde phosphate and fructose phosphate can both enter the glycolytic sequence either to be metabolised to pyruvic acid or to be used to regenerate glucose phosphate.

If the demand for ribose phosphate exceeds that for $NADPH_2$ then the reverse of the transketolase/transaldolase reaction can generate ribose phosphate from glyceraldehyde phosphate and fructose phosphate.

Wernicke-Korsakoff syndrome is a neuropsychiatric disorder caused by lack of dietary thiamin (see Chapter 10 for details); it is usually associated with thiamin deficiency brought on by alcoholism in industrialised countries. Some people seem to have a genetic predisposition to this syndrome because their transketolase enzyme has a low affinity for thiamin pyrophosphate, making them extremely susceptible to the ill-effects of thiamin deficiency. The symptoms of this syndrome are probably due to inadequate $NADPH_2$ synthesis leading to impaired synthesis of **myelin**, the fatty sheath that surrounds many neurones.

PART II
THE NUTRIENTS

6 Energy

Contents

Although the range of nutrients required by living organisms varies enormously, all organisms require some exogenous supply of energy. Fats, carbohydrates, proteins and, in some cases, alcohol are the sources of that energy in human diets.

Units

The Standard International unit of energy is the **joule**, which is defined as the energy expended when a mass of 1 kg is moved through a distance of 1 metre by a force of 1 newton. For nutritionists the **kilojoule – kJ** (a thousand joules) and the **megajoule – MJ** (a million joules) are more practical units. Traditionally, nutritionists have used a unit of heat, the **kilocalorie – kcal,** as their unit of energy (although strictly a thousand calories, most people, when dealing with nutrition, tend to use the terms calorie and kilocalorie as if synonymous). A kcal is defined as the heat required to raise the temperature of a litre of water by 1°C. In practice, the kilocalorie is still widely used both by nutritionists and by non-scientists. The kcal is a convenient unit both because its definition can be understood by those with a limited knowledge of physics and because nutritionists may use heat output as their method of measuring both the energy yields of foods and the energy expenditure of animals and people.

To interconvert kilocalories and kilojoules:

$$1 \text{ kcal} = 4.2 \text{ kJ}$$

Energy requirements

Table 6.1 shows selected UK EARs for energy and their corresponding American equivalents (RDAs). Differences between the two sets of values will partly reflect different assumptions about standard activity levels.

Table 6.1 Selected current UK EARs for energy and corresponding American RDAs. All values are kcal (MJ) per day. Data sources: COMA (1991) and NRC (1989a)

Age (years)	UK EAR	American RDA
1–3 boys	1230 (5.15)	1300 (5.44)
1–3 girls	1165 (4.86)	1300 (5.44)
7–10 boys	1970 (8.24)	2000 (8.37)
7–10 girls	1740 (7.28)	2000 (8.37)
15–18 men	2755 (11.51)	3000 (12.56)
15–18 women	2110 (8.83)	2200 (9.21)
19–50 men	2550 (10.60)	2900 (12.14)
19–50 women	1940 (8.10)	2200 (9.21)
75+ men	2100 (8.77)	2300 (9.63)
75+ women	1810 (7.61)	1900 (7.96)

It must be borne in mind when using figures such as those in Table 6.1 that these are estimates of average requirements under average circumstances – lifestyle differences, particularly levels of physical activity, and genetic variability will mean that the variation in individual energy requirements can be very large. The relative energy requirement (per unit body weight) of growing children is higher than that of adults – a two-year-old child may be only around a fifth of the weight of an adult but that child requires more than half of the adult energy intake. In the case of older teenagers, the absolute energy requirement is even higher. This relatively high energy requirement of growing children partly reflects the energy requirements for growth but, particularly in small children, it is also partly a manifestation of the general inverse relationship between the relative metabolic rate and body size (see Chapter 3). Both UK and US dietary standards imply that there is a considerable reduction in energy needs in the elderly.

Sources of energy in the UK diet

Dietary recommendations and survey reports often quote carbohydrate, fat, protein and even alcohol intakes as a percentage of total energy or total calories. This method of presentation allows meaningful comparison of the diet composition of persons with widely differing energy intakes. Quoting absolute values for intakes of these major nutrients (e.g. grams per day) may be of limited usefulness and may even on occasion be misleading.

For example, absolute *per capita* intakes of fat in the UK have dropped very sharply over the last couple of decades, yet this reduction is entirely accounted for by a reduction in total food intake rather than reflecting any switch to a lower fat diet. In order to calculate macronutrient intakes as a percentage of total energy, the following energy equivalents are used to approximate the metabolisable energy yields of each of the major classes of energy-yielding nutrients:

- 1 g of fat yields 9 kcal (37 kJ)
- 1 g of protein 4 kcal (17 kJ)
- 1 g of carbohydrate 3.75 kcal (16 kJ)
- 1 g of alcohol 7 kcal (29 kJ).

Therefore, to calculate the proportion of energy derived from one of these nutrients, the following formula is used:

$$\frac{\text{g of nutrient consumed} \times \text{energy equivalent (as above)}}{\text{total energy intake}} \times 100$$

For example to calculate the proportion of energy from fat in a 2700 kcal diet containing 100 g of fat:

$$\frac{100 \times 9 \times 100}{2700} = \frac{900 \times 100}{2700} =$$

33.3% of energy as fat.

Figures for the contribution of the various energy-yielding nutrients to total energy intake depend to some extent upon the way in which they are determined and expressed. They may be expressed as proportions of household food energy as traditionally defined by the UK National Food Survey,, i.e. excluding food eaten outside the home, alcoholic drinks, soft drinks (soda) and confectionery (candy). Below are recent UK values determined in this way (MAFF, 1993):

fat	41.7%
protein	13.5%
carbohydrate	44.8%

When calculated in this way, the fat figure has remained remarkably constant over the last 20 years whereas carbohydrate has dropped from 46.3% in 1969 and protein has risen from 11.6% in 1969 (Chesher, 1990). In 1992, the National Food Survey included for the first time a record of purchases of alcoholic drinks, soft drinks and confectionery for home consumption. When these are included in the above figures, they tend to have a diluting effect upon fat in particular, e.g. the proportion of energy in household food and drink (from MAFF, 1993 as above):

fat	39.9
protein	12.9
carbohydrate	45.9

Despite the recent extension in its scope, the National Food Survey remains an incomplete measure because it only considers household food and drink and it also measures composition of food purchases rather than food consumption (see Chapter 3 for more complete discussion). Table 6.2 shows estimates of the contribution of the various energy-yielding nutrients to the total energy supplies of adults in the UK as measured directly, using a weighed inventory of the intakes of a nationally representative sample of British adults (Gregory *et al.*, 1990).

Table 6.2 Sources of energy in the diets of British adults expressed as percentages of total energy. Data source Gregory *et al.* (1990)

Nutrient (%)	Men	Women
Fat	37.6	39.4
Protein	13.7	15.2
Carbohydrate	41.6	43.1
Sugars	17.6	19.2
Alcohol	7.1	2.3
Total (kcal/day)	2450	1680
(MJ/day)	10.26	7.03

Energy density and nutrient density

The **energy density** of a food or diet is the metabolisable energy yield per unit weight of food (e.g. kcal/100 g food). The values of the energy equivalents of the various nutrients that are listed above, indicate that variations in the fat content of foods or diets are likely to have particularly large effects upon their energy density – this is discussed at length in Chapter 9. High water and fibre content of foods or diets will also tend to reduce their energy density; foods with high fibre content are also usually low in fat.

It is now widely believed that the low energy density of children's diets, especially weaning diets, may be a major precipitating factor for malnutrition. It has been suggested that weaning diets in some developing countries may have energy densities that are so low that, even under optimal conditions, children may have difficulty in consuming sufficient volume of food to satisfy their energy needs. Children fed these low energy diets may be in energy deficit, i.e. starved, despite apparently being fed enough to satisfy their demands. These low energy diets are based upon starchy staples, are often practically fat-free and have large amounts of water added to produce a consistency considered suitable for babies. Children fed such low energy density diets may need to consume up to eight times the weight of food that children on a typical Western weaning diet would need to obtain the same amount of energy.

It is widely believed that a reduction in the energy density of adult diets in affluent, industrialised countries will assist people in balancing their energy intake more closely with their expenditures, thus reducing the tendency to adiposity. The cross population changes in diet that tend to be associated with increasing affluence also tend to increase the energy density of the diet, i.e. the partial replacement of starchy, fibre-rich foods with foods rich in fats and sugars but low in fibre. These compositional changes produce diets that as well as being more energy dense are also higher in palatability. This combination of high palatability and high energy density may increase the likelihood of energy intake exceeding expenditure and thus may help to precipitate becoming overweight and obese. If gut-fill cues (e.g. stomach distension) play any role at all in the regulation of energy intake, then one would expect high energy density of the diet to reduce the effectiveness of food intake regulating mechanisms. This may be particularly so if, as in many industrialised countries, there is also low and declining energy expenditure due to inactivity.

Diets high in fat, and therefore of high energy density, have often been used to induce obesity in rodents. According to Miller (1979), high energy density, rather than fat content *per se* is the primary obesifying influence; varying the energy density and the proportion of fat independently (by using an inert bulking agent) produced a strong correlation between adiposity of the animals and dietary energy density but not between adiposity and dietary fat content.

Nutrient density is another widely used term – it is the amount of nutrient per unit of energy in the food or diet (e.g. mg nutrient/100 kcal food). In the diets of the affluent, nutrient density is often almost a mirror image of energy density; adding ingredients to foods or diets which contain much energy but few nutrients (e.g. fats, sugar and alcohol) raises the energy density but reduces the overall nutrient density. Diets and foods high in nutrient density ensure nutritional adequacy, those low in nutrient density increase the possibility that energy requirements may be met without also fulfilling the requirements for all of the essential nutrients.

Those consuming relatively small amounts of energy (e.g. those on reducing diets or elderly, immobile people) may need to take particular care to ensure that their diet is nutrient dense. It is possible to predict the likely adequacy of a combination of foods for any particular nutrient by multiplying the nutrient density of the mixture by the Estimated Average Requirement (or RDA) for energy:

Nutrient density × energy EAR =

amount of nutrient consumed by subjects meeting their energy needs

If this figure exceeds the RNI (RDA) for that nutrient, then that diet is probably adequate for that nutrient.

Similar calculations are also often made for individual foods in order to illustrate their value as a source of particular nutrients; this is illustrated by examples in Table 6.3, which is on the next page.

Clearly milk and potato crisps (chips) are relatively poor sources of vitamin C, especially if the milk has been stored for a

Table 6.3 The number of calories (kJ) of various foods that would need to be con obtain the UK adult RNI for vitamin C (40 mg)

Food	Amount	
	kcal	(k
Fresh whole milk	1700*	(7120)
Potato crisps (chips)	1250	(5230)
Avocado pear	600	(2510)
Boiled old potatoes	230–800†	(960–3350)
Banana	320	(1340)
Orange	28	(117)
Green pepper (capsicum)	6	(25)

* doubles within 24 hours of storage † depends upon length of storage
Compare with the UK energy EAR for an adult male of 2550 kcal/day (10.6 MJ/day)

few days whereupon its vitamin C content may be negligible. Oranges and peppers are clearly good sources of the vitamin and potatoes may be an important source because they regularly contribute a large amount of energy to many British diets.

Energy balance

The concept

The concept of balance between energy intake and energy expenditure is a useful and widely used one:

Energy in – energy out =
energy balance

The "energy in" is the sum of the metabolisable energy yields of all of the food and drink consumed, it will normally only be influenced by the nature and amount of food and drink consumed. The "energy out" can be directly measured by determining the heat output of the individual in a calorimeter or, as is more usual, by predicting the heat output from measurements of oxygen consumption and carbon dioxide evolution (see Chapter 3). This output figure will be influenced by a number of factors that raise heat output above the

resting level, i.e. factors that have a thermogenic (heat producing) effect:

1 *The thermogenic effect of exercise* – The sweating and increased skin temperature induced by exertion are clear manifestations of this thermogenesis.

2 *Thermoregulatory thermogenesis* – The increase in metabolic rate, and therefore heat output associated with shivering or non-shivering mechanisms used for heat generation in a cold environment.

3 *Drug-induced thermogenesis* – The increase in heat output brought about by certain drugs (e.g. caffeine) that have a stimulating effect upon metabolic rate.

4 *The thermic effect of feeding or diet-induced thermogenesis* – The increase in metabolic rate and heat output that follows feeding. This is at least partly attributed to energy expended in digesting, absorbing and assimilating the food, and this component is usually referred to as the thermic effect of feeding or postprandial thermogenesis. The term diet-induced thermogenesis is usually used to describe the longer term effects (e.g. the suggested adaptive increase in metabolic rate in response to overfeeding) although it can be used more generally to encompass the thermic effect of feeding.

a healthy adult whose weight is stable, then, over a period of time, the energy intake and output must be matched. There is a zero balance, i.e. the energy content of the body remains constant. There is quite wide variation in the energy intakes that different individuals require to maintain balance, even when subjects are apparently matched for age, sex, size and physical activity.

If energy intake exceeds output then that individual is said to be in **positive energy balance**. Under these circumstances, body energy content must be increasing, because, according to the first law of thermodynamics "energy cannot be created or destroyed only changed from one form to another", the surplus energy is changed from chemical energy of food to chemical energy of body tissues. Increase in body energy content means either increase in lean body mass (growth) or increase in body fat deposition or both. Children, pregnant women, and those regaining weight after a period of illness or starvation would all properly be expected to show a positive balance. For most of the rest of the population, positive balance is due to increasing adiposity which, if unchecked, will ultimately lead to overweight and obesity.

If energy output exceeds intake, then that individual is said to be in **negative energy balance** and the shortfall must be made up from body energy stores. Individuals in negative energy balance must be losing body energy and this will almost certainly be reflected in weight loss. It is just possible that body energy content can fall without weight loss if fat loss is compensated by increased lean tissue and water content as might happen in someone starting a training or body building programme. Loss of body energy may be due to loss of lean tissue (protein) or loss of fat or, as is most likely, both. Persons who are starving or successfully dieting will be in negative energy balance, as will, for example many sick or seriously injured people, those losing large amounts of

nutrients, e.g. uncontrolled diabetics, and those whose expenditure is particularly high such as people with hyperactive thyroid glands or those undertaking intense physical activity for prolonged periods.

Regulation of energy balance

Regulation of energy balance could be achieved in one of three ways:

1 by regulating energy intake so that it matches expenditure
2 by regulating energy expenditure so that it matches intake
3 by a combination of these two.

The sensations of hunger and satiation are universally experienced manifestations of some energy intake regulating mechanism. Traditionally, therefore, studies on the regulation of energy balance have focused upon the mechanisms regulating food intake.

Regulation of energy intake

Studies that began during the 1940s showed that permanent obesity could be induced in rodents and a variety of other mammalian species by destroying small, discrete areas on each side of the brain, i.e. bilateral lesions in the ventromedial region of the hypothalamus. This surgically produced obesity has traditionally been attributed to overeating, although some reports have suggested that reduced energy expenditure is an important factor contributing to obesity. Conversely, lesions in the lateral region of the hypothalamus completely abolish feeding and drinking behaviour in animals.

These observations of the effects of hypothalamic lesions resulted in the widespread acceptance of a relatively simple and probably simplistic theory of food intake regulation known as the **dual-centre hypothesis** (Mayer, 1956); this hypothesis is summarised diagrammatically in Figure 6.1. A spontaneously active **feeding centre** is envisaged as being

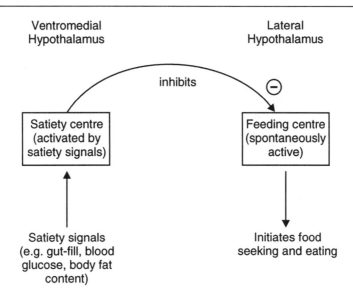

Ventromedial
Hypothalamus

Lateral
Hypothalamus

inhibits

Satiety centre
(activated by
satiety signals)

Feeding centre
(spontaneously
active)

Satiety signals
(e.g. gut-fill, blood
glucose, body fat
content)

Initiates food
seeking and eating

Figure 6.1 A diagrammatic representation of the dual-centre hypothesis of food intake regulation and the regulation of total energy balance

located in the lateral region of the hypothalamus. This feeding centre initiates food seeking and eating behaviour, and thus its destruction, by lateral hypothalamic lesions, results in a cessation of eating behaviour. This feeding centre is periodically inhibited by a **satiety centre** located in the ventromedial region of the hypothalamus. This satiety centre becomes active in response to certain **satiety signals** which strengthen after feeding and produce satiation. As time after feeding elapses one would envisage these satiety signals dying away; the satiety centre becomes quiescent, allowing the feeding centre to become active again and producing hunger. Destruction of this satiety centre, by ventromedial hypothalamic lesions, would reduce satiety and result in excessive food consumption and eventually obesity. Direct electrical stimulation of the lateral region of the hypothalamus evokes feeding behaviour in experimental animals and stimulation of the ventromedial region inhibits feeding. The hypothalamus is thus envisaged as acting like a meter or **"appestat"** that adjusts the feeding drive in response to a variety of physiological signals that reflect the short and long term energy status of the body – energy intake

is thus matched to output and energy balance is maintained.

This dual-centre hypothesis has had an enormous influence on thinking about energy balance regulation and obesity over the years. In the 1960s and 1970s several nutrition and physiology texts devoted whole chapters to hypothalamic regulation of feeding (e.g. Davidson and Passmore, 1963; Wohl and Goodhart, 1968; Bogert *et al.*, 1973). It was widely thought that human obesity might be due to some physiological defect in this regulatory system. References to the early experimental work on these hypothalamic mechanisms regulating food intake have been excluded, but interested readers will find detailed and well-referenced accounts of this work in editions of many texts published during the 1960s and 1970s or by reference to Mayer (1968), Mayer (1956) or Brobeck (1974), two of the most prolific and influential researchers in this field.

Human obesity due to hypothalamic injury had been suggested long before these experiments with hypothalamically-lesioned rodents (Gilbert, 1986), and experimental lesions produce obesity syndromes in a variety of species from mice to monkeys. Therefore, it is reasonable to expect that, whatever the mechanism, similar lesions in people would also produce similar syndromes of obesity. Elucidation of the roles of these regions of the hypothalamus in experimental animals will almost certainly provide useful indicators of their roles in man. Little, if any, evidence exists for the converse argument, that significant numbers of obese people are obese because they have visible hypothalamic lesions. Realistically, some defect, acquired or inherited, in nerve transmitter synthesis or receptor affinity that predisposes to obesity is more likely than morphological lesions.

Several factors have tended to undermine the view of energy balance being regulated solely by hypothalamic regulation of food intake involving a mechanism such as that shown in Figure 6.1. For example:

1 Ventromedial hypothalamic lesions in weaning rats (21 days old) produces obesity (i.e. increased fatness) but without either excessive weight gain or overeating – it results in short, fat rats.
2 It has been suggested that the concept of discrete satiety and feeding centres within the hypothalamus is a myth – ventromedial lesions have been said to interrupt neuronal pathways that happen to pass through this region rather than destroying a discrete satiety centre (Gold, 1973). It has been suggested that subtly different obesity syndromes can result from slightly different lesions in the region of the ventromedial hypothalamus (Peters *et al.*, 1979).

A detailed discussion of the anatomical locations and interconnections of the hypothalamic and other neural centres controlling energy balance is beyond the scope of this book, but the original dual centre theory is almost certainly an over-simplification of reality. Nonetheless this discussion of the dual centre hypothesis may still be conceptually useful for readers of this book. Any mechanism regulating energy intake must involve the key elements of this scheme, namely:

● a system for sensing parameters that reflect body energy status (satiety signals and sensors)
● integration of these satiety inputs within the brain (centres regulating the feeding drive)
● a response – a feeding drive that is modulated so that it is appropriate to the level of the satiety inputs.

Various satiety signals have been proposed and investigated over the years, e.g.: signals emanating from the alimentary tract and triggered by gut distension or chemical components of food; blood substrate levels, e.g. blood glucose – the **glucostat theory**; signals emanating from adipose tissue and indicating total body fat stores – the **lipostat theory**.

1 *Gut-fill cues* – We all experience the feeling of stomach fullness that occurs after a meal and the feelings of stomach emptiness and hunger contractions that occur after fasting. Feeding normally finishes before there have been detectable changes in blood substrate levels. These observations would suggest that signals from the alimentary tract play some part in signalling satiation, mediated either through sensory nerves in the gut directly affecting the hypothalamic centres or perhaps through the effect of hormones released from the gut by the presence of food.

Despite the temptation to assume that such a mechanism must have some influence, at least over short term appetite regulation, there is ample evidence that rats fed diluted diets are able to maintain their body weights by a compensatory increase in their volume of food intake. Even rats trained to receive all of their nourishment intravenously in response to their pressing a lever still regulate their body weight. These experiments do not show that alimentary signals do not usually play some role in regulating food intake. They merely demonstrate that they are not the sole factor regulating intake and that animals can adapt to energy dilution or even to the absence of alimentary signals.

The observations, noted earlier, that feeding diets of high energy density causes obesity in rats suggests that over concentration of the diet may reduce the effectiveness of the food intake control mechanisms. The current widespread belief that reducing the energy density of human diets will help in the treatment and prevention of obesity seems to be an implicit acceptance of there being some modulating effect of dietary bulk upon appetite. One could, for example, envisage alimentary signals playing an important role in signalling satiety at the end of a meal but being overridden or dampened by other physiological signals indicating the need for energy intake. Given the prevailing conditions for most people throughout history, then the evolutionary priority would be for a system that prevents undernutrition rather than overnutrition. One might therefore expect compensation for overdilution of the diet to be more efficient than for overconcentration of the diet. Human energy intake regulating mechanisms do indeed appear to be much more effective in preventing inadequate consumption than they are in preventing excess consumption.

2 *The glucostat theory* – This envisages glucose receptors or sensors in the hypothalamus (and probably elsewhere) that respond to blood glucose concentration – producing satiety when blood glucose concentration is high and hunger when blood glucose concentration is low. The occurrence of both high

blood glucose and hunger in uncontrolled diabetes was explained by suggesting that the glucoreceptor cells in the ventromedial hypothalamus needed insulin for glucose entry in the same way as say muscle cells do. In the absence of insulin (i.e. in diabetes), despite a high blood glucose concentration, the glucoreceptor cells are deprived of glucose resulting in hunger.

This theory was given a decisive boost in the 1950s by work that showed that a glucose derivative, **gold thioglucose**, produced both obesity and lesions in the ventromedial region of the hypothalamus of mice. No other gold thio compounds produced this effect, the glucose moiety appeared to be essential, thus providing strong support for the presence of glucoreceptors in this region that would bind the gold thioglucose and thus lead to accumulation of neurotoxic concentrations of gold in their vicinity (reviewed by Debons *et al.,* 1977). In the 1950s and 1960s, the brain was regarded as being exclusively dependent upon a supply of glucose in the blood, and thus hypothalamic glucoreceptors sensitive to fluctuating blood glucose seemed a logical homeostatic device. The brain is now known to be capable of using alternative substrates (see metabolic adaptation to starvation).

Although there is much evidence of the effects of blood glucose concentration on appetite in the short term, it is difficult to envisage such a regulatory mechanism being able to maintain long term energy balance and stable body weight.

3 *The lipostat theory* – This theory has been used to explain how body energy stores (i.e. fat) might be regulated in the long term by regulation of apparently short term phenomena like hunger and satiety. It is suggested that either a) some appetite regulating chemical

factor might partition between blood and fat so that its concentration in blood would reflect total amount of stored fat or b) that some regulatory factor might be released from adipose tissue and again its concentration in blood would reflect the total amount of stored fat. Such mechanisms would allow the total amount of body fat to have a modulating effect upon appetite control. On any given day, there may be great disparity between energy intake and output but over a period of weeks there is usually good regulation of energy balance.

In a recent report, Zhang *et al.*, (1994) describe the cloning of the mouse "obese (ob)" gene and its human equivalent. It is a mutation in this "obese" gene that is responsible for the extreme syndrome of inherited obesity seen in the "obese-hyperglycaemic" or "ob/ob" mouse described later in this chapter. They report that the product of this gene is a small protein that is produced specifically in fat cells and they speculate that this might be the putative satiety factor envisaged as being produced by adipose tissue in the lipostat theory. Rink (1994) gives a concise, referenced review of the evolution of the lipostat theory and the possible implications of the findings of Zhang *et al.*

Regulation of energy expenditure

In marked contrast to the universal acceptance of food intake regulation, the regulation of energy expenditure as a mechanism for the homeostatic regulation of energy balance is a controversial topic. There is no doubt that overfeeding of animals or human volunteers results in increased energy expenditure that will help to restore balance or at least help to reduce the imbalance. It is equally clear that starvation or caloric restriction results in reduced energy expenditure which will reduce or prevent the negative energy balance – people on reducing diets are usually all too aware that despite a considerable reduction in their usual energy intake they may not continue to lose weight. The point of controversy is whether any component of these changes in energy expenditure represent an adaptive regulatory response to the over or underfeeding.

Overfeeding inevitably results in increased energy expenditure because of:

- increased energy costs of digesting, absorbing and assimilating the extra food; this would include, for example, the energy costs of secreting digestive juices and chewing
- the energy costs of storing any surplus energy, e.g. the energy costs of fat synthesis
- if body weight increases, then increased energy costs of maintaining and moving a bigger body.

Underfeeding or starvation inevitably results in reduced energy expenditure because:

1 less energy is required to digest, absorb and assimilate food
2 as the body wastes, so the energy costs of maintenance and movement are reduced
3 most starving people markedly reduce their voluntary activity
4 if there were any reduction in the set point for body temperature, this would result in reduced energy expenditure. Hypothermia is often present in children with Protein Energy Malnutrition and in the malnourished infections often do not cause fever.

In 1902 the German scientist Neumann coined the term **luxoskonsumption** to describe an adaptive increase in energy expenditure in response to overfeeding. The term **diet induced thermogenesis (DIT)** is usually used today. This latter term describes the increase in metabolic rate and therefore heat output, that occurs after feeding. It can encompass the inevitable increases required to digest, absorb and assimilate the food, but it is usually used to imply some additional and adaptive homeostatic element, i.e. luxoskonsumption. Essentially, it is envisaged that some energy-wasting metabolic process is activated when people overeat and that this "burns off" the surplus calories in order to restore energy balance or, at least, to reduce the imbalance.

Experiments in rodents have produced very convincing evidence for the existence of adaptive DIT. Rothwell and Stock (1979) have even proposed a credible mechanism for this DIT in small mammals. Overfeeding is said to result in increased sympathetic nerve stimulation of a tissue known as **brown adipose tissue** that is the major site thermoregulatory heat production (non-shivering thermogenesis) in small mammals. The sympathetic stimulation of brown adipose tissue results in uncoupling of oxidative phosphorylation in the tissue, i.e. oxidation accelerates but does not result in ATP production. The chemical energy released during oxidation is released as heat which warms the body during cold exposure. Such a mechanism seems to be well-established for thermoregulatory thermogenesis in small mammals (and human babies) and it is suggested that essentially the same response occurs during overfeeding. The heat generated under these circumstances is dissipated from the relatively large surface of the small animal. One would expect the sympathetic control of brown adipose tissue, whether for thermoregulation or for regulation of energy balance, to be mediated through the hypothalamus. Perkins *et al.* (1981) have reported that stimulation of the ventromedial hypothalamus in rats increases the thermogenesis in brown adipose tissue, indicating perhaps, that this region may be involved in regulation of both energy intake and energy expenditure and thus perhaps offering an explanation for the claims of reduced energy expenditure in ventromedially lesioned animals.

It would be unwise to be too ready to extrapolate these findings in laboratory rats to people without considerable direct support from human studies. Adult human beings have very limited capacity for non-shivering thermogenesis, and brown adipose tissue has traditionally been regarded as vestigial in adult man; heat conservation supplemented by shivering are the predominant physiological strategies used by people, and other large animals, to maintain homeothermy in the cold. A large animal with a relatively small surface area to volume ratio is less able to dissipate large amounts of surplus heat generation, this might also make DIT a less advantageous strategy for maintenance of energy balance in people. See Webb (1990) and (1992b) for critical discussion of the applicability of these studies on small animal models of obesity to people.

Several groups of researchers have reported evidence for diet induced thermogenesis in overfed student volunteers or prisoners. Several other groups have failed to find evidence for DIT in people. Stock (1992) and Hervey and Tobin (1983) present the cases for and against DIT respectively. The major reasons for this controversy remaining unresolved are:

- the lack of precision in the measurement of energy expenditure and energy intake in human subjects; and,
- the difficulty of making precise estimates of the amounts that should be allowed for the previously discussed inevitable increases in expenditure that accompany overfeeding.

Subtle imbalances between expenditure and intake that are maintained over long periods of time will be enough to produce enormous variations in body energy stores and yet only relatively crude methods are available to measure intake and expenditure in free living subjects. Some experiments have used captive subjects (e.g. prisoners or hospital patients) but even in these experiments there have been questions raised about whether underfed subjects have received extra smuggled food supplies and whether overfed subjects have somehow deceived the experimenters and disposed of some of the extra food.

Let us consider the deceptively simple question "do obese people eat more than lean?". In the past, it would have been largely assumed that the obese ate more and that this, together with inactivity, would have been assumed to be the cause of their obesity. Measurements of intakes of lean and obese subjects by different investigators have produced variable answers to the question – some have suggested that the obese eat more, some that they eat less and some have found no differences between the two groups. In Chapter 3 it was argued that, for example, average salt intake or saturated fat intake could be important determinants of average population blood pressure and serum cholesterol respectively despite the absence of any significant correlation between the two associated variables within individuals of any given population. Perhaps energy intake and adiposity are another example of this phenomenon. Average population energy intake could be a major factor in determining the average level of population adiposity even if it were not the major determinant of the differences in adiposity between individuals within any population; large variations in population and individual activity levels would be a major complicating factor in this case.

Some of the possible reasons why it might be difficult to find a significant difference in the food intakes of lean and obese subjects are listed next:

1 A small but sustained positive energy balance may lead to obesity, but measures of intake are imprecise and difficult to validate – some subjects may consciously or unconsciously deceive researchers.

2 Large inherent variability exists in the maintenance requirements of even apparently matched people.

3 Activity is variable and markedly affects energy expenditure and requirements – it is extremely difficult to quantify.

4 Groups of lean subjects may contain active weight gainers, whereas some obese people may be stable in weight or even losing weight.

5 Some subjects may be dieting.

6 Bingeing may occur, food intake including or excluding the binges may be quite different. Subjects usually feel guilt about bingeing and may not admit to it if asked to recall food intake, or they may avoid it if asked to record intake prospectively.

7 Obese people and lean people are often treated as single groups and yet there are likely to be a variety of causes for obesity. If some people are obese because they eat more but some because they expend less energy, then the average intakes of lean and obese may not be different.

If an adaptive mechanism like DIT does occur, then one would expect that, under conditions of plentiful food supply, people would tend to consume more than their absolute minimum needs and they would maintain energy balance by burning off the excess. For example, if both intake and expenditure are regulated, then, by analogy with other physiological control systems, one would expect both to be contributing to maintenance of balance under these "normal" conditions. When food intake is restricted, then one would expect to see this DIT "switched off" and thus see an apparent adaptive increase in metabolic efficiency and reduction in energy expenditure.

Starvation

For most of the world population, starvation results from the lack of physical or economic availability of food. There is also the suggestion that some children may be unwittingly starved because they are fed foods of such low energy density that, under the prevailing conditions, they are unable to consume sufficient volume of the diluted food to meet their energy needs. Inadequate food intake usually results in hunger and, if food is available, in eating. In some circumstances, hunger may not occur or may be suppressed, and in some circumstances nourishment will not reach the tissues despite hunger and eating. In affluent countries, these other causes of negative energy balance may predominate, for example:

1 illness, injury or therapy may result in loss of appetite
2 illness may result in hypermetabolism or loss of nutrients, e.g. the "metabolic response to injury" or the glucose and ketones lost in the urine of diabetics (see Chapter 13)
3 psychological state or psychological illness may result in inadequate food intake, e.g. Anorexia Nervosa
4 some diseases may result in poor absorption of nutrients e.g. coeliac disease and cystic fibrosis (see Chapter 13).

The most obvious physiological response to energy deficit is wasting because any deficit of intake in meeting expenditure must be made up from body energy reserves. All tissues, with the exception of the brain, will waste during starvation – the most obvious wasting will be in body fat and muscle but other vital organs will also waste. After prolonged starvation, the heart may be only half its original weight, and this wasting of heart muscle can lead to death from circulatory failure. The intestines of starving people will atrophy – they become thin and have greatly reduced digestive and absorptive capacity – this may cause considerable problems in re-feeding people after prolonged starvation.

A healthy and well nourished non-obese man could expect to be able to lose around 25% of his initial body weight before his life is threatened. During such weight loss, the man would lose around 70% of his stored fat and around 25% of his body protein (Passmore and Eastwood, 1986). Total carbohydrate content of the body is small (say 500 g) even in well fed people, and so the small loss of carbohydrate during this prolonged period of weight loss would make an insignificant contribution to total losses of body energy. The energy yield of this 25% loss of body weight represents around 7 weeks' energy expenditure in a totally starved and sedentary man. Thus well nourished adults can survive several weeks of total starvation; this was strikingly illustrated by the IRA hunger strikers in the Maze prison in Northern Ireland during the 1980s. It took around two months of total starvation for these healthy young men to reach the point of death. This capacity of people to survive long periods of food shortage, or even complete starvation, clearly represents a very considerable aid to the survival of the species. If food runs short prior to harvest, then there is a good chance that many people will survive until that harvest is ready. Children are more vulnerable to starvation than adults; survival times of completely starved babies or children may be measured in days rather than weeks, depending upon age. Permanent stunting of children may result from prolonged periods of undernutrition; some permanent impairment of brain growth and intellectual development may occur and chronic undernutrition may increase the later risk of cirrhosis and other liver disorders.

Metabolic adaptation to starvation

Many cells of the body can utilise either glucose or fatty acids as an energy source. During fasting, because there is little stored carbohydrate in the body, these tissues will be switched to using fatty acids to produce their energy needs. The cells of some tissues, including the brain, lack the enzymes necessary for the oxidation of fatty acids and thus cannot be switched to the direct use of fatty acids as an alternative energy source. The glycerol released from stored fat can be used to make some glucose; amino acids released from muscle and other body protein can be converted to glucose in the liver (see gluconeogenesis in Chapter 5). This process of gluconeogenesis is energy expensive (i.e. wasteful), and supplies of amino acids are limited because they are being taken from lean tissue and essential organs. A maximum of around 5 kg of protein is available for gluconeogenesis in an adult man.

It was once thought that the brain relied exclusively upon glucose as its substrate for energy production. This would mean that, as there are no stores of carbohydrate in the brain, that it would rely entirely upon glucose produced from gluconeogenesis during prolonged fasting. The brain normally uses the equivalent of around 120 g of glucose per day, and unless some adaptation occurred, this would lead to rapid depletion of body protein reserves and the size of these protein reserves would limit the duration of survival during fasting. Starving people would be likely to die from depletion of body protein reserves before body fat stores were exhausted. If one monitors nitrogen excretion (i.e. protein breakdown) during fasting, then one finds that it declines during the first few days of fasting and eventually plateaus at a level some way below the initial rate of loss – some adaptation to starvation has occurred. Also, during the first days of

fasting the blood levels of substances called **ketone bodies** rise and it is now clear that these can act as alternative substrates for the brain during prolonged fasting. These ketones are synthesised in the liver from acetyl CoA that is produced during the oxidation of fatty acids (see Chapter 5):

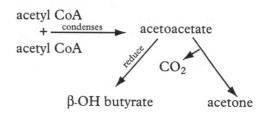

After prolonged fasting, more than half of the brains energy supply will be from b-OH butyrate – thus the brain is indirectly using fatty acids as an energy source and this represents a substantial brake upon the depletion of lean tissue during starvation.

For many years, these ketones were thought of as abnormal metabolic products produced during uncontrolled diabetes. In severe juvenile-onset diabetes, they are produced to excess and their concentrations build up to the point where they become highly toxic. They are toxic principally because they are acidic and produce a metabolic acidosis. These ketones are responsible for the "pear drops" smell on the breath of persons in a diabetic coma. Persons on very low calorie diets (VLCD) may also experience mild ketosis. VLCDs are commercial preparations that contain very low levels of calories but adequate amounts of the other nutrients. Their use amounts to virtual starvation, and although they may result in rapid short term weight loss, this weight loss will be of both lean and fat tissue.

Some other effects of starvation

There are derangements of endocrine function associated with starvation. Pituitary gonadotrophin secretion is greatly depressed in starvation and this manifests itself outwardly in a cessation of menstruation in starving women. Puberty is delayed by malnutrition.

Infection is often associated with starvation, and the concept of a cycle of infection and malnutrition is one that is frequently referred to. Malnutrition predisposes to infection and infection increases the severity of malnutrition or may precipitate malnutrition in areas where there is not overt food shortage. Sick children (or adults) may have reduced appetite and increased requirement for nutrients, they may be starved or fed a very restricted diet in the belief that this is the correct way to treat sick children. Malnutrition has very profound, specific and deleterious effects upon the functioning of the immune system; these are discussed at some length in Chapter 13. Cohort studies in malnourished children in which nutritional status has been related to subsequent death rate show that the risk of dying increases exponentially as one moves from the better nourished to the mildly, moderately and severely malnourished (Waterlow, 1979).

There may also be very pronounced psychological effects and personality changes produced by starvation. During the 1940s, in Minnesota a group of young male volunteers were subjected to a period of partial starvation that resulted in a 25% body weight loss (Keys *et al.*, 1950 see Gilbert, 1986 for summary). The feeding behaviour of these men changed markedly during their period of deprivation, including a dramatic decline in their speed of eating. They became preoccupied with food, it dominated their conversations, thoughts and reading. Personality tests conducted during the period of starvation showed a considerable movement towards the neurotic end of the scale as starvation occurred. Towards the end of the period of weight loss, the results from personality tests with these starved men became comparable with those of people with frank psychiatric disease. These men became introverted, selfish and made irrational purchases of unwanted items.

Eating disorders

Anorexia nervosa is the best known of the eating disorders. The condition was first described more than a century ago, but there is general agreement that the disease has become more prevalent in recent decades. It is characterised by an obsessive desire to be thin and an intense fear of being fat even though the victim may be severely emaciated. It seems probable that the disease is precipitated by social pressures upon young people to be thin, pressures that may be particularly acutely felt by young women. The average woman (and man) in many industrialised countries is getting fatter as judged by surveys of weight and height, but images of the ideal woman are apparently getting thinner. Many of the models used in classical painting of the female form would be overweight by present standards and studies on American winners of beauty contests and models for men's magazines indicated that the "ideal" body shape got thinner over the period 1959–1978. Anorexia seems to occur more often in girls and women for whom thinness is a career requirement, e.g. models, ballet dancers and airline stewardesses.

Sufferers from anorexia are usually females between the ages of 15–25 years. They are often from upper and middle class families and have good education and knowledge of nutrition. They are usually white. There are cases in males, older women and other racial groups, and it is suggested that the disease is radiating out from its traditional risk group. The disease has significant mortality and many sufferers appear to make only a partial recovery; they continue to eat very restricted diets and to maintain very low body weights. The disease requires specialist management, the non-specialist's role can only be to be able to recognise likely sufferers, appreciate that this is a "real" and potentially life-threatening illness and to direct them towards specialist help.

The diagnostic characteristics of the disease:

- low body weight – at least 15% below expected minimum
- intense fear of becoming fat even though underweight
- distorted body image – seeing themselves as fat even though alarmingly emaciated to the outside observer
- lack of menstrual periods
- frequently, use of purgatives, induced vomiting or emetics
- often intense physical activity, in marked contrast to other victims of starvation.

Victims of the disease may also go to great lengths to hide their restricted food intake and their physical emaciation from relatives and friends – they may wear loose clothing, avoid social eating situations, eat very slowly, choose only foods very low in calories, conceal food that they have pretended to eat and then dispose of it, or induce vomiting after they have eaten.

Bulimia is a related condition characterised by recurrent bouts of binge eating. Periods of restricted eating are interspersed with sometimes huge binges where massive quantities and bizarre mixtures of foods may be consumed in very short periods of time - the voracious eating may continue until abdominal pain, sleep or interruption trigger its end. Often the binge is followed by self-induced vomiting. People whose body weight is within normal limits may exhibit periods of bulimic behaviour. The morbid fear of fatness and distortion of body image seen in anorexia are also seen in this condition. Some surveys amongst college students and amongst more random samples of women in the UK and USA have suggested disturbingly high proportions of subjects exhibiting bulimic behaviour –

Gilbert (1986) concludes "that at any one time up to 2% of women up to the age of 40 may be experiencing problems with controlling their eating".

Over the years, many suggestions have been made as to the individual causes of anorexia nervosa and related eating disorders – social conditions may favour increasing prevalence of the disease, but what individual factors make some women develop the disease?

The effects of starvation on the men in the experiment of Keys and his colleagues, that were discussed earlier may be of relevance in understanding the development of anorexic behaviour (see Gilbert, 1986). The slowness of eating seen in these starving men is typical of anorexics. The men's unsociability, their obsessive interest in food and their curtailment of other activities are all recognised as traditional symptoms of anorexia nervosa. These men also developed personality profiles that were characteristic of people with frank psychiatric disease as they starved. During the period of re-feeding and rehabilitation of these men many of them showed a marked tendency to binge eat, behaviour in many ways similar to that found in bulimia. Some months after the re-feeding period a high proportion of the men had put themselves on a reducing diet; men who had previously had a normal interest in food became preoccupied with dieting after this bout of starvation.

These observations on starving individuals have encouraged the suggestion that anorexia and bulimia may be triggered by social and cultural conditions that require young women in particular to be thin. The dieting itself may, in susceptible individuals, cause some of the grossly aberrant and apparently irrational behaviour characteristic of anorexia nervosa and bulimia. Weight loss and leanness are generally admired and praised in our culture, and thus the initial positive reactions to the results of anorexic behaviour may serve as powerful reinforcement or reward and thus encourage learning of anorexic behaviour. In people whose self esteem is low and who feel that because of their family environment they lack control over their own lives, this initially praised ability to totally control some aspect of their lives may also act as positive reinforcement and encourage continuation and intensification of the anorexic behaviour.

There are numerous other theories as to the origins of anorexia. Some have suggested that there is some defect in the hypothalamic mechanisms regulating intake, but the frequent occurrence of binge eating suggests suppression of appetite rather than lack of appetite.

Some adherents to Freudian psychological theories have suggested that the subconscious goal of these women and girls is to avoid adult responsibility and sexuality by starving themselves; the cessation of menstruation, inhibition of sexual development and lack of adult female form found in anorexics are seen as the aims and rewards of anorexic behaviour. This theory has attracted much attention over the years and is probably the one theory about anorexia that non-specialists will have heard of. It would be fair to say that this theory has gone out of fashion as has, to some extent, the Freudian view of psychology.

Some have suggested that anorexia is a symptom of a frank affective psychiatric disorder like clinical depression. This is supported, to some extent, by claims of successful treatment of anorexics with anti-depressant drugs. One major problem of trying to investigate the psychological and physiological characteristics that bring about the disease is that by the time the disease is recognised, it will be impossible to decide which abnormalities are due to starvation and which are causes of the self-starvation. A detailed discussion of either the causes or treatment of eating disorders is beyond the scope of this book – the aim of this brief discussion has been to increase the awareness of non-specialists and to help them to recognise potential sufferers. The discussion may also give those in contact with anorexics some insight into the psychological consequences of anorexia/ starvation and thus help them to deal more sympathetically with difficult and incomprehensible behaviour. A detailed and well-referenced account of eating disorders may be found in Gilbert (1986).

Cancer cachexia

Severe emaciation and malnutrition are frequently associated with terminal malignant disease and starvation may, in many cases, be the immediate cause of death. There may be several readily identifiable causes for the loss of weight seen in these cancer sufferers: when malignancy affects the alimentary tract or where the disease otherwise makes eating difficult or painful; or when appetite is depressed in patients who are in great pain or extremely distressed; anti-cancer therapies may themselves induce nausea and anorexia. There are nonetheless occasions when patients with malignant disease may lose weight initially for no clearly apparent reason. Sometimes weight loss may be the symptom that triggers the investigation leading to the diagnosis of malignancy. Hypermetabolism (increased energy expenditure) seems to be partly responsible for such weight loss and this may be a reflection of the metabolic activity associated with rapidly dividing malignant cells. There is additionally thought to be an anorexic effect of tumour growth. It may be that some metabolic disturbance or metabolic by-product of tumour growth has a depressing effect upon appetite. It is an extremely difficult area to study because, once cancer is suspected or confirmed, the psychological reactions to the disease, the effects of any treatment, the pain and discomfort caused by disease or treatment and any more direct patho-physiological effects of the disease on feeding control will all interact and be difficult to differentiate.

Obesity

Nature and extent of the problem

Prevalence and consequences

In Chapter 3, body mass index (BMI) was seen to provide a simple means of categorising the severity of overweight and obesity, for example:

Weight/height²	Condition
less than 20 kg/m²	underweight
20–25 kg/m²	ideal range
25–30 kg/m²	overweight (grade I obesity)
30+ kg/m²	obese (obesity, grades II and III)

Table 6.4 Distribution (%) of a representative sample of English adults between four categories of Body Mass Index (BMI). Data source: White et al., 1993).

Category (BMI)	Men	Women
Underweight (under 20)	6	9
Ideal range (20–25)	42	47
Overweight (25–30)	40	29
Obese (30+)	13	16
Mean BMI (kg/m²)	25.6	25.4

There is little doubt that overweight and obesity are more common in the UK and USA than in previous generations and that the prevalence is still rising. Using the above cut-off points, around half of English adults are overweight (i.e. BMI 25+) and around 15% are obese (i.e. BMI 30+) (White *et al.*, 1993). The distribution of a representative sample of English men and women between the above four BMI categories is shown in Table 6.4. These figures in Table 6.4 represent substantial increases in the prevalence of overweight and obesity compared to values obtained in 1986/87 (in Gregory *et al.*, 1990).

American figures for the prevalence of obesity and overweight are probably at least as bad as those quoted for the UK. In 1976–80, 26% of all American adults were either overweight or obese (DHHS, 1992). However, the cut off points for being classified as overweight were a BMI of 27.8 for men and 27.3 for women. In order to be classified as overweight by these criteria a woman of 160 cm (5ft 3in) would have to weigh 70 kg (154 pounds) and a man of 178 cm (5ft 10in) would have to weigh 88 kg (194 pounds). Many people would consider themselves overweight even though they were some way below these thresholds. Given the British experience it is also quite probable that there will have been substantial increases in prevalence in the 15 years since these figures were current.

Studies conducted by life insurance companies have found that being overweight is associated with excess mortality and that this increase in mortality rises exponentially and is steep at body mass indices of over 30; mortality ratio is doubled at a BMI of around 35. According to COMA (1984) there is an increased risk of coronary heart disease in the overweight especially in overweight younger men; a 30% higher mortality from coronary heart disease in younger men with a relative weight excess of 19%. Other studies have indicated similar risks of even mild to moderate overweight in middle-aged women (e.g. Manson *et al.*, 1990). White *et al.* (1993) found a strong corellation between BMI and serum cholesterol in their sample of English adults. Serum cholesterol in men who were classified as underweight averaged 5.0 mmol/l (5.4 in underweight women) but averaged 6.1 mmol/l in men classified as obese (6.4 in obese women). Numerous other diseases and problems are associated with overweight and obesity (Passmore and Eastwood, 1993; Hamilton *et al.*, 1991), for example:

- maturity onset diabetes
- hypertension
- hernia
- increased surgical risk
- higher accident rate
- increased risk of complications during pregnancy
- gall bladder disease
- gout
- arthritis.

There are also numerous indications that on top of any excess morbidity and mortality associated with being over-weight, there are major social and economic disadvantages to being over-weight. In some cultures, obesity may be admired as a symbol of wealth and success and fatness regarded as physically attrac-tive. In most Western countries however, the obese have long been poorly regarded and discriminated against. In his book on obesity, Mayer (1968) devotes a whole chapter to largely literary examples of hostility towards the obese and Gilbert (1986) also includes a short, referenced review of negative attitudes towards the obese.

Several studies have been conducted in which children have been asked to rate the likeability of other children from pictures and to assign various character traits to them. They consistently rate the obese children in these pictures as less likeable than the lean and, in some studies, even less likeable than children with physical deformities; they attribute unpleasant character traits to the obese children. Basically similar attitudes are also wide-spread amongst adults of all social classes. Obese people are subject to practical discrimination as well; they are less likely to be accepted for university education and for employment (see Gilbert, 1986). These negative attitudes towards the obese even permeate into the caring professions – Maiman *et al.* (1979) surveyed partici-pants at a scientific conference on the causes and treatment of obesity and found that:

- 32% of those surveyed agreed that the obese lacked willpower
- 87% agreed that they were self indul-gent
- 88% agreed that eating was a compen-sation for the obese
- 70% agreed that emotional problems were the cause of obesity.

These results suggest that, even amongst those helping the obese professionally, obesity is widely regarded as a self-inflicted condition caused by overeating, and that this overeating is probably trig-gered by emotional problems in people who are weak and self-indulgent. Harris (1983) conducted a survey amongst psy-chology students in Australia. When asked how they would feel about being obese themselves, all of these students gave negative responses and around 60% said that they would dislike it intensely – the highest level of negative response offered. Obesity is something that people fear in themselves and are often desperate to avoid or "cure"; it is something that is very widely denigrated and despised in others.

These negative attitudes to the obese may well be rooted in the historically assumed association between overweight, excessive food intake and inactivity (i.e. obesity is widely assumed to be due to greed and laziness). The obese are seen as responsible for their own condition due to the presence of these two undesirable personality traits. These judgmental atti-tudes are likely to be particularly strong in societies with an underlying puritanical philosophy where hard work and frugality are admired. The presence of obesity in societies where some go hungry, would surely encourage denigration of the obese – the obese may be seen as partly responsible for the deprivation of others.

There is still debate about whether obesity is primarily caused by failing to regulate food intake or whether it is partly a result of metabolic susceptibility.

However, the earlier discussion of the question of "whether the obese eat more than the lean" illustrates that, whatever the eventual answer to the question, the difficulty encountered in answering it indicates that any differences are relatively small. The image of obese people indulging in continuous gorging is, at least for the majority of overweight and obese people, false. In the longer term, recognition of this might lessen the social stigma attached to obesity even if prevention and successful treatment are more difficult to realise.

Distribution of adipose tissue in relation to health risks of obesity

Studies in the early 1980s indicated that the **waist:hip ratio** was an important determinant of the health risks associated with obesity. The health risks seem to be greater if the obesity is associated with a high waist:hip ratio – the typically male pattern of fat distribution – but much lower if associated with a low waist:hip ratio – the typically female pattern. This research suggests that the health risks associated with obesity are primarily due to fat deposited in the abdominal cavity. The male sex hormones – androgens – are thought to play an important role in increasing deposition of fat in the abdominal cavity. These ideas on waist:hip ratio and distribution of fat have progressed to the point where specific recommendations on waist:hip ratio have been included in official health recommendations in the US and to the point where life insurance companies will soon incorporate waist:hip ratios in their premium calculations. Seidell (1992) gives a short, referenced review of this topic.

In their recent survey of English adults, White *et al.* (1993) found that, as one would expect, average waist:hip ratio was higher in men than in women and that this ratio increased progressively with age in both sexes. It is still difficult to say at what level of waist:hip ratio the risk of cardiovascular disease is increased, but standards

of 0.95 or 1.0 have been suggested for men and 0.8 for women. In this survey sample, 6% of all men had a ratio over 1.0 and 24% over 0.95; 42% of the women had values over the still very tentative standard of 0.8.

Models of obesity causation, implications for treatment

Population factors in obesity causation

Obesity is rare in peasant communities where the lifestyle demands hard physical work and where food supplies are limited in both amount and range. Obesity is common in countries like the USA and UK where a sedentary lifestyle is common and where food is varied and plentiful. Certain population factors can be said to be permissive to the development of obesity, such as:

- a plentiful energy supply
- wide variety of palatable food available
- an energy dense diet
- low requirement for physical activity.

At the population level, the declining need for physical activity seems to be strongly implicated in the increasing prevalence of obesity. In the UK and US, *per capita* energy intakes have dropped substantially over the last couple of decades. According to Durnin (1992) the average energy intake of teenagers were up to a third higher in the 1930s than they are now. According to the National Food Survey, *per capita* household food consumption has dropped by more than a quarter since 1950; a similar trend is seen using wider measures of energy consumption (COMA, 1984). Paradoxically, it was seen earlier in the chapter, that the UK population has also been getting steadily fatter. The most likely explanation for these opposing trends is that the fall in energy intake is as a result of an increasingly sedentary lifestyle and reduced energy expenditure. However, the fall in intake has lagged behind the fall in expenditure resulting in an increasingly positive population energy balance which has culminated in increased prevalence of overweight and obesity.

For most people in affluent countries, economic means do not impose major limitations on their ability to buy palatable and energy-rich foods – there is an abundance of such food available and more apparent variety than ever before. The laboratory rat has long been regarded as a model regulator of its energy balance – normal animals, under standard laboratory conditions, fed standard laboratory diets are not prone to obesity. However, if one offers adult animals a variety of palatable, energy-rich, human foods, in addition to their normal pellet diet (cafeteria feeding), many of them also overeat and become obese (Rothwell and Stock, 1979). When laboratory rats are exposed to conditions that are intended to model the lifestyle of affluent people, they show the same increased prevalence of adiposity – i.e. when they are no longer required to forage or work for food, and when there is a wide variety of highly palatable and energy dense foods freely available.

Individual factors in obesity causation

Given that most people in the USA and UK are exposed to these population factors that are permissive to the development of obesity, why do some get fat whilst others remain lean? It is certainly not a simple matter of variations in individual ability to take advantage of these permissive opportunities – obesity is more prevalent in these countries amongst the lower socioeconomic groups. Obesity is most prevalent amongst those with the more limited economic means and a higher probability of their occupation involving manual labour. This is illustrated by Table 6.5 which shows social class differences in the BMIs of a representative sample of people in England (White *et al.,* 1993); rates of obesity are 50% higher in men in social classes IV and V than in those in classes I and II, in women the rates are doubled between the two groupings.

There are two basic paradigms or models of obesity causation. *The traditional model of obesity* is that, when these permissive population conditions prevail, those who become obese are the ones who take most advantage of them.

Table 6.5 Differences in Body Mass Index (BMI) of people in different social classes in England. Data source: White *et al.* (1993)

| | Social class of head of household | | | |
	I and II	III non-manual	III manual	IV and V
Men				
Mean BMI (kg/m²)	25.6	26.0	25.5	26.0
% BMI 25+	49	60	53	55
% BMI 30+	12	10	11	18
Women				
Mean BMI (kg/m²)	24.6	25.0	25.8	26.9
% BMI 25+	37	44	50	53
% BMI 30+	11	13	18	23

The obese are those most prone to overeat and underexercise when given the opportunity and this is why they get fat. Obese people have traditionally been regarded as greedy and lazy – gluttony and sloth has been the traditional model of obesity causation. The etymology of the word obese betrays this general prejudice about obesity causation – it is of Latin derivation from *ob* – completely and *esum* from the past participle of the Latin verb *edere* – to eat. Any survey of early medical or nutrition texts would show an almost unanimous acceptance of this model of obesity causation, for example:

• Corpulence ... is promoted by a diet too rich in fat-forming materials, fats, starches and sugars, bodily inactivity, tranquillity of mind.
  The modern cyclopedia (1899), London: The Gresham Publishing Company.
• ...99% of cases are due to wrong eating or lack of exercise.
  Bogert, L.J. (1931) *Nutrition and physical fitness*. Philadelphia: W.B. Saunders.
• Almost invariably imbalance between intake of food and output of work, either or, more usually, both may be at fault. Rare cases of metabolic obesity may occur.
  Hutchinson, R. and Mottram, V.H. (1933) *Food and the principles of dietetics*. London: Edward Arnold.
• Obesity in adults is often a result of over indulgence in food and of sedentary habits and should not be explained and excused by pronouncing the persons victims of glandular deficiencies.
  Cooper, L.F., Barber, E.M. and Mitchell, H.S. (1943) *Nutrition in health and disease*. 9th edn. Philadelphia: J.B. Lippincott.
• The result of excessive calorie intake or, in other words greed, is obesity.
  Akroyd, W.R. (1937) *Human nutrition and diet*. London: Thornton Butterworth Limited.

• Abnormality in weight is due to dietary indiscretion.
  Hawley, E.E. and Carden, G. (1944) *The art and science of nutrition*. London: Henry Kimpton.

A metabolic predisposition to obesity is the other model of individual obesity causation. Given the population conditions that favour obesity, then it is suggested that most people tend to reduce their activity and to eat more than their minimum energy requirement. There is, however, individual variation in the ability of individuals to homeostatically regulate expenditure to match output; lean people overeat but remain lean by "burning off" the surplus calories – obese people are less able to "burn off" the excess and thus more of these excess calories are deposited as body fat. This model was given a considerable boost by animal studies that convincingly demonstrated considerable capacity for diet induced thermogenesis in rats and pigs fed on low protein diets (e.g. Miller and Payne, 1962) and in cafeteria fed rats (e.g. Rothwell and Stock, 1979). One type of genetically obese mouse (obese-hyperglycaemic or ob/ob) has apparently profound defects in its ability to thermoregulate: it has a reduced body temperature; it dies when subjected to cold stress; and, has a low capacity for thermogenesis (Mayer, 1960). These observations have been widely interpreted as supporting a metabolic causation for obesity, i.e. a defect in the ability to "burn off" calories by increasing thermogenesis (e.g. Rothwell and Stock, 1979). As previously discussed, Rothwell and Stock (1979) suggested brown adipose tissue as a possible site for this "burning off" of surplus calories, i.e. of diet-induced thermogenesis. They suggested that the sympathetic nerves activate a "futile, heat generating metabolic cycle." The sympathetic drive to this tissue would be regulated by the hypothalamus.

Many experimental studies of obesity have used animal models with some inherited or induced lesion that produces extreme obesity. This has tended to encourage the view that obese and lean are two distinct categories. In real people, it is much more likely that obesity is due to a variety of influences and rather than a simple "all or none" categorisation, there is likely to be a continuum of susceptibilities ranging from very resistant to very susceptible. There is also no need to regard these two models as mutually exclusive; there could well be a range of susceptibilities to the temptation to overeat and underexercise and a range of metabolic susceptibilities to obesity – the precise combination of these two variables would determine the degree of expression of obesity under the prevailing environmental conditions.

There has been considerable debate over the years about the relative importance of genetic and environmental factors in the genesis of obesity. Clearly, certain environmental conditions are necessary for the expression of any genetic tendency to obesity, but equally some individuals do seem to be more susceptible than others; generations of animal breeders have been able to very successfully manipulate the fatness of animal carcasses by selective breeding. There is undoubtedly some genetic element in the predisposition of individuals to obesity; it is the relative importance of genetics (nature) and environmental influences (nurture) that is in doubt.

There are significant correlations between the fatness levels of parents and children and between siblings, but it is difficult to dissect out how much of this is due to common environmental factors and how much to shared genes. Several lines of enquiry point towards a considerable genetic component in this tendency of obesity to be familial. There is a much higher correlation between the fatness of monozygotic (identical) twins than between dizygotic (non-identical) twins.

Studies performed using adopted pairs of monozygotic twins who have been reared apart also strongly support there being a major inherited component in susceptibility to fatness. Large studies on adopted children in Denmark suggest that correlations between the Body Mass Index of adopted children and their natural first degree relatives (parents and siblings) are about the same as in natural families – suggesting that family resemblances in adiposity are mostly due to genetic factors. Sorensen (1992) gives a concise, referenced review of these genetic aspects of obesity.

Implications for treatment

It is sometimes considered that evidence for inheritance of obesity susceptibility favours the metabolic view of obesity, but inheritance of behavioural traits seems just as probable as inheritance of metabolic similarities.

Changes in the popularity of the two models of obesity causation could have considerable practical implications for the treatment of obesity. Perhaps most significantly, wide acceptance of a major metabolic component to obesity causation might increase sympathy for obese people who would then be seen as less to blame for their condition and more as victims of their biochemistry. This might increase the social standing of the obese and reduce discrimination against them – it might not help in their treatment, but it might make living with their condition less unpleasant.

If one believes in the traditional gluttony/sloth model of obesity, then one would focus efforts at treatment upon helping patients to improve their inefficient intake control mechanisms; behavioural therapy to correct aberrant control of eating behaviour and perhaps appetite suppressing drugs would be logical consequences of this model of causation. Bulkier diets might be expected to help by increasing feedback effects from the alimentary tract upon appetite. Increased expenditure by increased activity would seem to be consistent with either model especially given the strong evidence of the importance of inactivity as a population factor in obesity causation and the other health benefits of regular exercise.

If one believes in the metabolic model of obesity, then in the short term this might make relatively little difference to the approach to therapy. The aim would probably still be to reduce calorie intake below expenditure by the use of low calorie diets. One's expectation of success from this approach might be less and this might well be a self fulfilling prophecy. In the longer term, research would be concentrated upon ways of increasing energy expenditure by searching for behavioural modifications, dietary changes and pharmacological agents that would increase thermogenesis. Animal studies have shown that the sympathetic activation of brown adipose tissue is mediated through a previously unknown adrenergic receptor – the β-3 receptor. There is currently active research upon the development of drugs that stimulate these receptors (β-3 agonists) for possible use in the treatment of obesity (Stock, 1992). The notion of a pill that could cure obesity by increasing expenditure without the need for dieting is superficially attractive. However, production of a drug that is effective but nonetheless safe enough for long term use by the high proportion of the population with mild to moderate obesity seems like a very distant prospect.

Some specific theories of obesity causation and treatment

The fat cell theory

Knittle and Hirsch (1969) reported that early overfeeding of young rats predisposed them to obesity as adults. Early overfeeding increased the number of fat cells in the rat's epididymal fat pad (fat around the testis). Hirsch and Han (1969) suggested that prior to six weeks of age that these fat pads grew by cell division (hyperplasia) and by increased cell size (hypertrophy) but that, after this critical period, the number of fat cells was fixed and further growth could only occur by hypertrophy. Thus, overfeeding prior to six weeks increased the number of fat cells and made the animals permanently susceptible to obesity. These observations have had immense impact, encouraging the belief that overfeeding of children prior to their "critical period" increases cellularity in their adipose tissue and thus predisposes them to obesity as adults – **the fat cell theory**. According to this theory, plump children are highly likely to become obese adults.

Pond (1987) published a critical review of this theory and concluded that this fat cell theory is dependent upon the assumption that the growth of the rat epididymal fat pad is a reasonable model for the growth of human adipose tissue. As a result of a comparative study of adipose tissue in different species she has concluded that it is, in fact, a poor model. She found that human adipose tissue has more cells than non-primate adipose tissue. In adult primates, there is relatively little capacity for increases in fat cell size but that the capacity for hyperplasia is not limited as it is in older rats. She suggests that in human beings changes in fat cell numbers are important in the growth of adipose tissue throughout life rather than, according to the fat cell theory, being fixed in early childhood and determining the individual's lifelong propensity for obesity. Hausberger and Volz (1984) have suggested that, even in rats, adult feeding was of more importance than early feeding in determining the adult rat's level of adiposity – early overfeeding did not appear to predispose nor did early underfeeding protect against the later obesifying effect of a high fat diet.

The internal/external hypothesis

This theory essentially suggests that lean people regulate their food intake primarily in response to their internal physiological hunger mechanisms whilst obese people are much more responsive to external, non-physiological influences upon their feeding behaviour. In the obese, the internal physiological regulatory mechanisms may be overridden by these external influences with resultant poor regulation of energy balance. External factors like time of day, palatability of food, ease of access to food, sight and smell of food or emotional state are the major determinants of eating behaviour in the obese. This theory was proposed by Schachter (1968) and is reviewed in Gilbert (1986).

Schachter and Rodin (1974) identified certain behavioural characteristics of obese rats and then, in an ingenious series of experiments, demonstrated very similar behavioural characteristics in obese people. For example:

1 obese rats and people consumed more food than leans when it was readily available but less than leans when they were required to work for the food
2 the obese consumed more than leans when the food was palatable but less when it was made unpalatable, e.g. by the addition of quinine – they were more finicky
3 the feeding behaviour of the obese was much more affected by their anxiety state than was that of the lean.

Although obese rats (and people) ate more than the lean controls under normal conditions, they seemed to have a reduced hunger drive – a "hunger motivation deficit". They concluded that the feeding behaviour of obese rats and obese people was motivated primarily by **appetite** (the learned, hedonistic desire to eat food) rather than by **hunger** (the physiological need to eat food). This theory has lost favour in recent years but has, nonetheless,

had a great practical influence on the treatment of obesity. Much behavioural treatment of obesity is based upon this concept of external orientation of food intake regulation in obese people.

Behaviour is envisaged as being initiated by certain cues or antecedents, and then, if the behaviour results in pleasure that acts as a reward or reinforcement, then that behaviour is learned. If the behaviour has unpleasant consequences, then this acts as negative reinforcement and discourages repetition of the behaviour:

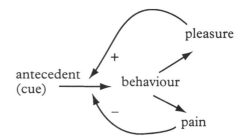

Thus obese people are triggered into inappropriate eating behaviour by certain circumstances or cues and their inappropriate behaviour is rewarded, and thus learned, because of the hedonistic pleasure or relief of anxiety that results from the inappropriate eating behaviour. **Behaviour therapy** seeks to identify and then to devise means to avoid the cues or antecedents to inappropriate behaviour (e.g. eating high calorie foods) and to reinforce or reward appropriate behaviours (e.g. taking exercise or achieving weight loss targets) so that they are "learned".

In order to identify the antecedents or cues that trigger inappropriate eating behaviour, patients are often asked to keep a diary of when and what they eat, and in what circumstances they eat it. They are then encouraged to modify their habits and environment to reduce these cues, for example:

1 they may be encouraged to avoid the temptation to buy high calorie foods on impulse by shopping strictly from a list

2 they may reduce casual, impulse consumption of high calorie snacks by making them less accessible, e.g. keeping them on a high shelf or in a locked cabinet so that this snacking has to be a premeditated act

3 they may reduce the temptation to pick at food they are preparing by encouraging other family members to prepare their own snacks

4 they can reduce the temptation to eat leftovers by throwing them away

5 they can even be encouraged to modify the process of eating by allowing a set number of mouthfuls per minute.

An extreme version of behaviour therapy is aversion therapy. The aim is to train the patient to associate painful electric shocks with food or to associate images of food with other unpleasant images. In this way, it is hoped that the patient may develop learned aversions to "problem foods". The fact that people have voluntarily agreed to undergo such therapy says much about the desperation of many obese people to be "cured". A thorough and referenced review of the behavioural methods employed to treat obesity may be found in Gilbert (1986).

The nibbling theory

Rats and mice are naturally nibblers; they spend long periods of time foraging and feeding. They can be experimentally induced to feed intermittently, to gorge, either by feeding them through a stomach tube or by allowing them access to food for only a short period each day and thus training them to eat their daily food in short, discrete meals. Under these "gorging" conditions rodents become metabolically more efficient, i.e. they accumulate more body energy for a given intake and fat deposition rather than growth of lean tissue is favoured (Fabry, 1969).

Nibbling regimes have been widely used to aid in the treatment of human obesity – the designated calorie intake is split up into many small meals in the expectation that this will reduce metabolic efficiency and reduce the tendency to synthesise fat. There has been relatively little direct testing of the effects of nibbling and gorging regimes in humans.

Final comments on the treatment of obesity

A crash diet may result in spectacular short term weight losses – perhaps as much as 3 kg within a week. However, much of this initial weight loss is artefact and does not represent much loss of body fat. During fasting, there is initially depletion of body carbohydrate and protein with considerable resultant loss of water; there will also be reductions in the weight of gut contents. Such instant losses will tend to be replaced equally quickly. One kilogram of adipose tissue represents around 7000 kcal (29.4 MJ), and so even a negative energy balance of 1000 kcal (4.2 MJ) per day could only be expected to result in loss of 1 kg of adipose tissue per week.

Long term treatment of obesity is notoriously unsuccessful – very few patients reach and maintain their target weights. Many treatments achieve considerable numbers of short term successes. Sometimes even very overweight patients reach their target weights, but few people maintain this weight loss in the longer term. All of the treatments that seriously address the problem of overweight will involve extended periods of discomfort if large amounts of weight need to be lost. Some of these treatments may involve very considerable discomfort and even danger to patients, e.g. surgical by-pass of a large part of the small intestine (jejuno-ileal by-pass), jaw wiring, very low calorie diets (virtual starvation) and drugs. If weight losses that are only achieved at great cost to the patient are not maintained in the longer term, then one must question whether these sacrifices are justified. There is considerable evidence that repeated bouts of weight loss and regain actually favours replacement of lean tissue by fat and accumulating evidence that cycles of weight loss and regain are associated with increased mortality.

Garrow (1992) argues that one major reason why some people remain relatively lean whilst others get very fat, is that the lean are more vigilant. The lean monitor their body weight more closely and take steps to correct any weight gain (i.e. eating less and exercising more) before it has become a major problem. He argues that the obese, on the other hand, are less vigilant and therefore do not initiate corrective steps until the condition has progressed to the point where the person cannot cope with the magnitude of weight loss that is required to restore normal body weight. This idea has been used to explain the social class differences in the incidence of obesity; it has been suggested that people in the lower socioeconomic groups tend to be less vigilant in monitoring their body weight and this is why they are more prone to becoming obese. This class difference in body weight vigilance would be consistent with the general trend for the upper social groups to be more likely to choose foods with "healthy images" noted in Chapter 2.

Similar lack of vigilance, it has been argued, allows regain of weight after successful slimming – the weight creeps back on unnoticed by the patient until it is not readily correctable. Once the weight loss or re-loss required is high then the patient feels unable to control the situation, becomes disheartened and no longer makes any sustained effort to reduce or even to maintain body weight. Garrow has used an adjustable waist cord to increase the vigilance of his patients – the patient is only able to adjust the length of this cord by an amount that allows for normal day to day fluctuations in waist size. Any increase in waist size above the adjustable range would make the cord uncomfortable to the patient and immediately signal the need for corrective measures. Such a cord can be used to reduce the risk of weight regain after slimming. It can be used during weight loss – it can be shortened by the physician as slimming proceeds and it could also be used as a preventative measure. A cherished or expensive item of clothing that becomes uncomfortably tight may serve as a similar early warning signal for many of us who struggle to keep our weight within certain tolerance limits.

Dietary changes that are in line with current nutrition education guidelines would increase the bulk of the diet (lower its energy density). This may increase the efficiency of intake regulating mechanisms, most obviously by increasing satiety signals associated with distension of the gut. There are also many reasons for strongly recommending increased levels of physical activity (see Chapter 14) as well as strong indications that inactivity is an important factor serving to increase the population prevalence of overweight and obesity. There is thus a good probability that simultaneous implementation of these dietary and activity changes would reduce the prevalence of overweight and obesity. This does not mean, however, that such measures will be effective in the short term treatment of individual obesity. Whilst regular exercise and a bulkier diet are important elements in treating obesity (and maintaining weight loss), the loss of considerable amounts of stored fat is additionally going to require an extended period when energy intake is reduced to less than expenditure, i.e. dieting. Most conventional and many unconventional treatments for obesity represent different strategies for making dieting more effective or more acceptable.

7 Carbohydrates

Contents

Introduction

Carbohydrates have traditionally supplied the bulk of the energy in most human diets. They still provide the bulk of the energy intake for the majority of the world's population, the diet of which is based upon cereals or starchy roots. Dietary carbohydrates are almost exclusively derived from the vegetable kingdom and the carbohydrate content of most foods of animal origin is dietetically insignificant. The only major exception is lactose or milk sugar, which provides around 40% of the energy in human milk and 30% of the energy in cow milk. In the main, it is thus only in populations consuming large amounts of foods derived from animal sources where the dominance of carbohydrates as the principal source of dietary energy is challenged by increased fat consumption; some affluent vegetarian populations may also derive relatively large proportions of their energy supply from extracted vegetable oils.

In some Third World countries, carbohydrates account for well over 75% of the total energy intake, and this carbohydrate will be predominantly starch. In the affluent countries of Western Europe, Australasia and North America, carbohydrates are likely to provide only around 45% of the calories, with close to half of this percentage in the form of simple sugars in some countries. These affluent populations are currently being advised to increase their proportion of energy derived from carbohydrates to 55–60% of the total and yet, at the same time, to substantially reduce their consumption of simple sugars, perhaps limiting "extracted" sugars to no more than 10% of the total energy intake.

Nature and classification of carbohydrates

Carbohydrates are monomers or polymers of simple sugar units or **saccharides**. Carbohydrates may be described according to the number of saccharide units they contain, i.e. the **monosaccharides** (one), the **disaccharides** (two), the **oligosaccharides** (a few), and the **polysaccharides** (many). Although there are likely to be a range of monosaccharides present in human diets, three of them make up the bulk of monosaccharide that is released for absorption and utilisation during the digestion of most human diets, namely glucose, galactose and fructose. These three monosaccharides each contain six carbon atoms and are termed **hexoses**.

Carbohydrates must be broken down (digested) to their component monosaccharide units before they can be absorbed in the small intestine. Saliva and pancreatic juice contain an enzyme known as **alpha(α)-amylase** that breaks up digestible polysaccharides into oligosaccharides and disaccharides. A range of specific enzymes, that are localised on the absorptive surface of the small intestine, complete carbohydrate digestion by cleaving these disaccharides and oligosaccharides into their component monosaccharides.

Dietary carbohydrates are usually classified into three major subdivisions – the **sugars**, the **starches** and the **non-starch polysaccharides (NSP)**, summarised in Figure 7.1. Sugars and starches are readily

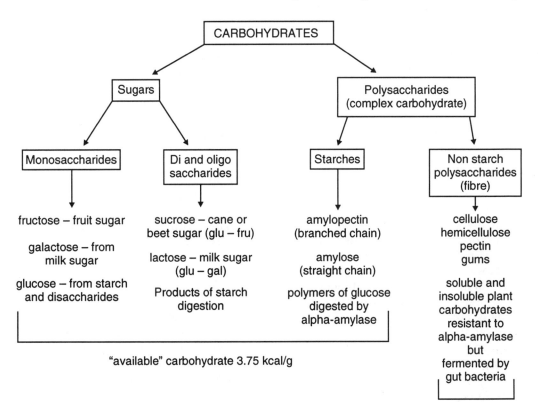

Figure 7.1 A summary of carbohydrate classification

digested and absorbed in the human small intestine; they thus clearly serve as a source of dietary energy and are sometimes termed the **available carbohydrates**; they all yield around 3.75 kcal (16 kJ) per gram. The non-starch polysaccharides are resistant to digestion by human gut enzymes and are thus referred to as the **unavailable carbohydrate**.

Sugars

Sugars may be monosaccharides, disaccharides or oligosaccharides; they are characteristically soluble in water and have a sweet taste. The monosaccharides glucose and fructose are present in some fruits and vegetables and in honey. Fructose is three times as sweet as glucose and is largely responsible for the sweet taste of fruits and some vegetables. Sucrose (relative sweetness 100) is used as the standard against which the sweetness of other sugars and also of artificial sweeteners is measured. The relative sweetness of the other major dietary sugars is: lactose 30; glucose 50; and, fructose 170.

Lactose or milk sugar

Lactose is a disaccharide found exclusively in milk and is the least sweet of the major dietary sugars. It is comprised of one unit of glucose and one of galactose; lactose is the only significant source of galactose in the diet. Although galactose is essential in several synthetic biochemical processes, it is not an essential nutrient; humans, even babies, have the capacity to manufacture galactose from glucose.

On rare occasions, babies may inherit an enzyme deficiency which renders them unable to metabolise dietary galactose. If such babies are fed with breast milk or lactose-containing infant formula, then galactose accumulates in their blood (**galactosaemia**). This galactosaemia results in a range of symptoms (e.g. vomiting,

weight loss and jaundice) and if untreated it may result in death or permanent disability (e.g. cataracts, retarded physical and mental development). Infants with this condition must be fed on a lactose-free formula and will need to continue to avoid milk and milk-containing foods after weaning.

Some babies are born deficient in the enzyme **lactase** that cleaves lactose into its component monosaccharides in the small intestine (lactase insufficiency). This insufficiency results in a failure to digest and absorb dietary lactose. Such infants will fail to thrive. They will suffer from diarrhoea because of the osmotic effect of undigested lactose causing retention of water within the gut and bloating because of fermentation of lactose by intestinal bacteria causing gas production. These infants also need to be fed on a lactose-free formula.

In many human populations, and in many other mammals, lactase activity in the small intestine declines after weaning, reducing the capacity to digest, and therefore to absorb, dietary lactose. Such **lactose intolerant** individuals experience symptoms of diarrhoea and bloating at varying levels of severity after consuming milk. Lactose intolerance may also occur as a secondary consequence of other degenerative changes in the gut, e.g. as a result of the changes in the intestine associated with coeliac disease (Chapter 13) or severe malnutrition.

Sucrose

Sucrose is a disaccharide composed of one unit of glucose and one unit of fructose; the terms sucrose and sugar are often used as if they are synonymous. Sucrose is found in several fruits and vegetables and is present in large quantities in sugar beet and sugar cane from which it is extracted and purified on a vast industrial scale. Sucrose is readily available in highly purified or partly purified forms (e.g. white sugar, brown sugars, treacle or syrup). It is also very widely used by food processors to sweeten, preserve and to texturise a variety of foods.

High sucrose consumption has, at one time or another, been blamed for many of the illnesses that afflict affluent populations. The poor health image of sucrose was encapsulated in the phrase "Pure, white and deadly". Its poor health image has led many food manufacturers to use other sugars, or sugar-containing extracts, in their products so that they can imply in advertising claims that their product is "healthier" because it has reduced levels of sucrose. The term extrinsic non-milk sugar has been used to cover all of the dietary sugars (still principally sucrose) that are not present as natural components of the fruit, vegetable and milk in the diet. Sucrose is a natural plant sugar that happens to be present in large enough amounts in readily cultivatable plants to make it convenient for extraction in industrial quantities. It seems reasonable to suppose that if sucrose is indeed harmful as it is used in affluent countries, then other sugars used in the same ways and quantities are also likely to be harmful. Substitution of sucrose by other extracted sugars that have not yet acquired the poor health image of sucrose does not appear to offer a high probability of dietary "improvement". Extrinsic non-milk sugars comprise between about 10% and around 20% of the total calorie intake in most affluent populations. US and UK intakes are towards the top end of this range.

Sucrose and other sugars have a very high, almost addictive, sensory appeal and may therefore encourage overconsumption of food energy and thus predispose to obesity. Offering sugared water to rats and mice has been used as an experimental means of inducing obesity. In these experiments with rodents, increasing sugar consumption depresses intake of solid food (and therefore nutrients) but not by enough to compensate for the extra calories in the sugar

(Kanarek and Hirsch, 1977).

There is little convincing evidence that, at levels typical of UK and US diets, added sugars are directly implicated in the aetiology of cardiovascular diseases, diabetes or hypertension. At very high intakes, 30% or more of total calories, they may elevate serum cholesterol levels and lead to insulin resistance which is important in the aetiology of the maturity onset form of diabetes (COMA, 1991).

When extracted sugars are added to foods, they add calories but no nutrients. They reduce the nutrient density of the diet; the phrase "empty calories" has been coined. The significance of this reduction in nutrient density will depend upon the general level of nutrient adequacy; in populations or individuals with high nutrient intakes it will be of less significance than those whose nutrient intake is more marginal. Some nutrient-rich foods may only become palatable if sugar is added, e.g. some sour fruits and fruit juices.

Artificial sweeteners

Artificial, non-sugar, sweeteners have been developed and manufactured to satisfy our craving for sweetness without the consumption of sugars. Saccharin was the first of these artificial sweeteners and has been in use for much of this century. It is around 400 times as sweet as sucrose, and it has no calories. It is absorbed and excreted unchanged in the urine and has been reported to increase the incidence of bladder tumours in rats; despite this, it is still a permitted sweetener in most countries including the US and UK because, at practical intake levels, it is not thought to represent a significant hazard. Saccharin has a bitter after-taste and, as it is destroyed by heating, it cannot be used as a substitute for sugar in cooking; this limits its usefulness to food manufacturers. Aspartame is a relatively recent addition to the sweetener range, it is a dipeptide made up of the amino acids aspartic acid and glutamic acid. Aspartame is around

200 times as sweet as sucrose so, despite being digested to its constituent amino acids and absorbed, it has a negligible calorific yield because so little need be used. Although both compounds mimic the sweetness, of sugar they do not have the preservative or textural effects of sugar.

Diet and dental health

The notion that sugar is implicated in the aetiology of dental caries (tooth decay) stretches back to the Ancient Greeks. The evidence that sugars, and sucrose in particular, have some effect on the development of dental caries is overwhelming; only the relative importance of sugar as compared to other factors, like fluoride intake and individual susceptibility, is really disputed. There is a strong correlation across populations between average sugar consumption and the number of **decayed, missing and filled (DMF)** teeth in the children. In populations with low sugar consumption (less than 10% of energy intake) dental caries are uncommon. Observations with island populations have shown strong correlations between changes in the sugar supply and changes in the rates of tooth decay.

In Britain during World War II, rates of tooth decay fell when sugar was rationed. Low rates of tooth decay have been found in diabetic children living in institutions whose sugar intake would have been kept very low as part of their diabetic management. In a study conducted more than 40 years ago in Swedish mental hospitals, the Vipeholm study, groups of patients were exposed to not only differing levels of sugar intake but also differences in the form and frequency of that sugar intake. Not only was the amount of sugar important in determining rates of tooth decay but form and frequency had an even greater impact: sugar taken between meals was found to be the most cariogenic; frequent consumption of small amounts

of sugar was more harmful than the same amount consumed in large infrequent doses; and, the most cariogenic foods were those where the sugar was in a sticky form that adhered to the teeth, e.g. toffees. COMA (1989a) and Binns (1992) give referenced reviews of the role of sugars in the aetiology of dental caries; most of the uncited references used in this section are listed here.

The key event in the development of dental caries is generally agreed to be the production of acid by the bacteria *Streptococcus mutans* in dental **plaque** – plaque being a sticky mixture of food residue, bacteria and bacterial polysaccharides that adheres to teeth. These bacteria produce acid by fermenting carbohydrates, particularly sugars, in foods. When the mouth becomes acidic enough (i.e. pH drops below 5.2) demineralisation of the teeth begins. The demineralisation of teeth induced by the acid can lead to holes in the hard outer enamel layer of the tooth, exposing the softer under layers of dentine and thus enabling decay to proceed rapidly throughout the tooth. This is not a one-way process, between periods of demineralisation, there will be phases of remineralisation or repair; it is the balance between these two processes that will determine susceptibility to carie formation.

The key role of oral bacteria in the development of caries is highlighted by experiments with germ-free animals; rats born by caesarean section into a sterile environment and maintained germ-free throughout their lives do not develop dental caries even when their diets are high in sucrose. Tooth decay is considered to be a bacterial disease that is promoted by dietary sugar. Sugars are ideal substrates for the acid producing bacteria of the plaque. When sugar is consumed as part of a meal then other constituents of the food can act as buffers that "soak up" the acid and limit the effects on mouth pH of any acid produced. High saliva production also reduces acid attack by buffering and diluting the acid. The more frequently sugar containing snacks or drinks are consumed, and the longer that sugar remains in the mouth, the longer the period that the overall pH of the mouth is below the level at which demineralisation occurs. In the UK, there is a target for reducing extrinsic non-milk sugars to around half of current intakes. Reducing between meal sugar in drinks and sugary snacks is regarded as the priority in the prevention of dental caries. Prolonged sucking of sugary drinks through a teat by infants and young children is particularly damaging to teeth and manufacturers of such drinks recommend that they be consumed from a cup.

In a review of the role of sugars in caries induction from the sugar industry viewpoint, Binns (1992) emphasises the importance of other factors in determining caries frequency and shows evidence of a substantial reduction in caries frequency in industrialised countries since the late 1960s – see Table 7.1. During the period covered by Table 7.1 sugar consumption has not changed substantially and Binns suggests that consumption of sugary snacks between meals may even have increased.

The decline in the prevalence of caries in children, seen in Table 7.1, may be attributed in large part to the effect of increased fluoride intake. In some places, water supplies have been fluoridated, some parents give children fluoride supplements and, most significantly, almost all toothpaste is now fluoridated (95% of the UK toothpaste market). The evidence that fluoride has a protective effect against the development of dental caries is very strong. There is an inverse epidemiological association between the fluoride content of drinking water and rates of decayed, missing and filled teeth in children. These epidemiological comparisons suggest that an optimal level of fluoride in drinking water is around 1 part per million (1 mg per litre). At this level, there seems to be good protection against tooth decay without the risk of the mottling of

Table 7.1 *Changes in the rates of decayed, missing and filled (DMF) teeth in 12-year-old children over the period 1967 to 1983. All values are average numbers of DMF teeth per child. Data source: Binns (1992)*

Country	1967 rate	1983 rate
Australia	4.8	2.8
Denmark	6.3	4.7
Finland	7.2	4.1
Netherlands	7.5	3.9
New Zealand	9.0	3.3
Norway	10.1	4.4
Sweden	4.8	3.4
United Kingdom	4.7	3.0
United States	3.8	2.6

teeth that is increasingly associated with levels above this. Intervention studies (see example in Chapter 3) and experimental studies have also confirmed the protective effects of fluoride.

The major effect of fluoride in preventing tooth decay is thought to be by its incorporation into the mineral matter of the tooth enamel; incorporation of fluoride into the calcium/phosphate compound hydroxyapatite to give fluorapatite renders the tooth enamel more resistant to demineralisation. This means that fluoride is most effective in preventing dental caries when administered to young children (under 5s) during tooth formation. Fluoride in relatively high doses also inhibits bacterial acid production and inhibits bacterial growth; it may concentrate in plaque to produce these effects even at normal intake levels, (Binns, 1992).

Several expert committees have made specific recommendations to ensure adequate intakes of fluoride, especially in young children (e.g. COMA, 1991; NACNE, 1983; and, NRC, 1989b). COMA (1991) give a "safe intake" of 0.05 mg/kg body weight for fluoride in infants only, NRC (1989a) give a range of safe intakes for all age groups.

Despite the very strong evidence for a beneficial effect of fluoride upon dental health, there has been limited fluoridation of water supplies in the UK in contrast to the US where water fluoridation is widespread. This is because of strong opposition from some pressure groups. Opposition to fluoridation has been partly on the grounds that addition of fluoride to the public water supply amounts to mass medication without individual consent. There have also been persistent concerns expressed about the long-term safety of this level of fluoride consumption; it is very difficult, for example, to prove beyond any doubt that there is no increased carcinogenic risk associated with lifetime consumption. The difference between the therapeutic levels proposed and the dose associated with early signs of fluoride overload (mottling of the teeth) is also relatively small (2–3 fold). There may also be a relatively small number of people who are fluoride sensitive.

Starches

Plants use starches as a store of energy in their roots and seeds. Animals also manufacture and store a form of starch, **glycogen**, in their muscles and livers but the amounts present in most flesh foods is dietetically insignificant.

Starches are polymers of glucose. The glucose may be arranged in straight chains (**amylose**) or, more frequently, in branched chains (**amylopectin**). The glucose residues in starches are joined together by linkages that are able to be broken (hydrolysed) by human digestive enzymes. These linkages are mainly α 1-4 linkages with some α 1-6 linkages that cause the branching of the glucose chain in amylopectin.

The dimers and oligomers of glucose that are produced as a result of digestion by α-amylase are then finally cleaved by enzymes on the mucosal surface of the small intestine to yield glucose.

Starches provide approximately the same energy yield as sugars (3.75 kcal/g);

they have low solubility in water, and they do not have a sweet taste. As starches are bland, then starchy foods also tend to be bland. This is one reason why affluent populations, whose wealth affords them the opportunity, tend to select foods with more sensory appeal; they tend to reduce the proportion of their dietary energy that is supplied by starch and replace it with fats and sugars. If both sugar and fat intakes are to be reduced in line with the recommendations discussed in Chapter 4 then this must inevitably involve a large increase in starch consumption, perhaps a doubling of current intakes.

Non-starch polysaccharide

Halliday and Ashwell (1991) have written a concise, referenced review of this topic, many of the uncited references used for this discussion are listed here. Non-starch polysaccharides (NSP) are structural components of plant cell walls (cellulose and hemicellulose) and viscous soluble substances found in cell sap (pectin and gums); they are resistant to digestion by human gut enzymes. Animal-derived foods can be regarded for dietetic purposes as containing no NSP. NSP contains numerous different sugar residues, but it passes through the small intestine and into the large bowel undigested. The term non-starch polysaccharide is essentially synonymous with the term **dietary fibre** although the latter term would also include resistant starch and lignin, the principle component of wood, that is not carbohydrate.

Americans and Britons are currently being advised to substantially increase their consumption of NSP or fibre – current recommendations suggest increases over current intakes of 50–100%. NSP and starches are usually found within the same foods (cereals, fruits and vegetables). So, increasing NSP and starch intakes are likely to go hand in hand. The milling of cereals so that all or part of the indigestible outer layers of the cereal grains (**bran**) is removed, substantially reduces the NSP and micronutrient content of the end product, but without removing significant amounts of starch. Whole grain cereals therefore contain substantially more NSP than refined cereals, for example:

Food	NSP content g/100 g
Wholemeal bread	5.8
White bread	1.5
Brown rice	0.8
White rice	0.2

Current average intakes of NSP in the UK are around 12 g/day with a wide individual variation (5–25 g/day); around 40% of this UK total comes from cereals, 50% from vegetables and the remainder from fruits (Gregory *et al.*, 1990).

NSP is frequently categorised into two major fractions – the soluble substances that form gums and gels when mixed with water (the gums and pectins) and the water insoluble fraction (cellulose and hemicellulose). The NSP in the UK diet is made up of similar proportions of **soluble** and **insoluble NSP**. The insoluble forms of NSP predominate in the bran of wheat, rice and maize, but oats, rye and barley contain higher proportions of soluble NSP. The proportions of soluble and insoluble NSP in fruit and vegetables varies, but they generally contain a substantially higher proportion of soluble NSP than wheat fibre, the principle cereal NSP in the British diet. Table 7.2 shows the proportion of the total NSP that is soluble in a number of common foods.

Many starchy foods, particularly heat processed foods such as bread, cornflakes and boiled potatoes, contain starch that is resistant to digestion by α-amylase *in vitro*. If resistance to α-amylase digestion is used in the chemical determination of NSP in food then this **resistant starch**

Table 7.2 The soluble NSP content of some common foods. Data source: Halliday and Ashwell (1991)

Food	Total NSP g/100 g	% soluble NSP
Wholemeal bread	5.8	17
Brown rice	0.8	12
Oatmeal (raw)	7.0	60
"All-Bran"	24.5	17
Cornflakes	0.9	44
Potatoes	1.2	58
Apples	1.6	38
Oranges	2.1	66
Bananas	1.1	64
Carrots	2.5	56
Peas	2.9	28
Sprouts	4.8	52
Cabbage	3.2	50
Baked beans	3.5	60
Roasted peanuts	6.2	31

would be classified as part of the NSP. Studies upon patients with ileostomies (i.e. whose small intestines have been surgically modified so that they drain externally into a bag rather than into the large intestine) suggest that a large proportion of this resistant starch also resists digestion by gut enzymes *in vivo*. Most resistant starch thus enters the large intestine undigested and behaves physiologically like NSP. This resistant starch, although usually only a small component of total starch in any food, may make a considerable contribution to the apparent NSP content of some foods, e.g. resistant starch represents around 30% of the NSP in white bread, 33% in boiled potatoes and 80% in boiled white rice. The amount of resistant starch in any given food may vary quite a lot depending upon slight differences in preparation, e.g. in freshly cooked potatoes around 3–5% of the starch is not digested in the small intestine but this rises to 12% when potatoes are cooked and cooled before being eaten; in greenish under ripe bananas as much as 90% of the starch is in the form of granules that are not digested in the small intestine and reach the large intestine. Resistant starch is just one of a number of factors that complicate the measurement of dietary fibre intakes of a population – estimates of fibre intake will vary widely according to the definition of dietary fibre used and the analytical methods used. This clearly represents a major hindrance to epidemiological investigations of the effects of NSP/fibre on health. For example, several oriental populations with rice-based diets (e.g. Japanese) have lower fibre intakes than the British because of the very low NSP content of white rice. These oriental diets are, however, very high in starch and inclusion of resistant starch with NSP would change the fibre position of these diets very substantially. Resistant starch has been reviewed by Berry (1988).

Although NSP is resistant to digestion by human gut enzymes and passes through the small intestine largely intact, in the large intestine, most of the components of NSP are to some extent fermentable by gut bacteria. The fermentability of the components of NSP varies according to the type; the pectins are very readily fermentable but cellulose remains largely unfermented in the human colon. NSP thus acts as a substrate for bacterial growth within the large intestine; the by-products of this fermentation are intestinal gases and short chain fatty acids (acetate, butyrate and propionate). The short chain fatty acids thus produced can be absorbed from the gut and can serve as a human energy source so that the typical mix of NSP in British and American diets may contribute around 2 kcal (8 kJ/g) to dietary energy.

Note that in ruminating animals like sheep and cattle, the short chain fatty acids produced by the fermentation of starches and NSP by microorganisms in the rumen are the animal's principal energy source. Even in pigs, whose gastrointestinal physiology is much more like that of humans, such fermentation in the large intestine, and the resulting short chain fatty acids, can make up a substan-

tial proportion of the total dietary energy.

Increasing levels of NSP in the diet can be convincingly shown to have a number of physiological effects in the short term:

1 Increased NSP content of foods slows down the rate of glucose absorption from the gut and thus reduces the postprandial peak concentrations of glucose and insulin in blood. This effect is attributed primarily to the soluble components of NSP and it is thought to be largely due to the mechanical effect of the viscous NSP components in reducing the contact of dissolved glucose with the absorptive surface of the intestinal epithelium. Guar gum (a soluble NSP that forms a viscous solution when mixed with water) has been shown to reduce the outflow of dissolved glucose even *in vitro* experiments using a dialysis bag made from synthetic materials. The NSP can only produce this effect if taken with the glucose or digestible carbohydrate – it cannot work if taken a few hours before or after the ingested glucose. Increased intakes of dietary fibre have been shown to improve glucose tolerance; diabetics, in particular, may benefit from this improvement. Dietary guidelines for diabetics now include a recommendation to ensure good intakes of high NSP foods.

2 Increased intakes of NSP increase the volume of stools produced and reduce the **transit time** (i.e. the time it takes for an ingested marker to pass out in the faeces). The fermentable components of NSP lead to increased proliferation of intestinal bacteria and thus increase the bacterial mass in the stools. The short chain fatty acids produced during fermentation also tend to acidify the colonic contents and may act as substrates for the intestinal cells. The unfermented components of NSP hold water and thus they also increase the stool bulk and make the stools softer and easier to pass. The increased bulk

and softness of stools, together with more direct effects on gut motility, produced by the products of fermentation, combine to accelerate the passage of faeces through the colon.

These effects of fibre/NSP on the gut are often presented as being only relatively recently recognised, but they do in fact have a very long history. The following are quotes from a booklet published by the Kellogg company in 1934:

- It is imperative that proper bulk be included in the foods that are served. Otherwise, the system fails to eliminate regularly. Common constipation, with its attendant evils, sets in.
- This bulk is the cellulose or fibre content in certain natural foods.
- Within the body, it (bran) absorbs moisture and forms a soft mass which gently helps to clear the intestines of wastes.

Way back in the 1880s, Dr. Thomas Allinson was championing the cause of wholemeal bread. He suggested many benefits of wholemeal over white bread (i.e. of bran) that are widely accepted today, e.g. prevention of constipation and the prevention of minor bowel disorders like haemorrhoids (piles).

3 NSP and some of the substances associated with it (e.g. phytate) tend to bind or chelate minerals and probably also vitamins and thus may hinder their absorption. In compensation, foods rich in NSP tend also to have higher levels of micronutrients than refined foods. Levels of NSP likely to be consumed by most Britons or Americans are thought unlikely to pose a significant threat to micronutrient supply.

4 In recent years, there has been considerable interest in the possible effects that increased intakes of soluble NSP may have in reducing the serum cholesterol concentration. A number of controlled studies have indicated that consumption of relatively large quanti-

ties of oats, which are rich in soluble NSP, can have a significant cholesterol-lowering effect in subjects with either elevated or normal cholesterol levels. The most widely promulgated explanation for this effect is that the soluble NSP binds or chelates both dietary cholesterol and bile acids (produced from cholesterol), and this reduces their absorption or reabsorption in the small intestine and thus increases the rate of faecal cholesterol loss. Most of the considerable quantity of bile acids and cholesterol secreted in the bile each day are reabsorbed and recycled (see enterohepatic recycling of bile acids in Chapter 9); high NSP intake may interfere with this process.

5 High fibre diets tend to be high in starch and low in fat, and thus the energy density of such diets tends to be low. There is a widespread belief that such dietary bulking may contribute to maintaining energy balance and thus to reducing overweight and obesity. Blundell and Burley (1987) review evidence that NSP may also have a satiating effect and thus may be a useful aid to regulating energy balance in those prone to overweight and obesity (another effect of bran proposed by Allinson in the 1880s). It is suggested that this might be because high NSP foods slow eating speed; slow gastric emptying and contribute to feelings of fullness; and, because they slow down the absorption of nutrients and reduce the insulin response to absorbed nutrients. A large insulin response to absorbed nutrients may cause blood glucose concentration to fall below resting levels (the rebound effect), triggering feelings of hunger.

Does dietary fibre/NSP protect against bowel cancer and heart disease?

Bingham (1990) has reviewed the role of NSP in bowel cancer and lists most of the uncited references used here; see also the general review of Halliday and Ashwell (1991).

In the UK, the bowel is the second most common site for cancer in both men (after lung cancer) and women (after breast cancer). Age standardised rates for bowel cancer are even higher in the US than in Britain. There are very large international variations in the incidence of bowel cancer, with generally high rates in Western Europe, Australasia and North America but low rates in, for example, Japan, India, China and rural Africa. As a general rule, populations with high rates of coronary heart disease also tend to have high incidence of bowel cancer. Also as a general rule, high fibre diets tend to be low fat diets and low fibre diets, high fat diets. This means that much of the evidence, to be discussed in Chapter 9, that implicates fat in the aetiology of coronary heart disease could also be used to implicate fat in the aetiology of bowel cancer. Likewise much of the evidence described below linking low fibre diets to increased risk of bowel cancer could equally well be used to implicate high fat diets. This recurring problem of confounding variables that plagues the epidemiologist is once again highlighted.

The recent preoccupation with the possible protective effects of dietary fibre against large bowel diseases, including diverticular disease, appendicitis, haemorrhoids and especially cancer, can be traced back to the work of Burkitt, Trowell, Painter and others in the 1960s and 1970s. These workers noted the rarity of these bowel diseases in rural African populations consuming high-fibre diets and their much greater frequency in populations consuming the "Western" low-fibre diet. Burkitt (1971) suggested that dietary fibre might protect against colonic cancer by diluting potential carcinogens in faeces and speeding their elimination so that the intestine is exposed to them for less time. Human faecal extracts often contain substances that induce mutation in bacteria (mutagens) and such mutagens are known to be likely carcinogens in animals and people. In controlled experimental studies in which animals are exposed to known chemical carcinogens then bran has been consistently reported to reduce the number of tumours; bran appears to protect against these chemically initiated cancers. It has also been suggested that increased fibre intake might reduce the production of mutagens within the bowel, perhaps by changing the metabolism of bile acids within the large bowel. In experimental studies, bran fibre has been reported to reduce the mutagenicity of faeces produced by human subjects. Another proposed mechanism is that the butyric acid produced by bacterial fermentation of NSP and resistant starch in the large bowel might not only act as a substrate for the mucosal cells of the intestine but might also regulate cell division and thus directly inhibit their differentiation and proliferation into cancerous tumours.

There is a general trend for populations with high-fibre intakes to have low rates of bowel cancer but the negative relationship between fibre intake and incidence of bowel cancer is very sharply reduced when this relationship is corrected for differences in fat and meat consumption. The factors correlating most strongly and positively with rates of bowel cancer are meat consumption and animal fat consumption. Time trends within the Japanese population whose diet has shifted very much towards the Western pattern over the last 30 years show that this has been accompanied by major increases in the incidence of colon cancer (doubled since

1960). During this period there has been no significant change in overall fibre intakes but major increases in consumption of meat, dairy produce and wheat as well as a large decrease in rice consumption. Note, however, that, although fibre intakes of the Japanese may not have changed over this period, there has been a very substantial decline in the proportion of calories derived from starch and most of the functional NSP in white rice is resistant starch. Measures of the fibre intake that have taken no account of residual starch may thus be misleading. The reduction in the amount of carbohydrate in the Japanese diet over this period has been offset by increased fat consumption; consumption of animal fat has more than doubled over this period.

Migrations studies, together with these time trends for populations like the Japanese, clearly indicate the predominance of environmental factors in the aetiology of bowel cancer. The international differences in prevalence of this disease are largely due to environmental influences, probably dietary influences, rather than genetic differences between the races concerned.

Vegetarian groups, like Seventh Day Adventists in the USA, have lower rates of bowel cancer than other Americans and higher intakes of dietary NSP. Once again low meat and fat intakes or even high intakes of antioxidant vitamins in fruits and vegetables make it impossible to finally attribute these low cancer rates to a direct protective effect of dietary NSP.

According to Bingham (1990) a large majority of case-control studies indicate that cases of bowel cancer ate less vegetable fibre than controls. According to Willett *et al.* (1990) most case-control studies also indicate a significant positive association between total fat intake and bowel cancer. The limitations of case-control studies have been discussed in Chapter 3. As Bingham points out, diseases of the large bowel produce pain and altered bowel function. So, one of the

effects of bowel disease may be to make patients change their diets in order to avoid the symptoms; the low-fibre intakes of the cases in these case-control studies might be a consequence of the disease rather than an indication of its cause.

Willett *et al.* (1990) have reported results from a six year follow-up using a cohort of almost 90 000 American nurses. They found no significant association between total fibre intake and risk of developing colon cancer over the six year period. They also found no significant associations when they used subdivisions of the fibre from different food sources, i.e. vegetable, fruit or cereal fibre (although there was a non significant trend with fruit fibre). They did find significant positive associations between total fat intake and colon cancer risk and an even stronger association with animal fat intake (illustrated in Chapter 3 Figure 3.9); "red meat" (beef, pork and lamb) consumption was also positively associated with bowel cancer risk. They confirmed the expected negative association between fibre intake and animal fat intake in their population; this perhaps explains the apparent contradiction between these results and the fibre results from case-control studies. Their results provide rather weak support for the proposition that low intakes of fruit fibre might contribute to the risk of colon cancer but much stronger evidence in favour of the proposition that high animal fat intake is linked to increased risk of colon cancer. It should nonetheless be borne in mind that, despite the apparently very large sample size, the analysis is based upon only 150 total cases and only 103 cases when those developing cancer within the first two years of follow-up were excluded.

Other cohort studies amongst Seventh Day Adventists in California and 265 000 Japanese gave some indications of lower fibre and vegetable intakes in those later developing bowel cancer (Bingham, 1990)

The overall conclusion from the current evidence is that there is strong support for the proposition that a diet higher in fibre/NSP containing foods (cereals, vegetables and fruit) will reduce the incidence of bowel cancer in countries like the UK and US. Such dietary change would be consistent with the nutrition education guidelines in both the UK and US. Such a diet would not only have more fibre than current US and UK diets but would also have less fat, less animal fat, more starch and more antioxidant vitamins. The evidence supporting a direct protective effect of dietary fibre, or any individual component of the non-starch polysaccharides, is much weaker than the evidence supporting this more generalised change. The current evidence may be interpreted in several ways, for example:

- that high dietary NSP/fibre directly protects against bowel cancer
- that high dietary fat/animal fat promotes bowel cancer and thus that any apparent protective effect of high intake of complex carbohydrates is an artefact due to the inverse relationship between fat and complex carbohydrate intakes
- that NSP protects against the cancer promoting effects of high dietary fat in the bowel.

A very similar conclusion could be made about the possible relationship between NSP intakes and coronary heart disease – the evidence supporting the beneficial effects of dietary changes that would increase NSP intake are very much stronger than the evidence for a direct link between NSP intake and coronary heart disease. Possible mechanisms by which NSP might have a specific influence on coronary heart disease risk are:

- lowering the serum cholesterol concentration by interfering with the enterohepatic recycling of cholesterol and bile acids
- improving glucose tolerance and reducing insulin secretion (diabetes greatly increases the risk of coronary heart disease)
- indirectly, by lowering the energy density of the diet and thus reducing the risk of obesity.

These conclusions mean that the consumption of more foods naturally rich in complex carbohydrates has a much higher probability of reducing the risk of these diseases than adding extracted fibre to foods or the use of foods in which the fibre content has been greatly "amplified" by food manufacturers.

8 Protein and amino acids

Contents

Traditional scientific aspects of protein nutrition

Introduction

Experiments stretching back over the last two centuries have demonstrated the principle that all animals require an exogenous supply of protein. In humans, and in other non-ruminating mammals, these must be present in the food that they eat. For example, when dogs were fed experimental diets devoid of nitrogen-containing foods, they lost weight and their muscles wasted, and they recovered when nitrogen-containing foods were added back to their diets. Adequate amounts of nitrogen-containing foods were shown to be essential to allow growth in experimental animals. Such experiments demonstrated the need for nitrogen-containing foods (i.e. protein) even before the chemical nature of dietary protein was known.

Chemistry and digestion

Protein is the only major nitrogen containing component of the diet; it is composed of chains of up to 20 different **amino acids** that are linked together by **peptide bonds**. Figure 8.1 illustrates the chemical nature of amino acids and proteins. The amino acid side chain (the R group in Figure 8.1, which is on the next page) is the group that varies between amino acids; some examples of the R groups in particular amino acids are shown in Figure 8.1. The way in which amino acids are linked together by peptide bonds is also illustrated; the nitrogen atom in the **amino group** of one amino acid is linked to the carbon atom of the **carboxyl group** in the adjacent amino acid. A protein may be comprised of hundreds of amino acids linked together in this way; each protein will have a free amino group at one end (the **N-terminal**) and a free carboxyl group at the opposite end (the **C-terminal**).

Dietary proteins are digested to their constituent amino acids prior to absorption in the small intestine; some dipeptides and other very small peptide fragments may also be absorbed. **Protease** and **peptidase** enzymes in gastric and pancreatic juice break (hydrolyse) the peptide bonds between specific amino acids in dietary proteins yielding small peptides, dipeptides and free amino acids. The digestion of these small protein fragments is continued by peptidase enzymes located on the mucosal surface of the small intestine.

Figure 8.1 The chemical nature of proteins and amino acids

Generalised chemical formula of amino acids

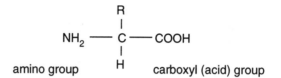

amino group $\qquad$ carboxyl (acid) group

Examples of amino acid side chains

R = H   amino acid = glycine
R = CH$_3$ amino acid = alanine
R = CH$_2$SH   amino acid = cysteine
R = (CH$_2$)$_4$NH$_2$ amino acid = lysine
R = CH$_2$OH   amino acid = serine

Two amino acids linked by a peptide bond

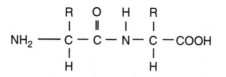

Diagramatic representation of a protein

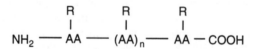

N-terminal   C-terminal

Protein quality

The observation that all proteins contain approximately 16% by weight of nitrogen (see Chapter 3) enabled early workers to determine the protein contents of diets and thus to match diets for protein content by matching them for nitrogen content. Using such nitrogen-matched diets, it soon became clear that all proteins were not of equal nutritional value, i.e. that both the amount and the quality of protein in different foods was variable. For example, pigs fed on diets based upon lentil protein grew faster than those fed barley-based diets even though the diets were matched in terms of their nitrogen content and thus also their crude protein content; lentil protein was apparently of higher nutritional quality than barley protein.

Essential amino acids

It is now known that the quality differences between individual proteins arise because of variations in their content of certain of the amino acids. In order to synthesise body protein, an animal or person must have all 20 amino acids available. If one or more amino acids is unavailable, or in short supply, then the ability to synthesise protein is generally compromised irrespective of the supply of the others. Proteins cannot be synthesised, leaving gaps or using substitutes for the deficient amino acids. Each body protein is synthesised with a genetically-determined and unalterable, precise sequence of particular amino acids.

About half of the amino acids have carbon skeletons that can be synthesised by people and these amino acids can therefore be synthesised by transferring amino groups from other surplus amino acids, **transamination** (see Chapter 5). The remaining amino acids have carbon skeletons that cannot be synthesised by people and they cannot, therefore, be made by transamination – these are termed the **essential amino acids** and have to be obtained pre-formed from the diet. The protein gelatine, lacks the essential amino acid tryptophan and so dogs fed on gelatine, as their sole nitrogen source, exhibit symptoms similar to those of dogs fed on a protein-free diet. Despite a surplus of the other amino acids, the dog cannot utilise them for protein synthesis because one amino acid is unavailable. Under these circumstances, the amino acids in the gelatine will be used as an energy source and their nitrogen excreted as urea. The essential amino acids in humans are:

- histidine (in children)
- isoleucine
- leucine
- lysine
- methionine
- phenylalanine
- threonine
- tryptophan
- valine.

The amino acids cysteine and tyrosine are classified as non-essential even though their carbon skeletons cannot be synthesised. This is because they can be made from methionine and phenylalanine respectively.

Establishing the essential amino acids and quantifying requirements

Rats have been shown to grow normally if synthetic mixtures of the 20 amino acids are given as their sole source of dietary protein. Growth is not affected if one of the non essential amino acids is left out of the mixture because the rats are able to produce this missing amino acid endogenously by transamination. Growth ceases, however, if one of the essential ones is left out. In this way the essential amino acids for the rat have been identified and the amount of each one that is required to allow normal growth has also been determined.

Such experiments with children were ruled out on ethical grounds. However, adults have been shown to maintain nitrogen balance (i.e. protein balance, see below) if fed mixtures of the 20 amino acids, and like the rats, adults can cope with removal of certain amino acids and still maintain this balance; these are the non-essential amino acids. When one of the essential amino acids is left out, then there is a net loss of body nitrogen, i.e. a depletion of body protein. The requirement for each of the essential amino acids has been estimated from the minimum amount necessary to maintain body protein content and prevent net loss of body nitrogen when the others are present in excess. The range and relative needs of the essential amino acids in rats and people are found to be similar, and the rat has been widely used as a model for humans in biological assessments of protein quality.

Limiting amino acid

In any given dietary protein, one of the essential amino acids will be present in the lowest amount relative to human requirements, i.e. a given amount of the protein will contain a lower proportion of the requirement for this essential amino acid than for any of the others. The availability of this amino will "limit" the extent to which the others can be utilised if that particular protein is fed alone and in amounts that do not fully supply the needs for the amino acid. This amino acid is called the **limiting amino acid**. The amino acid is limiting because, if supplies of this essential amino acid are insufficient, then the use of the others for protein synthesis will be limited by its availability – protein cannot be made leaving gaps where this missing amino acid should be. For example, if only half of the requirement for the limiting amino acid is supplied then, in effect, only about half of the protein requirement is being supplied; surpluses of the others will be used as energy sources and their nitrogen excreted. In many cereals the limiting amino acid is lysine, in maize it is tryptophan and in beef and milk it is the sulphur

containing amino acids; one of these three is the limiting amino acid in most dietary proteins. In the past, lysine-supplementation of cereal-based diets or developing "high lysine" strains of cereals has been widely advocated, and sometimes used, as means of improving the protein quality of diets based upon cereals.

Complete and incomplete proteins

Whatever measure of protein quality is used, the proteins of animal origin have high values. Meat, fish, egg and milk proteins contain all of the essential amino acids in good quantities; they have been termed first class proteins or **complete proteins**. Many proteins of vegetable origin, however, have low measured quality; this is true of many staple cereals and starchy roots; they have been termed second class or **incomplete proteins** because they have a relatively low amount of one or more of the essential amino acids. Pulses (peas and beans) are a major exception to this general rule and have good amounts of high quality protein. Some examples of the relative quality values of common dietary proteins are shown in Table 8.1.

Mutual supplementation of protein

In human nutrition, and certainly in affluent countries, this concept of a limiting amino acid producing large variations in protein quality may have limited practical

Table 8.1 The relative qualities of some proteins commonly found in human diets as illustrated by their Net Protein Utilisation (NPU) values. Data source: Passmore and Eastwood, 1986

Food	NPU (%)
Maize	36
Millet	43
Wheat	49
Rice	63
Soya	67
Cow milk	81
Egg	87
Human milk	94

relevance. First, because the human requirement for protein is low, both in comparison to other species and also in comparison to the protein content of many dietary staples. Secondly, because affluent people seldom eat just single proteins, rather they eat diets containing mixtures of several different proteins.

The probability is that the different proteins consumed over a period of time will have differing limiting amino acids, and thus any deficiency of one will be compensated for by a relative surplus of that amino acid in another. Thus the quality of the total protein in different human diets will tend to equalise even though the nature and quality of the individual proteins in those diets may vary very considerably. This is called **mutual supplementation of proteins** and it means that any measure of protein quality of mixed human diets, as opposed to individual proteins, tends to yield a fairly consistent value.

Measurement of protein quality

The simplest method of assessing the quality of a protein is to chemically compare its limiting amino acid content with that of a high quality reference protein; this is called the **chemical score**. Egg protein has traditionally been used as the reference protein in human nutrition. In the protein under test, the limiting amino acid is identified and the amount of this amino acid in a gram of test protein is expressed as a percentage of that found in a gram of egg protein.

Chemical score =

$$\frac{\text{mg limiting amino acid/gram of test protein}}{\text{mg this amino acid/gram of egg protein}} \times 100$$

This chemical score does not necessarily give an accurate guide to the biological availability of the amino acids in the protein. Thus, for example, if a protein is poorly digested, then the chemical score could greatly overestimate the real biological quality of the protein.

Net protein utilisation (NPU) is a widely used biological measure of protein quality; it is a particularly important measure in agricultural nutrition but is nowadays considered to be of much less significance in human nutrition. To measure NPU the protein to be tested is fed to an animal (or person) as the sole nitrogen source at a level below the minimum requirement for growth or balance. The amount of nitrogen retained under these circumstances is corrected for the nitrogen losses that occur even on a protein-free diet, and then this figure is expressed as a percentage of the intake.

$$\text{NPU} = \frac{\text{amount of retained nitrogen}}{\text{nitrogen intake}} \times 100$$

Retained nitrogen =
intake − (loss − loss on protein-free diet)

The NPU values for some proteins were shown in Table 8.1. The NPU of diets as well as those of individual proteins may be determined, and because of the mutual supplementation effect, the NPU of most human diets comes out within a relatively narrow range even though the qualities of the individual constituent proteins may vary widely. An NPU of around 60–70 would be typical of many human diets and would be largely unaffected by, for instance, the proportion of animal protein in the diet. The NPU is only likely to be of significance in human nutrition if a single staple with low amounts of poor quality protein makes up the bulk of the diet and is the source of most of the dietary protein.

Nitrogen balance

The concept

Intakes and losses of nitrogen are used as the measure of protein intake and protein breakdown respectively; the difference between intake and total losses is the **nitrogen balance**. Thus:

nitrogen balance =
          nitrogen input – nitrogen losses

The nitrogen input is from food protein. Nitrogen losses arise from the breakdown of dietary and endogenous protein; most of these losses are in the urine but with small amounts also lost in faeces and via the skin.

Negative nitrogen balance

A negative balance indicates that body protein is being depleted. Injury, illness, starvation (including dieting) or inadequate protein intake *per se* may lead to negative nitrogen balance. The minimum amount of protein, in an otherwise complete diet, that enables an adult to achieve balance indicates the minimum requirement for protein. A deficit in energy supplies would be expected to lead to negative nitrogen balance for two reasons:

- because a diet that is inadequate in energy will also tend to have a low protein content
- because under conditions of energy deficit, the protein that is present will tend to be used as an energy source rather than being used for protein synthesis.

Requirements for balance

Adults who are put onto a protein-free, but otherwise complete diet, excrete a low and relatively constant amount of nitrogen after the first few days – this is termed the **obligatory nitrogen loss** and represents the minimum replacement requirement. Studies using radioactively labelled amino acids indicate that around 300 g of protein is broken down and re-synthesised in the body each day – the **protein turnover**. Under these circumstances, most of the amino acids released during the breakdown of body protein re-enter the body amino acid pool and are ultimately re-cycled into new protein

synthesis, but a proportion (say 10%) are not re-used and become the obligatory nitrogen loss. Several amino acids have additional functions to that of protein building and are irreversibly lost from the body amino acid pool, e.g. for synthesis of non-protein substances such as pigments or transmitters and for conjugation with substances to facilitate their excretion. When amino acids are lost from the pool for such reasons, then some other amino acids have to be catabolised to retain the balance of the body's pool of amino acids. Some protein will be also lost as hair, skin, sloughed epithelial cells and mucus, etc. Such obligatory losses explain why adults have a requirement for dietary protein even though their total body protein content remains constant.

Positive nitrogen balance

A positive nitrogen balance indicates a net accumulation of body protein. Healthy adults do not go into positive nitrogen balance if dietary protein intake is stepped up. Instead they utilise the excess protein as an energy source and excrete the associated nitrogen as urea. Growing children would be expected to be in positive nitrogen balance, as would pregnant women, those recovering after illness, injury or starvation, and those actively accumulating extra muscle, such as body builders. It would be reasonable to expect these groups, particularly rapidly growing children, to have a relatively higher protein requirement than other adults, i.e. they would be expected to require more protein per kilogramme of body weight. Note also the extra requirement for the synthesis of milk protein in lactating women.

Dietary adequacy for protein

Table 8.2 shows some of the current UK Reference Nutrient Intakes for protein; in addition to the absolute values, the RNI is also calculated as a percentage of the Estimated Average Requirement for energy. To put these values into context, the average UK diet currently contains around 14-15% of the energy as protein (Gregory *et al.*, 1990). This suggests that primary protein deficiency is highly improbable in the UK and indeed in other industrialised countries.

To give these values in Table 8.2 an international perspective, rice has around 8% of energy as protein and hard wheat around 17%; the other major cereal staples lie between these two extremes; only finger millet (*Eleusine corocana*) is below this range (7%). Some starchy roots, which are important staples, do fall substantially below this range for cereals, for example:

cassava   3%
plantains (cooked bananas) 4%
yam   7%
sweet potato   4%.

Table 8.2 Some UK Reference Nutrient Intakes (RNIs) for protein. Values are expressed both in absolute terms and as a percentage of the Estimated Average Requirement (EAR) for energy. Data source: COMA (1991)

Age (years)	RNI g/day	% energy
1–3	14.5	4.7
7–10	28.3	5.7
male		
11–14	42.1	7.7
19–50	55.5	8.7
65–74	53.3	9.2
female		
11–14	41.2	8.9
19–50	45.0	9.3
pregnancy	+6	9.5–10.5*
lactation	+11	8.9–9.4*

* varies as energy EAR varies during pregnancy and lactation

Table 8.3 shows the protein content of some common British foods. A comparison of these values with those in Table 8.2 suggests that people meeting their energy needs and eating a mixed diet, even a mixed vegetarian diet, would seem to run

Table 8.3 The protein content of some British foods expressed both in absolute terms and as a percentage of energy. Values are generally for raw food. Data source: Paul and Southgate (1979)

Food	g protein/ 100 g food	protein (% energy)
Whole milk	3.3	20.3
Skimmed milk	3.4	41.2
Cheddar cheese	26.0	25.6
Human milk	1.3	7.5
Egg	12.3	33.5
Wholemeal bread	8.8	16.3
Sweetcorn	4.1	12.9
Cornflakes	8.6	9.3
Beef (lean)	20.3	66.0
Pork (lean)	20.7	56.3
Chicken (meat)	20.5	67.8
Cod	17.4	91.6
Herring	16.8	28.7
Shrimps	23.8	81.4
Peas	5.8	34.6
Broad beans	4.1	34.2
Baked beans (tin)	5.1	31.0
Lentils	23.8	31.3
Potatoes	2.1	9.7
Mushrooms	1.8	55.4
Broccoli	3.3	57.4
Carrots	0.7	12.2
Peanuts	24.3	17.1
Peanut butter	22.4	14.5
Almonds	16.9	12.0
Apple	0.3	2.6
Banana	1.1	5.6
Orange	0.8	9.1
Dried dates	2.0	3.2

little practical risk of protein deficiency. This is generally true even though fats, oils, alcoholic drinks, soft drinks and sugar-based snacks contain little or no protein and will thus tend to have a diluting effects reducing the proportion of total calories that are derived from protein.

The significance of protein in human nutrition?

Introduction

The change in attitude to protein deficiency as a suspected key cause of human malnutrition represents perhaps the single most striking change in human nutrition over the last 50 years.

The author has previously reviewed this topic (Webb, 1989) and this discussion is a development of that review; it is recommended as a case-study to illustrate a number of important general points discussed earlier in the book:

1 the potential costs of premature and ineffective "health promotion" intervention; these costs may be very real and substantial even if an unhelpful intervention does not do direct physiological harm (Chapter 1)
2 the potential dangers of overestimating dietary standards by "erring on the safe side" (Chapter 3)
3 the dangers of hasty and ill-considered extrapolation of results obtained in animal experiments to people (Chapter 3).

Most of the uncited references used for this discussion are listed in Webb (1989).

Historical overview

For more than two decades (the 1950s and the 1960s) the belief that primary protein deficiency was "the most serious and widespread dietary deficiency in the world" (Waterlow *et al.*, 1960) dominated nutrition research and education. The consensus of nutrition opinion considered it likely that "in many parts of the world the majority of young children suffered some protein malnutrition" (Trowell, 1956). The relative protein requirements of young children compared to adults were generally considered to be very high, perhaps five times higher on a weight-for-weight basis. Even where diets contained apparently adequate amounts of total protein it was believed that protein availability might still be inadequate unless some high quality protein (usually animal) was taken with each meal. Calculations of the amount of protein required by the world population when compared with estimates of protein availability gave the impression of a large and increasing shortfall in world protein supplies – **the protein gap.** Jones (1974) suggested that an extra 20 million tons of protein were required each year; this figure implied that many hundreds of millions of people were protein deficient. This protein gap was so large that a whole new field of research was initiated to try and close it – the mass production of protein from novel sources such as leaves and microbes. An agency of the United Nations "The Protein Advisory Group" was set up specifically to oversee these developments. As late as 1972 the chairman's opening address to an international scientific conference contained the following statements:

- Every doctor, nutritionist or political leader concerned with the problem of world hunger, has now concluded that the major problem is one of protein malnutrition.
- The calorie supply (of developing countries) tends to be more or less satisfactory, but what is lacking is protein, and especially protein containing the essential amino acids.

Gounelle de Pontanel, 1972.

As estimates of human protein requirements were revised downwards, this protein gap disappeared "at the stroke of a pen" with no significant change in protein supplies. The above quotations from Gounelle de Pontanel contrast very sharply with the conclusions of Miller and Payne (1969): that almost all dietary staples contain sufficient protein to meet human needs and that even diets based upon very low protein staples are unlikely to be specifically protein deficient. In the 25 years since 1969 this view has become the nutritional consensus. Despite this revolutionary change of mind, the greatly reduced emphasis on protein in human nutrition has been slow to permeate beyond the ranks of the specialists. Even amongst nutrition educators there may still be some ambivalence towards protein; these quotations from a well-respected American nutrition text seem to sum up that ambivalence:

- *Most people* in the United States and Canada would find it *almost impossible* not to meet their protein requirements.
- Protein is at the heart of a good diet. Menu planners build their meals around the RDA for protein. (Hamilton *et al.*, 1991).

This exaggerated importance attached to protein in the past led to a huge concentration of research effort, physical resources, educational effort and political priority into protein nutrition and into efforts to close the protein gap. It now seems almost certain that much of this effort was wasted; directed towards solving an illusory problem. McClaren (1974) and Webb (1989) have discussed some of these costs of exaggerating human protein needs, and McClaren was moved to entitle his article "The great protein fiasco".

Origins of the "protein gap"

Three assumptions seem to have been critical in creating the illusion of a massive world protein shortage:

1 that children required a high protein concentration in their diets, i.e. that the proportion of total dietary energy derived from protein should be substantially higher for children than in adults
2 that the nutritional disease known as **kwashiorkor** was due to primary protein deficiency, i.e. due to a diet in which the proportion of energy derived from protein was too low
3 that this nutritional disease kwashiorkor was the most prevalent form of worldwide malnutrition and yet these cases of frank clinical kwashiorkor were thought to represent only the "tip of the iceberg" with many more children impaired to some extent by lack of protein.

There are now good grounds for suggesting that each of these three assumptions is either dubious or improbable.

Past exaggeration of protein requirements?

Figure 8.2 illustrates the changes in the American RDAs for protein over the past 50 years; in 1943, the protein RDA for a two-year-old child was substantially more than double its current value (also more than double the current UK RNI). When expressed as a proportion of the energy allowance, the child's protein RDA was well above the adult value in 1943 but is now well below the adult value. The current value suggests that children can manage on a lower minimum concentration of protein in their diets than adults. This conclusion seems at first sight to be inconsistent with the notion that growing children have higher relative protein needs than adults. It has always been, and still is assumed that children need more protein on a weight-for-weight basis than do adults, only the assumed scale of this difference has declined. In the past, figures of up to five times higher weight-for-weight requirements in children have been suggested (e.g. Waterlow *et al.*, 1960), nowadays a figure of around double is considered more reasonable. Table 8.4 shows why this higher relative requirement is not inconsistent with need for a lower dietary protein concentration, as suggested by Figure 8.2. Children not only require relatively more protein than adults but also more energy. Table 8.4 on

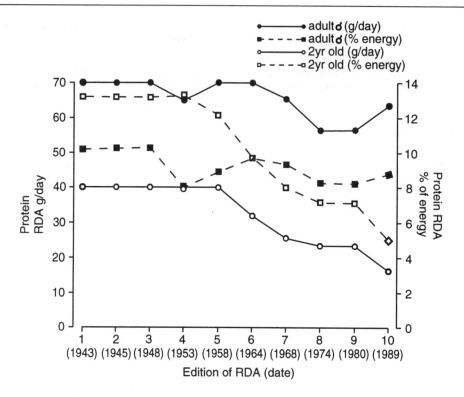

Figure 8.2 Changes in the American RDA for protein for an adult man and a two-year-old child over ten editions (1943–1989). Expressed both in absolute terms (g/day) and as a percentage of the energy RDA
Source: Webb, G.P. (1994) *Journal of Biological Education* 28(1), 104

page 175 shows the current UK RNIs for protein and the EARs for energy expressed per kilogramme of body weight. A two-year-old child requires almost three times as much energy as an adult on a weight-for-weight basis but only about one-and-a-half times as much protein. Therefore, the need for increased energy or increased total food intake is far greater than the increased relative need for protein. For all ages of children the increased energy need cancels out or, in most cases, greatly exceeds the increased need for protein.

Inappropriate extrapolation from animal experiments to humans may have been a factor in encouraging the early inflated estimates of protein requirements in children. Primates have slower growth rates than most animals and much lower rates than most common laboratory animals (see Table 8.5, which is on the next page). The relative protein requirements of these rapidly growing species are thus likely to be higher than those of human infants and children, and this seems to be borne out by the comparison of milk composition of the species shown in Table 8.5. Up to 80% of the nitrogen requirements of a growing rat are for growth (Altschul, 1965); this perhaps gives some hint of the origin of the belief that a child's relative protein requirements was up to five times that of an adult. As four-fifths of the requirement of young rats is for growth and only one-fifth for maintenance, then, by direct analogy, it might well suggest a five-fold difference in the requirements of children (for growth and maintenance) compared to those of adults (for maintenance only).

Table 8.4 Selected EARs for energy and RNIs for protein expressed per kg body weight and as a percentage of the adult value. Data source: COMA, 1991

Age	Energy EAR		Protein RNI	
	kcal/kg (kJ/kg)	% adult value	g/kg	% adult value
0–3 months	92 (385)	271	2.12	287
4–6 months	90 (377)	265	1.65	220
7–9 months	93 (389)	274	1.54	205
10–12 months	94 (394)	276	1.52	203
1–3 years	98 (410)	288	1.15	153
4–6 years	96 (402)	282	1.11	148
7–10 years	70 (293)	206	1.00	133
11–14 years	52 (218)	153	0.98	131
15–18 years	43 (180)	126	0.86	115
19–50 years	34 (142)	100	0.75	100
75+ years	30 (126)	88	0.75	100

Animal experiments also probably played their part in exaggerating the importance of low protein quality as a practical problem in human nutrition. When a diet containing 10% egg protein as the sole nitrogen source is fed to growing rats under test conditions, then one gram of egg protein will bring about an increase in weight of 3.8 grams in the animals – egg protein has a **protein efficiency ratio** of 3.8. Around 80% of the consumed protein is retained as body protein. Wheat protein has a protein efficiency ratio of only 1 and just 20% of the wheat protein would be retained as body protein (Altschul, 1965). Such demonstrations of the apparently very low quality of many cereal and vegetable proteins would have encouraged the view that, unless some high-quality protein was present, then protein deficiency would have seemed almost inevitable – 4 grams of wheat protein is only equivalent to 1 gram of egg protein in growing rats. Of course, most human diets are mixtures of proteins and mutual supplementation can occur. It was for some time thought, however, that this mutual supplementation could only occur within a meal, but it is now thought that such supplementation can occur over an extended time-scale. If a meal lacking in one amino acid is consumed, then the

Table 8.5 Growth rates and milk composition of seven species

Species	Double birth weight (d)	Protein in milk (g/l)	Milk energy (kcal/l)	Energy as protein (%)
Man	120–180	1.1	710	6
Calf	47	3.2	660	19
Sheep	10	6.5	1090	24
Cat	7	10.6	1570	27
Rat	6	8.1	1290	25
Mouse	5	9.0	1690	21
Chimp	100	1.2	670	7

Source: Webb, G.P. (1989) *Journal of Biological Education* 23(2), 121

liver will donate the deficient amino acid to allow protein synthesis to continue and will replenish its complement of this amino acid at a later meal. This makes it rather unlikely that protein deficiency will occur due to unbalanced amino acid composition except under very particular conditions.

Low concentration of dietary protein causes kwashiorkor?

The nutritional disease kwashiorkor was first described in the medical literature in the 1930s and a very tentative suggestion was made at that time that it might be due to dietary protein deficiency. Over the next 35 years it became generally accepted that two diseases known as kwashiorkor and **marasmus** represented different clinical manifestations of malnutrition in children, with differing aetiologies. Marasmus was attributed to simple energy deficit (starvation) whereas kwashiorkor was attributed to primary protein deficiency. The marasmic child is severely wasted and stunted and the clinical picture is generally consistent with what might be expected in simple starvation. Several of the clinical features of kwashiorkor, however, are not superficially consistent with simple starvation but are consistent with protein deficiency (see Table 8.6). Many children suffer from a mixture of these two diseases and the two conditions were thus said to represent opposite extremes of a spectrum of diseases with the precise clinical picture depending on the precise levels of protein and energy deficit. The general term **Protein-Energy Malnutrition (PEM)** was used to describe this spectrum of diseases.

A number of studies over the last 25 years have seriously challenged this assumption that kwashiorkor is necessarily due to primary protein deficiency. Comparisons of the diets of children developing kwashiorkor or marasmus have reported no difference in their protein concentrations. Detailed analyses of the diets of children in the Third World have indicated that primary deficiency of protein is uncommon and that protein deficiency is usually a secondary consequence of low total food intake. The symptoms of kwashiorkor listed in Table 8.6 are nonetheless persuasively consistent with protein deficiency rather than energy deficit. Acute shortage of energy would, however, lead to use of protein as an energy source. Thus dietary energy deficit could well precipitate a physiological deficit of amino acids for protein synthesis and to fulfil other amino acid functions. Symptoms of protein deficiency might be triggered by energy deficit. Why starvation should sometimes result in marasmus and sometimes kwashiorkor is, as yet, still unclear.

Table 8.6 Some clinical features of kwashiorkor that are consistent with primary protein deficiency

Symptom	Rationale
Oedema – excess tissue fluid	lack of plasma proteins?
Hepatomegaly – liver swollen with fat	lack of protein to transport fat?
"Flaky paint syndrome" depigmented and peeling skin	lack of amino acids for skin protein and pigment production?
Mental changes - anorexia and apathy	lack of amino acids for transmitter synthesis?
Subcutaneous fat still present	inconsistent with simple energy deficit?
Changes in colour and texture of hair	similar causes to skin changes?

Kwashiorkor – the most common nutritional disease in the world?

McClaren (1974) suggested that the widespread assumption that kwashiorkor was the most prevalent manifestation of Protein Energy Malnutrition was caused by faulty extrapolation from a World Health Organisation survey of rural Africa in 1952. This survey did indeed find kwashiorkor to be the most prevalent form of PEM in this region, but the assumption that this was an accurate reflection of the worldwide pattern is now thought to be false.

Concluding remarks

Over the last 50 years, opinions as to the significance of protein in human nutrition have undergone some dramatic changes. For a time, protein adequacy was top of the list of international nutritional priorities. Nowadays primary protein deficiency is generally considered to be a relatively uncommon occurrence, not because of an improved supply, but rather because of a change of nutritional opinion. In the current editions of both the UK and US dietary standards (COMA, 1991 and NRC, 1989a) there are concerns voiced about the possible health risks of high protein intakes. Both of the panels suggest that it would be prudent to regard a value of twice the RNI/RDA as the safe upper limit for protein intake.

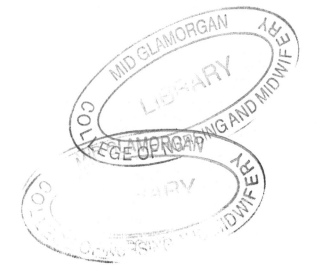

9 Fat

Contents

Nature of dietary fat

Dietary fats and oils are largely in the form of **triglyceride**; this is also the principal form in which fat is stored in the body. Triglyceride is composed of three **fatty acids** attached to the simple molecule glycerol; the three fatty acids in any triglyceride may be the same or different. A triglyceride molecule is represented diagrammatically in Figure 9.1a.

If the third fatty acid in Figure 9.1a is replaced by a phosphate containing moiety then this produces the family of compounds known as **phospholipids**.

Types of fatty acids

Fatty acids are of three major types – **saturated, monounsaturated** and **polyunsaturated**.

Saturated fatty acids

Carbon atoms have the potential to each form four bonds (i.e. they are tetravalent). In saturated fatty acids there is a variable-length chain of carbon atoms with an acid (carboxyl) group at one end; the carbon atoms in the chain are all joined together by single bonds, and all of the remaining bonds of the carbon atoms are occupied by bonding to hydrogen atoms as shown in Figure 9.1b. These fatty acids are termed saturated because all of the available bonds or valencies of the carbon atoms are occupied or "saturated" with hydrogen atoms.

The chemical structure of fatty acids is often represented schematically as shown in Figure 9.1c. Each angle represents a carbon atom, and the carbon atoms are numbered starting with the carbon furthest away from the carboxyl or acid

a) Schematic representation of a triglyceride molecule

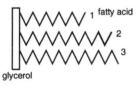

b) General chemical formula of a saturated fatty acid

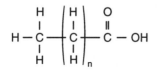

c) Diagramatic representation of a saturated fatty acid (palmitic acid – 16:0)

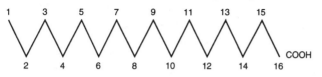

d) Diagramatic representation of a monounsaturated fatty acid (oleic acid – 18:1$_{\omega}$9)

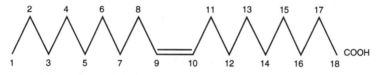

e) Diagrammatic representation of linoleic acid (18:2$_{\omega}$6)

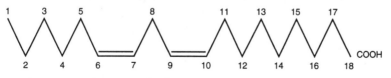

f) Diagramatic representation of eicosapentaenoic acid EPA (20:5$_{\omega}$3)

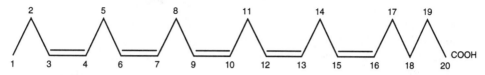

g) Diagram to illustrate the *cis* and *trans* configurations of unsaturated fatty acids

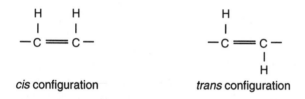

Figure 9.1 The chemical nature of fats

group. The fatty acid depicted in this diagram is called palmitic acid – it has 16 carbon atoms and no double bonds and therefore it can be written in shorthand notation as 16:0.

Monounsaturated fatty acids

These are fatty acids with a single point of unsaturation: two of the carbons in the chain are joined together by a double bond and thus there are two fewer bonds available to bond with hydrogen atoms than would be true in a saturated fatty acid of the same length. Oleic acid is depicted in Figure 9.1d; it is an 18 carbon monounsaturated fatty acid that is widely found in nature in both animals and plants (it is the principal acid in olive oil). The double bond in oleic acid is between carbons 9 and 10 in the sequence – the shorthand notation for this acid is $18:1_{\omega 9}$ (i.e. 18 carbons; 1 double bond; and, omega-9, the double bond is between carbons 9 and 10).

Polyunsaturated fatty acids

These are fatty acids that have two or more double bonds in the carbon chain i.e. they have more than one point of unsaturation. Figure 9.1e shows linoleic acid, this has 18 carbons, two double bonds and the first of these double bonds is between carbons 6 and 7 and thus its shorthand notation is $18:2_{\omega 6}$. Knowing the position of the first double bond makes it possible to predict the position of any further double bonds because they are normally separated by a single saturated carbon atom (i.e. are methylene interrupted). In linoleic acid, the first double bond is between carbons 6 and 7, carbon 8 is saturated and the second double bond lies between carbons 9 and 10. To give a slightly more complex example, eicosapentaenoic acid (EPA) has 20 carbons, 5 double bonds and the first double bond is between carbons 3 and 4; hence its shorthand notation is $20:5_{\omega 3}$;

in EPA, the second double bond is between carbons 6 and 7, the third between 9 and 10, the fourth between 12 and 13 and the fifth between 15 and 16 as shown in Figure 9.1f.

Cis/trans isomerisation

Different positional isomers as shown in Figure 9.1g are possible wherever a fatty acid has a double bond; either both hydrogen atoms can be on the same side, the *cis* form, or the hydrogen atoms can be on opposite sides, the *trans* form. Most naturally occurring fats contain almost exclusively *cis* isomers although small amounts of **trans fatty acids** are found in butter and other fats from ruminating animals.

It is possible to convert any unsaturated fatty acid into a saturated one through reaction with hydrogen in the presence of an activating agent or catalyst. This process is called hydrogenation and is used in the production of margarines and solid vegetable shortening, i.e. **hydrogenated vegetable oils** (or hydrogenated fish oil). The process of hydrogenation can result in the production of relatively large amounts of *trans* fatty acids in the final product, particularly in the cheaper, "hard" margarines in the UK.

Distribution of fatty acid types in dietary fat

All fat sources contain mixtures of the three types of fatty acid but the proportions vary considerably from fat to fat. Table 9.1 shows the variation in proportion of saturates, monounsaturates and polyunsaturates in eight types of fat.

The two animal fats in Table 9.1 are both high in saturates and low in polyunsaturates – this is generally true for fat from farm animals. Fat from ruminating animals (e.g. milk, beef and lamb) is the most saturated and the least amenable to manipulation by alterations in the diet

Table 9.1 Typical proportions(%) of saturated (S) monounsaturated (M) and polyunsaturated (P) fatty acids in different types of fat. Calculated from: Paul and Southgate (1979)

Fat	%S	%M	%P	P:S Ratio
Butter	64	33	3	0.05
Lard	47	44	9	0.2
Sunflower oil	14	34	53	4
Soyabean oil	15	26	59	4
Rapeseed*(canola)	7	60	33	5
Olive oil	15	73	13	0.8
Coconut oil	91†	7	2	0.02
Palm oil	48	44	8	0.2
Oil in salmon	28	42	30	1
Oil in mackerel	27	43	30	1

   * low erucic acid variety
   † includes large amount of short chain saturates

of the animal. The fatty acid composition of the fat from other animals can be manipulated by altering their diets, although this may affect the palatability and the texture of the meat.

Soya oil and sunflower oil are two vegetable oils that are typical of many vegetable oils in that they are low in saturates and high in polyunsaturates; the **omega(ω)-6 polyunsaturated fatty acids** usually predominate in vegetable oils, i.e. the first double bond of which lies between carbons 6 and 7. Olive oil and rapeseed (canola) oil are both particularly high in monounsaturates and low in saturates. The composition of the two tropical oils shown in Table 9.1 (coconut and palm oil) show that there are exceptions to this general observation that vegetable oils are low in saturates and high in polyunsaturates. Coconut oil contains a particularly high proportion (around 78%) of short chain saturated fatty acids (less than 16 carbons) that make up only a very small proportion of the fatty acids in most fats.

The oils in the two types of fish shown in Table 9.1 are typical of wild fish; they are much higher in polyunsaturates and lower in saturates than fat from farm animals. This fish oil is particularly rich in

omega(ω)-3 polyunsaturated fatty acids, i.e. the first double bond of which lies between carbons 3 and 4. When fish are farmed there may be substantial differences in their fatty acid composition compared to wild fish, differences which reflect the differing diets of farmed and wild fish.

The physical nature of fats may give some indication of their constituent fatty acids. Unsaturation increases the fluidity of a fat and thus highly saturated animal fats tend to be solid at room temperature whereas more unsaturated vegetable oils are usually liquid at room temperature.

P:S ratio and its significance

The **P:S ratio** of a fat is the ratio of polyunsaturated fatty acids to saturated. In the examples shown in Table 9.1 this ratio ranges from 0.02 in coconut oil to around 5 in rapeseed (canola) oil. More than 30 years ago, Keys *et al.* (1959) showed that, in short term experiments with young men, total serum cholesterol levels were significantly affected by the degree of saturation of fat in the diet even when the diets were matched for total fat content. As a result of such experiments, saturated fat has acquired a very negative health image; it raises serum cholesterol in such experiments and, of course, high serum cholesterol has been associated with an increased risk of coronary heart disease. In experiments of this type, polyunsaturated fats are cholesterol-lowering when used to replace saturated fat. As a result of such observations, some vegetable oils and soft margarines, because of their high P:S ratio, have, at times, been almost regarded as "health foods". In the experiments of Keys *et al.* (1959) switching from a diet very high in saturates (P:S 0.16) to one very high in polyunsaturates (P:S 2.8) resulted in a rapid, but variable, reduction in an individual's serum cholesterol concentration when the total fat intake was kept constant (illustrated in Figure 3.10 in Chapter 3).

These early experiments suggested that monounsaturated fatty acids were practically neutral in their effects on blood cholesterol level. Saturated fatty acids were about twice as potent in raising serum cholesterol as polyunsaturated fatty acids were in lowering it. Keys *et al.* (1965a) produced an equation which enabled the change in serum cholesterol of a group to be fairly well predicted in response to specified changes in its dietary fats.

Change in serum cholesterol

$$= (2.7 \times \text{change in S})$$
$$- (1.3 \times \text{change in P})$$

where:

serum cholesterol is in mg/100 ml

S = % of calories derived from saturated fat

P = % of calories from polyunsaturated fat

Current "health images" of different dietary fats

Effects on LDL and HDL cholesterol

It is now known that different fractions make up the total serum cholesterol (see later for details). The largest component of the serum cholesterol is the **low density lipoprotein** or **LDL** fraction. High levels of LDL cholesterol are positively associated with cardiovascular disease and high levels of LDL continue to be viewed negatively by health educators. The smaller component of plasma cholesterol is the **high density lipoprotein** or **HDL** fraction. High HDL cholesterol is negatively associated with cardiovascular disease and thus positively viewed by health educators. Taking such narrow measures at face value, it would seem desirable to lower the LDL cholesterol and raise the HDL cholesterol. The LDL cholesterol is generally considered to be rather readily responsive to dietary manipulation while the HDL is rather unresponsive. Current views on the ways in which the different dietary fat fractions affect the serum cholesterol and their current "health image" is summarised below.

The saturates

These raise the LDL cholesterol although short chain saturated fatty acids (e.g. found in high amounts in coconut oil) may not have this apparently detrimental effect. They have been and continue to be viewed very negatively by health educators.

The monounsaturates

As a result of the early experiments of Keys *et al.* (1959), these were regarded as neutral in their effects upon serum cholesterol concentration. More recent work suggests that these have a lowering effect on the LDL fraction and are neutral in their effects on the HDL fraction (e.g. Mattson and Grundy, 1985). These monounsaturates are very much "in fashion" at present, accounting for the current positive image of olive oil and, in the US, canola (rapeseed) oil.

One particular monounsaturated fatty acid is much less favourably viewed, the long chain monounsaturate **erucic acid**

($22:1_{\omega9}$) found in large amounts in some varieties of rapeseed oil although not in canola oil. When this erucic acid is fed to rats in large amounts it causes transient deposition of lipid in the heart muscle cells – **transient myocardial lipidosis**. Once enzyme systems are induced that are able to metabolise the erucic acid, then this lipidosis disappears although fibrotic changes in heart muscle may appear at a later stage. New varieties of low erucic acid rape (LEAR) have been developed. Within the EC rapeseed oil must contain no more than 5% erucic acid. Canola oil is low erucic acid rapeseed oil which also has a relatively high ratio of ω-3 to ω-6 polyunsaturates. Some fish oils contain similar long chain monounsaturates gadoleic acid ($20:1_{\omega11}$) and cetoleic acid ($22:1_{\omega11}$). These latter acids make up over 30% of the total fatty acid content of herring; these might be a potential cause for concern if there were to be widespread use of large doses of concentrated fish oil supplements.

The polyunsaturates

Polyunsaturates of the ω-6 series (the bulk of polyunsaturates in most vegetable oils) are still thought to lower LDL cholesterol when used to replace saturated fat in the diet. More recent evidence suggests that they also lower HDL cholesterol (see Crouse, 1989; Ashwell, 1992). Results from some of the early intervention trials using diets very high in polyunsaturates also suggested that very high intakes of these acids might have other detrimental effects including an increased cancer risk (see Oliver, 1981). Their high susceptibility to peroxidation (see Chapter 10) is one possible mechanism by which high intakes might produce detrimental effects (COMA, 1991). Populations that consume both high fat diets and have a high dietary P:S ratio have been rare because widespread use of large amounts of most extracted vegetable oils is a relatively recent phenomenon. Safety concerns, together with this lack of historical precedent have led a number of expert committees (e.g. COMA, 1991) to recommend that it would be prudent to limit individual consumption of polyunsaturated fatty acids to no more than 10% of total calories. There is little hard evidence of deleterious effects of high polyunsaturated fat intake, but, nonetheless, it would be fair to say that they are now much less positively viewed by health educators than they were in the 1960s, 1970s and even the 1980s.

The ω-3 series of acids is found in large amounts in marine oils and in variable amounts in different vegetable oils, e.g. 11.4% of total fatty acids in walnut oil, 7% in soya oil, 10% in canola oil but only 0.29% in sunflower seed oil. It is thought that they may lower blood triglycerides and LDL cholesterol without lowering the HDL cholesterol. They are also thought to have other apparently beneficial effects such as reducing inflammation and the tendency of blood to clot and therefore reducing the risk of thrombosis. They are very much "in fashion" at present. Fish oils, the sole dietary source of the long chain members of this series, are discussed more fully at the end of this chapter.

Trans fatty acids

Diets containing only naturally occurring fatty acids would be low in *trans* fatty acids; just small amounts from butter and other fat derived from ruminating animals. However, certain types of hydrogenated oils (margarine and vegetable shortening) may contain quite large amounts of *trans* fatty acids, particularly cheaper, hard margarines. *Trans* fatty acids are also generated when vegetable oils are heated, so frying adds some *trans* fatty acids to foods. There has naturally been concern about whether there are any health implications in consuming relatively large amounts of these *trans* fatty acids because of their low levels in unprocessed foods. In particular, it has been suggested that they may have similar unfavourable effects on blood lipoproteins as do saturated fatty acids. The precise health implications of consuming large amounts of *trans* fatty acids is still unclear, but COMA (1984) suggested that *trans* fatty acids should be regarded as equivalent to saturated fatty acids in their effects upon blood lipids. In short term experiments, using both men and women, Mensink and Katan (1990) compared the effects of diets that were matched except for their *trans* fatty acid content. They concluded that *trans* fatty acids are at least as unfavourable as saturated fatty acids in their effects upon blood lipids, tending not only to raise the LDL levels but also to lower HDL levels. Willett *et al.* (1993) in a large cohort study of American nurses reported a highly significant positive association between risk of coronary heart disease and dietary intake of *trans* fatty acids. In 1989 average intakes of *trans* fatty acids in the UK were around 5 g per day (2% of calories) but with very wide variation; some individuals consuming as much as five times this average value (COMA, 1991). COMA (1991) recommended that levels should not rise above current UK intakes; they have in fact been declining in recent years as consumption of the harder margarines has declined and they have been replaced by softer margarines containing much less *trans* fatty acids. See Ashwell (1993) for a short, referenced review of recent developments in this field.

Dietary cholesterol

In short term experiments, dietary cholesterol does tend to raise the LDL cholesterol level but, at usual intakes, this effect is small compared to the effects caused by altering the proportions of the various fatty acid fractions in the diet. Usual intakes of cholesterol are relatively small when compared to the normal rate of endogenous synthesis (around 10–20%). Keys *et al.* (1965b) calculated that a change in cholesterol intake from the top

to the bottom of the range in ordinary American diets of the time (i.e. from 1050 mg/day to 450 mg/day in a 3000 kcal diet) would lower serum cholesterol by only 0.23 mmol/l if all other factors remained constant. They concluded that dietary cholesterol should not be ignored in cholesterol-lowering but that changing it alone would achieve very little. Most current dietary recommendations in the US give reduced priority to specifically lowering dietary cholesterol intake for most people and in the UK they usually contain no specific recommendations concerning dietary cholesterol. Note however, that lowering saturated fat intake will almost certainly result in a consequential fall in cholesterol intake because cholesterol is found only in animal products. Some still argue that specific restriction of dietary cholesterol is important and this may be particularly so for individuals who are genetically prone to hypercholesteraemia (Brown and Goldstein, 1984).

Twenty-five years ago dietary cholesterol was widely believed to be of predominant importance in the genesis of high blood cholesterol and atherosclerosis (e.g. Frantz and Moore, 1969); the contribution of experiments with herbivorous rabbits to this belief was critically discussed in Chapter 3. Since the 1960s, the evidence linking high serum cholesterol levels with increased risk of atherosclerotic disease has strengthened, but the view of dietary cholesterol as a major influence upon serum cholesterol concentration has declined greatly.

Imai *et al.* (1976) have suggested that even much of the apparent atherogenic effect of cholesterol seen in some rabbit experiments could be due to the presence of highly atherogenic cholesterol oxides in the cholesterol used in these studies. Some old bottles of chemical cholesterol contain very large amounts of oxidised cholesterol. Oxidised cholesterol is many times more toxic to vascular endothelial cells than purified cholesterol. How much of the atherogenic effect of cholesterol in these earlier animal experiments was artefact, due to the presence of these highly atherogenic cholesterol oxide impurities? In fresh foods, cholesterol oxide concentrations might be expected to be low, but such oxides would be generated if these foods were subjected to prolonged heating and/or exposure to air, e.g. powdered eggs, powdered whole milk and some cheeses might be expected to contain much more oxide than fresh eggs or milk. Jacobsen (1989) reported that ghee (clarified butter used in Indian cooking) has high levels of cholesterol oxides whereas fresh butter does not. Jacobsen speculated about whether these cholesterol oxides in ghee might contribute to the high levels of coronary heart disease found in British Asians.

Sources of fat in the diet

The principal sources of fat in the human diet are:

1 *Milk fat* – in whole milk and yoghurt, cream, butter and cheese. These are almost inevitably highly saturated.
2 *Meat fat* – including (often especially) meat products like sausages and burgers; also including cooking fats of animal origin such as lard. This fat also tends to be highly saturated.
3 *Seeds and nuts* – which provide a concentrated source of energy for germination. These are also the source of the vegetable oils and soft margarines. They usually have a relatively high P:S ratio; the ω-6 acids usually predominate amongst the polyunsaturates. The tropical oils are clearly an exception to these generalities (see Table 9.1).
4 *Oily fish* – such as mackerel, herring, trout, mullet and salmon. The flesh of white fish (e.g. cod and haddock) is very low in fat although considerable amounts of fat may be stored in the livers of such fish (hence cod liver oil). Fish oils tend to have a high P:S ratio:

the ω-3 acids are generally abundant and they are the only significant dietary source of the long chain ω-3 polyunsaturates.

Any food that contains any of the above as an ingredient will also contain fat. Fat is a major ingredient of cakes, pastries, biscuits (cookies), and chocolate, and thus these foods contribute significantly to total fat intake. Any foods cooked with these fats will also be rich in fat. Thus, potatoes contain almost no fat but when fried or roasted, they absorb the cooking fat.

Table 9.2 shows the sources of fat and of saturated fat in household food purchases in the UK. Dairy produce (including butter) provides only 16% of total energy but almost a quarter of total fat and more than a third of saturated fat. Fats and oils, other than butter, contribute more than a quarter of all fat and around a fifth of saturated fat; meat and meat products together contribute around a quarter of both total and saturated fat; cakes and biscuits (cookies) provide much of the saturated fat that is not accounted for in these other foods. Much of the fat in milk and fresh meat can be avoided by choosing lower fat milk and lean meat and by trimming surface fat from meat.

Several different sources suggest that the contribution of fat to the UK diet has remained practically constant for more than two decades at around 40% of calories (e.g. COMA, 1984; Chesher, 1990; MAFF, 1993). Total fat consumption has dropped, but only in proportion to the decline in total energy intake that has occurred over the same period, leaving the proportion of fat unaltered. There have been quite significant changes in the composition of the dietary fat in the UK over the same period – according to the National Food Survey, the P:S ratio of the British diet was 0.17 in 1959, still only 0.23 in 1979 but by 1993 it had risen to almost 0.4. This change in P:S ratio has been brought about principally by

Table 9.2 The percentage contribution of various foods to the energy, fat and saturated fat content of UK household diets. Data source: MAFF (1993).

Food	%Energy	%Total fat	%Saturated fat
Milk and milk products*	13.8	16.7	26.7
Fats†	13.3	31.6	26.2
Meat and meat products	15.2	24.9	24.7
All dairy products‡	16.1	22.3	36.3
Carcase meat and poultry§	7.1	11.9	11.6
Other meat and meat products¶	8.1	13.0	13.1
Cakes, pastries and biscuits (cookies)	8.5	7.9	9.5
All cereals	32.2	14.1	14.0

* includes cheese and yoghurt but not butter
† includes butter, dairy spreads, margarine, oils and low fat spreads
‡ as * but including butter
§ All meat purchased raw and unprocessed including poultry
¶ includes bacon, cooked meats and pates, sausages, burgers,

replacement of butter, hard margarine and animal-based cooking fats by soft margarine and vegetable oils.

Roles of fat in the diet

Fat as an energy source

A gram of fat yields more than twice the amount of metabolisable energy of either carbohydrate or protein. Vegetable oils and animal-derived cooking fats are essentially 100% fat, and thus some yield close to the theoretical maximum metabolisable energy of any food, i.e. 9 kcal/g; this compares, for example, with less than 4 kcal/g for 100% pure sugar. These figures may even understate the real difference in metabolisable energy between fats and carbohydrates. For example, if surplus dietary calories are in the form of fat, then the energy costs of body fat synthesis may be less than if they are from carbohydrate; more of the surplus fat calories than surplus carbohydrate calories are likely to be retained in body fat stores.

Altering the fat content of foods profoundly affects their energy content. Table 9.3 shows some examples of how adding relatively small amounts of fat to portions of food profoundly changes the energy content and also makes a disproportionate (i.e. relative to the weight change) effect on the proportion of total calories that are derived from fat: adding 8 g of butter or margarine to a slice of bread increases the energy content by around 80%; adding a 35 g portion of double cream to a slice of fruit pie increases the energy content of the dish by 70%; adding 20 g of mayonnaise to a 210 g mixed salad results in a six-fold rise in the energy yield. Consumers should be wary of claims that a product is low fat simply because the percentage of fat by weight is low.

Altering the fat content of a diet profoundly affects its bulkiness or energy density. A high fat diet is a concentrated

Table 9.3 The effect of adding typical portions of fats to typical portions of some foods. Portion sizes and composition are from Davies and Dickerson (1991).

Food	kcal	% increase	% fat by weight	% kcal as fat
Slice bread	75		2.5	11
+ butter/margarine	134	79	17	61
Jacket potato	147		Tr	0.5
+ butter/margarine	221	50	5.5	34
Boiled potatoes	120		Tr	1.5
chips/french fries	379	216	11	39
Pork chop – lean	180		6.3	42.5
lean and fat	348	93	19	65.5
Lean steak	260		6	32
lean and fat	338	68	19	50
Skimmed milk	64		Tr	3
whole milk	129	102	4	53
Chicken meat	121		4	25
meat and skin	184	52	23	58
Fruit pie	223		8	38
+ double cream	380	70	17	62
Mixed salad	28		Tr	3
+ oil/vinegar	87	211	5	70
Mixed salad	28		Tr	3
+ mayonnaise	166	493	6.5	82.5

Tr = trace

diet and a low fat diet inevitably bulkier. For those requiring higher energy intake for sustained heavy physical work then a reasonably concentrated diet may be desirable if they are not to have to eat inordinate quantities of food to meet their high energy needs. On the other hand, it was suggested in Chapter 6 that increasing the bulkiness of a diet (including a reduction in the proportion of fat) may be helpful in the treatment and prevention of obesity. Finally, it was also suggested in Chapter 6 that the low energy density of some weaning diets might be a significant factor in precipitating Protein Energy Malnutrition; these bulky weaning diets are characteristically almost devoid of fat.

Palatability

The proportion of the total dietary energy that is derived from fat tends to increase with increasing affluence of a population. It has proved exceedingly difficult to persuade affluent populations to reduce their fat consumption. Despite prolonged and intensifying health education exhortations to reduce fat intake there has been no measurable fall in the fat level in the UK diet. Human beings when given free access (through affluence) to fatty foods tend to consume them at a level which current evidence suggests may be detrimental to maximum health and longevity. This is because fat increases the sensory appeal of foods; it enhances the flavour, colour, texture and smell of food.

Many volatile flavour compounds are fat soluble and are naturally concentrated in the fat portion of unprocessed foods. Flavour materials develop when food is cooked in fats and oils even though some processed oils may be devoid of any inherent flavour. Fat also changes the texture of solid foods and the viscosity of liquids; butter or margarine spread onto bread not only changes the taste but also the texture; full fat milk has a higher viscosity than low fat milk, a difference readily discernible to the human palate. Fat also affects the appearance of some foods; skimmed milk has noticeably less whitening effect than whole milk when used in tea or coffee. Volatile, fat soluble materials contribute to the smell of food as well as to its taste.

In the examples seen in Table 9.3 the addition of fat to these foods and dishes is associated, for most people, with an increased sensory appeal as well as an increase in energy yield. Boiled potatoes are essentially bland (especially if cooked without salt) whereas chips (french fries) have much more sensory appeal to most people, and there will be subtle differences in flavour depending upon which fat is used for the frying. Adding fat to boiled mashed potatoes enhances their flavour, texture, smell and appearance. Adding oily dressing to salads or cream to fruit pie is considered by many people to enhance the sensory appeal of these foods. Many people remove the surface fat from meat because they find such concentrated fat nauseating, nonetheless, a small amount of fat greatly improves the taste and texture of meat; connoisseurs of beef look for meat with some fat marbled into the flesh.

Granules that mimic the flavours of fats like butter and cheese have been available for some years and some artificial fats have been developed that mimic the textural effects of fats in foods. The use of such synthetic chemical substitutes for natural components of food is, however, likely to generate considerable controversy given the great suspicion with which other artificial additives to food are viewed. Intuitively, one might well be more inclined to trust a product of nature that has been eaten (and therefore tested) for many generations than a product of the synthetic chemist in spite of extensive laboratory tests.

Church (1979) suggested that fat was a key element in the production of weaning foods of appropriate viscosity for young children. Children require food of appropriate viscosity for their stage of development. In the first few months after birth they require a liquid feed, then after weaning (say 6–12 months) they need to be fed with a semi-solid gruel, and by 2 years they should be feeding themselves on mixed family foods; during any period of illness there is likely to be regression and the child may require food of lower viscosity. Low-fat and starchy staples when they are cooked require the addition of large amounts of water in order to produce foods of suitable viscosity for newly-weaned children; they may only become edible if 70–80% of their total weight is water and they may require 95% water to make them liquid. Their viscosity may increase sharply as they cool. Thus thick family pap made from maize may yield 1000 kcal (4.2 MJ) per kilogramme but as much as 4 kg of a typical maize gruel suitable for a newly-weaned child might be required to supply the same amount of energy. Church suggests that fat adds concentrated energy to weaning foods and also affects their viscosity such that they become palatable to young children over a wider range of water contents; at the other extreme from starchy staple foods is milk which remains drinkable even when evaporated to a water content of only 20%.

Satiation

It has traditionally been said that fat makes an important contribution to the satiating effects of a meal. Fat slows down the process of digestion and delays stomach emptying and thus is widely believed to extend the period of satiation after consumption of the meal. Other more recent studies (e.g. Tremblay et al., 1989) suggest that, in fact, quite the opposite may be true, i.e. that carbohydrate rather than fat may have the greater satiating effect. It has been suggested that people may become satiated only when they have obtained a given amount of carbohydrate. If this theory withstands the test of time, then clearly it provides extra motivation for the overweight or obese to moderate their fat intakes. Not only does fat increase the palatability and energy density of the diet but calorie for calorie fat may also have less satiating effect than carbohydrate, thus favouring weight gain and obesity still further.

Fat soluble vitamins

The fat soluble vitamins (A,D,E and K) are found mainly in the lipid fraction of fat-containing foods and they are also absorbed along with dietary fat in the gut. Dietary deficiency of vitamin A is a major international nutritional problem even today (see Chapter 10). Vitamin A, retinol, is found only in certain fats of animal origin although humans can convert the pigment carotene, from brightly coloured fruits and vegetables, into retinol. Dietary fat facilitates the absorption of carotene, and so extreme fat deprivation increases the risk of vitamin A deficiency in children even when the diet contains marginally adequate amounts of carotene.

Essential fatty acids

People and experimental animals require small amounts of polyunsaturated fatty acids, the **essential fatty acids**, to be present in their diets. These essential fatty acids have certain structural functions, and they are necessary for the synthesis of a group of important regulatory molecules, the **eicosanoids**, which include the **prostaglandins**, the thromboxanes and the prostacyclins. These acids are required in the diet even though we can synthesise fatty acids from other substrates. This is because we do not have the biochemical capability to insert double bonds between any of the first seven carbons of fatty acid molecules. The mini-

mum requirement for these essential fatty acids is, however, so small that the practical risks of overt fatty acid deficiency in humans is remote.

In the 1920s, an essential fatty acid deficiency disease was induced in rats by feeding them on a fat-free diet; this disease was cured by the addition of small amounts of fat. Fatty acids of the linoleic acid series (ω-6) are known to cure all of the symptoms of this deficiency disease, those of the linolenic acid series (ω-3) give only partial relief of symptoms; saturates and monounsaturates are not effective. The minimum human requirement for these essential polyunsaturates is extremely small (around 1% of calories) and it has not been possible to reproduce the symptoms of this deficiency disease of rats in deprivation studies with human volunteers. The extremely low requirement for these essential fatty acids, the presence of considerable reserves of polyunsaturates in body fat and the difficulty of eliminating all traces of fat from the diet, compound to make this disease difficult to induce experimentally in people (even fruits, vegetables and cereals regarded as essentially fat-free do contain small amounts of highly unsaturated fat). There have been some reports of essential fatty acid deficiency in humans. In the 1950s, some low birth weight babies fed on skimmed milk developed eczema which was reportedly cured by small amounts of essential fatty acids. In the early 1970s an adult developed a dermatitis when fed intravenously for three months with a fat-free preparation; this dermatitis was shown to be due to essential fatty acid deficiency and has since been reported in other patients maintained on intravenous fat-free nutrition. It took more than four decades after the first demonstration in the rat to demonstrate essential fatty acid deficiency in an adult human being and then only under very unusual circumstances. Rivers and Frankel (1981) have reviewed essential fatty acid deficiency.

Fatty acids of both the ω-6 and ω-3 series are metabolised to longer chain and more highly polyunsaturated acids as shown in Figure 9.2. The linoleic acid ($18:2_{\omega 6}$) or linolenic acid ($18:3_{\omega 3}$) first has a double bond inserted at the end of the existing sequence of double bonds, i.e. it undergoes desaturation by an enzyme known as a desaturase. This desaturated product then has an extra two carbon acetate unit added to the carboxyl end, i.e. is elongated by an elongase enzyme system; two further desaturations and one further elongation complete these pathways.

The long chain highly polyunsaturated acids at the end of these sequences in Figure 9.2 are essential components of cell membranes. The EPA and DHA of the ω-3 series are normal components of membranes and it is thought that ω-3 acids are probably essential in very small quantities in their own right not just as partial substitutes for ω-6 acids. The long chain products of the ω-3 series, EPA and DHA, can be made from the shorter acids in the series, but the principal dietary source of these longer acids is from fish oil or in some populations from the fat of marine mammals (fish oils are discussed later in the chapter).

Very high intakes of ω-6 acids will tend to competitively inhibit the conversion of shorter chain ω-3 acids to their longer chain derivatives and vice versa. Diets with very high concentrations of ω-6 fatty acids from nuts, vegetable oils and soft

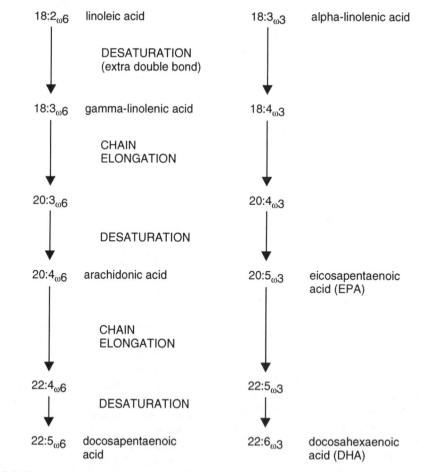

$18:2_{\omega 6}$　　linoleic acid

DESATURATION
(extra double bond)

$18:3_{\omega 6}$　　gamma-linolenic acid

CHAIN
ELONGATION

$20:3_{\omega 6}$

DESATURATION

$20:4_{\omega 6}$　　arachidonic acid

CHAIN
ELONGATION

$22:4_{\omega 6}$

DESATURATION

$22:5_{\omega 6}$　　docosapentaenoic
acid

$18:3_{\omega 3}$　　alpha-linolenic acid

$18:4_{\omega 3}$

$20:4_{\omega 3}$

$20:5_{\omega 3}$　　eicosapentaenoic
acid (EPA)

$22:5_{\omega 3}$

$22:6_{\omega 3}$　　docosahexaenoic
acid (DHA)

Figure 9.2 The metabolism of the essential fatty acids

margarine might thus lead to inadequate rates of production of EPA and DHA despite the presence of significant amounts of linolenic acid in the diet (Sanders *et al.*, 1984). This might be of practical significance in vegans consuming very large amounts of ω-6 polyunsaturates (e.g. from soft margarine and sunflower oil) or perhaps those on cholesterol-lowering diets; long chain ω-3 acids are not found in plant foods.

Arachidonic acid ($20:4_{\omega6}$) (see Figure 9.2) is the precursor for a range of local regulatory molecules, the eicosanoids or prostaglandins. The involvement of eicosanoids in the regulation of numerous physiological processes is well documented including, for example: the initiation of labour; blood platelet aggregation; blood vessel constriction/dilation; inflammation. Most of the symptoms of essential fatty acid deficiency in experimental animals are attributed to impaired prostaglandin production and are relieved only by linoleic acid or arachidonic acid. The second acid on the omega-6 pathway is called gamma(γ)- linolenic acid ($18:3_{\omega6}$) and it is the "active" ingredient in **oil of evening primrose**. It is suggested by advocates of this product that direct supply of this acid overcomes some block in this step, which is the rate limiting step in the pathway. Another interpretation could be that consumption of high amounts of γ-linolenic acid overrides the natural regulatory mechanism!

Blood lipoproteins

Fats are, by definition, insoluble in water, in order to transport them around the body in aqueous plasma they have to be associated with protein carriers and transported as lipid/protein aggregates, the **lipoproteins**. There are several subdivisions of lipoproteins in blood plasma which can be conveniently separated according to their density – the higher the proportion of fat in a lipoprotein then the lower its density because fat has low density.

The subdivisions of the plasma/serum lipoproteins are:

- chylomicrons
- very low density lipoproteins VLDL
- low density lipoproteins LDL
- intermediate density lipoproteins IDL
- high density lipoproteins HDL.

Chylomicrons are the form in which ingested fat is transported to the liver and tissues after its absorption from the intestine. They are normally absent from fasting blood, and so blood lipid determinations are ideally measured in fasting blood samples to avoid any distortion due to variable amounts of transitory chylomicrons. IDL normally represents only a very small fraction of total lipoproteins. The principal lipoproteins in fasting blood are VLDL, LDL, and HDL.

VLDL is rich in triglyceride and thus measures of blood triglycerides are taken to indicate the amount of VLDL. LDL is the major cholesterol containing fraction and thus measures of serum cholesterol are taken to indicate the LDL. The normal function of VLDL is to transport endogenously produced triglycerides from their site of synthesis (the liver) to their sites of storage (adipose tissue) or of use as an energy source. LDL acts as an external source of cholesterol for cells unable to synthesise sufficient supplies for use in membranes or as a precursor for steroid hormone synthesis. HDL serves to transport excess cholesterol from tissues back to the liver.

Epidemiological evidence and evidence from people with familial hyperlipidaemias suggest that high plasma LDL cholesterol concentrations are associated with an increased risk of coronary heart disease and that the association is probably causative. High HDL cholesterol concentrations seem to be protective against coronary heart disease, and the LDL to HDL ratio may be a better predictor of coronary heart disease risk than LDL concentration alone (Oliver, 1981). Raised VLDL is associated with obesity, glucose intolerance and high alcohol consumption; whether high VLDL is a significant independent risk factor for coronary heart disease is still a matter of debate.

Digestion, absorption and transport of dietary lipids

A summary scheme for the digestion and absorption of dietary fats is shown in Figure 9.3. Dietary fat is emulsified by the action of bile salts in the intestine. This emulsified fat is then partially digested by the enzyme **lipase** which is secreted into the gut in the pancreatic juice. Lipase splits off (hydrolyses) fatty acids from the glycerol component of triglyceride. This

process does not result in total breakdown of triglyceride, the major end products in the gut are monoglycerides and free fatty acids. This partially digested fat can now be absorbed into the mucosal cells that line the small intestine. Inside the mucosal cells the products of fat digestion are reassembled into triglycerides, coated with protein and the chylomicrons formed. Chylomicrons are essentially droplets or packets of triglyceride surrounded by a thin protein coat. These chylomicrons enter the lymphatics vessels that drain the small intestine and pass into venous blood via the thoracic duct which drains into the right subclavian vein.

Figure 9.3 A scheme to illustrate the digestion, absorption and transport of dietary triglyceride (TG)

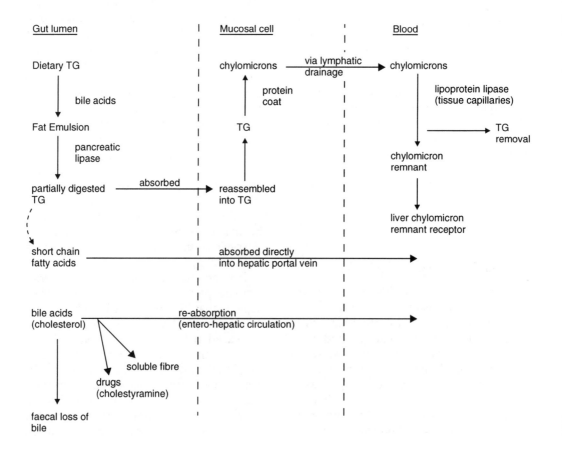

In the liver and adipose tissue, the triglyceride is removed from the chylomicrons by an enzyme called **lipoprotein lipase** that is located on the inner surface of the capillary. The products of this second digestion will be absorbed into the cells and once again re-assembled into triglyceride for storage. The fat-depleted remnants of the chylomicrons are cleared from the plasma by liver cells; they bind to a specific hepatic chylomicron remnant receptor. Some shorter chain fatty acids will by-pass this process; they will be absorbed directly from the gut into the hepatic portal vein and are transported directly to the liver.

Large amounts of cholesterol and cholesterol-derived bile salts are secreted into the intestine each day in the bile. Most of this cholesterol and bile salt is reabsorbed in the intestine and re-cycled to the liver – **entero-hepatic circulation**. Some substances are thought to exert a lowering effect on plasma cholesterol by interfering with this entero-hepatic re-cycling, leading to increased faecal losses of cholesterol and its derivatives. Soluble fibre may exert such an effect, and the cholesterol-lowering drug cholestryramine is a resin that binds or chelates bile acids in the intestine, preventing their re-absorption.

Transport of endogenously produced lipids

Figure 9.4 gives a summary of the origins and interrelationship of the non-chylomicron lipoproteins. Triglyceride-rich VLDL is the form in which fat that has been endogenously synthesised in the liver is transported to the tissues for storage and metabolic use. The enzyme lipoprotein lipase, in the tissue capillaries, hydrolyses

Figure 9.4 The relationship between the various lipoprotein fractions involved in endogenous lipid transport. After Brown and Goldstein (1984)

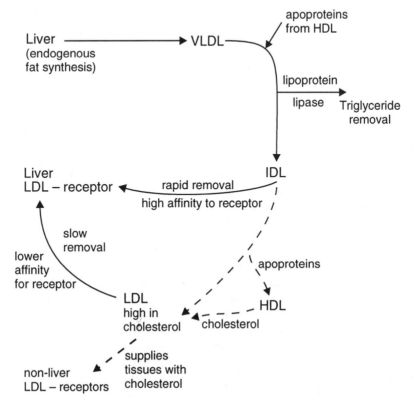

the triglyceride in VLDL, enabling it to be transported into the tissue cells. The triglyceride-depleted VLDL is now termed IDL. This IDL is then either rapidly cleared from the plasma by binding with a liver receptor, or some of it is modified within the blood to become LDL.

LDL and IDL both bind to a common receptor, called the **LDL receptor**, but this receptor has a higher affinity for IDL than for LDL and so LDL is cleared more quickly (2–6 hours) than LDL (2–3 days). More than 75% of LDL receptors are found in the liver; other tissues are supplied with cholesterol via binding of cholesterol-rich LDL to their LDL receptors (Brown and Goldstein, 1984). The perceived importance of the LDL receptor may be judged by the fact that its discoverers, Brown and Goldstein, were awarded the Nobel prize for physiology and medicine in 1985.

The diet-heart hypothesis

Introduction

Brown and Goldstein (1984) concluded that the high serum LDL cholesterol concentrations of many people living in the Western industrialised countries were due to reduced LDL receptor synthesis – protecting cells from cholesterol overload but also leading to elevated serum cholesterol levels. They suggested that dietary and other environmental factors that tend to raise serum LDL (e.g. high saturated fat intake) induce their effect by suppressing LDL-receptor synthesis.

Reduced LDL-receptor synthesis would be expected not only to increase the lifespan of LDL but also to lead to an enhanced rate of production because less IDL would be cleared and more would be converted within the blood to LDL. Reduced LDL-receptor synthesis

is seen as initiating a chain of events that can lead to increased atherosclerosis and ultimately increased risk of coronary heart disease and other atherosclerosis-linked diseases – the **diet-heart hypothesis.** The diet-heart hypothesis is outlined in Figure 9.5.

This diet-heart hypothesis could be reasonably described as the predominant theme of most nutrition education campaigns in the UK. Dietary measures that would lead to lowered serum cholesterol are widely seen as central to nutrition education for health promotion. A figure of 5.2 mmol/l has been widely suggested as an ideal maximum for individual serum cholesterol levels and yet the majority (around two-thirds) of the populations of both the UK and US exceed this level.

In Chapter 1, it was seen that in men the individual risk of coronary heart disease increases exponentially as the serum cholesterol concentration rises above this target value. However, in Chapter 1 it was also argued that most of the apparent excess population risk from high blood cholesterol seems to be concentrated in those men whose blood cholesterol levels are only slightly to moderately elevated. There are vast numbers of men (the majority of the population) who are apparently at some relatively small increased individual risk due to slight to moderate cholesterol elevation but only a small proportion at greatly increased risk due to very high serum cholesterol concentrations (refer back to Figures 1.1 and 1.2 and see Table 9.4).

The thrust of nutrition education has been to direct cholesterol-lowering dietary advice at the whole population with the aim of shifting the whole distribution downwards. Additionally, intensive dietary counselling and perhaps cholesterol-lowering drugs may be used on those individuals identified as having substantially elevated serum cholesterol levels or existing coronary heart disease. Some arbitrary cut off points for serum

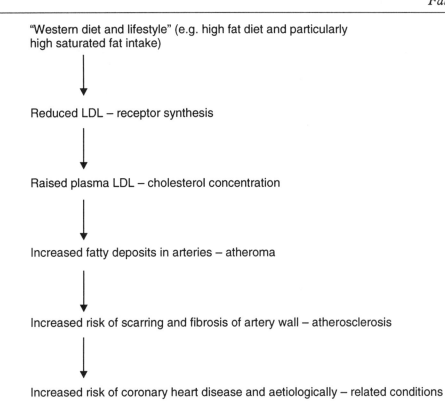

"Western diet and lifestyle" (e.g. high fat diet and particularly high saturated fat intake)

↓

Reduced LDL – receptor synthesis

↓

Raised plasma LDL – cholesterol concentration

↓

Increased fatty deposits in arteries – atheroma

↓

Increased risk of scarring and fibrosis of artery wall – atherosclerosis

↓

Increased risk of coronary heart disease and aetiologically – related conditions

Figure 9.5 The diet-heart hypothesis

cholesterol concentration:

< 4.1 mmol/l	low
4.1–5.2	desirable range
5.2–6.5	above optimal – encompassing a high proportion of the US and UK populations but regarded as higher than desirable
6.5–7.8	high
7.8+	hypercholesteraemic – regarded as abnormal or pathological because only a relatively small proportion of the population fall within this category.

White *et al.* (1993) measured serum cholesterol concentrations in a representative sample of English adults; some of their findings are summarised in Table 9.4. About 70% of men and 71% of women had values above the optimal range (i.e. above 5.2 mmol/l); 4% of men and 9% of women were above the 7.8 mmol/l threshold. There was a very pronounced trend in both sexes for serum cholesterol to increase with increasing age. In 18–24 year-old men and women the mean value was 4.8 mmol/l but in 65–74 year-olds this had rise to 6.2 mmol/l for men and 7.0 mmol/l for women. As discussed in Chapter 6, mean serum cholesterol also rose with increasing Body Mass Index.

Review of evidence supporting the diet-heart hypothesis

The general evidence linking raised serum cholesterol levels with increased risk of coronary heart disease is substantial and impressive. Not least of this evidence are

Table 9.4 Distribution (%) of serum cholesterol concentrations in a representative sample of English adults. Data source: White et al., 1993

Group	Serum cholesterol concentrations (mmol/l)				
	below 5.2	5.2–6.5	6.5–7.8	7.8+	mean
Men %					
All	31	43	23	4	5.8
18–24 years	66	30	2	3	4.8
65–74 years	16	43	36	5	6.2
Women %					
All	30	39	23	9	5.9
18–24 years	70	24	6	–	4.8
65–74 years	7	38	41	14	6.7

studies on people with **familial hyperc-holesteraemia**, an inherited condition in which there is a defect in the gene for the LDL receptor. Even persons who are heterozygous for this condition (i.e. one normal and one abnormal gene) become hypercholesteraemic, and they have a markedly increased probability of dying prematurely from coronary heart disease, particularly if they are male. Those few people who are homozygous for this condition fail to produce any functional LDL receptors and rely entirely upon other inefficient methods to clear LDL-cholesterol from blood; the serum cholesterol concentrations of such individuals may be up to six times normal, and they are likely to die from coronary heart disease in childhood. Injections of radioactively-labelled LDL into such individuals confirms that it remains in the circulation about two and a half times as long as in unaffected people and that the rate of endogenous LDL production is about doubled because of reduced IDL clearance (Brown and Goldstein, 1984).

Population comparisons

When comparing population diets with death rates from CHD there is a general trend for CHD mortality to rise with increased saturated fat consumption, although there are a number of interesting exceptions to these general trends, for example:

1 The Masai of East Africa eat a diet based upon milk, meat and blood which is high in saturated fat and cholesterol and yet they are free of advanced atherosclerosis and their rates of coronary heart disease are very low. The traditional Masai are a fit and lean population which could be used to explain their protection from the effects of their apparently atherogenic diet; it has also been suggested that the presence of large amounts of fermented milk (yoghurt) may be significant (McGill, 1979 contains a referenced summary of early studies on the Masai).

2 Some studies have reported that farmers have lower levels of CHD than non-farmers living in the same locality despite having similar fat intakes and higher serum cholesterol concentrations. These studies suggest that farmers are more active, fitter and smoke and drink less than non farmers (e.g. Pomrehn et al., 1982).

3 More recently, the low rates of coronary heart disease in France have attracted attention. Rates of coronary heart disease in France are less than a third of those in the UK and yet the French have quite high intakes of saturated fat (14–15% of calories) and

have similar serum cholesterol concentrations to those of Britons. A protective effect of the high wine consumption in France has been offered as an explanation for these findings (Renaud and de Lorgeril, 1992) – many would hope that this hypothesis is confirmed!

4 McKeigue *et al.* (1985) noted high rates of coronary heart disease amongst British Asians despite their having lower saturated fat and cholesterol intakes and lower serum cholesterol concentrations than the white population.

Experimental studies

Numerous short term experimental studies have shown that serum cholesterol concentration, primarily the LDL fraction, is alterable by manipulating intake of dietary lipids (e.g. Keys *et al.*, 1959, 1965a and 1965b; Mattson and Grundy, 1985; Mensink and Katan, 1990). There is general agreement that increases in total dietary fat and increased saturated fat tend to increase the plasma cholesterol whereas replacement of saturated with polyunsaturated fat tends to lower the cholesterol concentration. The probable effects of dietary cholesterol, monounsaturated fatty acids and *trans* fatty acids were discussed earlier in the chapter. Susceptibility to dietary manipulation of plasma cholesterol concentration varies between individuals, and there is a general trend for those with the higher baseline levels to be more responsive to dietary change (Keys *et al.*, 1959). Longer term dietary intervention studies aimed at lowering plasma cholesterol concentration have also generally produced significant reductions in plasma cholesterol in the test group (Oliver, 1981). However, according to Oliver (1981), plasma cholesterol is usually reduced by less than 10% in free-living subjects despite some very major dietary modification and even drug use in many of these studies.

Cohort studies

Cohort studies whether within or between population generally indicate that, at least for young and middle-aged men, high serum cholesterol concentration is predictive of subsequent risk of death from coronary heart disease over the succeeding 5–20 years. The classic cross cultural cohort study (the Seven Countries Study) showed high correlation between dietary saturated fat intake and both plasma cholesterol concentration and incidence of coronary heart disease (summarised in Oliver, 1981).

Summing up the evidence

The weakest point in the chain of evidence for the diet-heart hypothesis has been the failure to find any significant association between measures of dietary fat/saturated fat intake and serum cholesterol concentration in most within population studies. Oliver (1981) uses data from the Tecumseh study to illustrate this general finding; dietary intakes of fat, saturated fat, cholesterol and dietary P:S ratio were not significantly different when those in the highest, middle and lowest **tertiles** (thirds) for serum cholesterol concentrations were compared. In their more recent dietary and nutritional survey of British adults, Gregory *et al.* (1990) found no significant correlation between any measures of dietary fat and serum LDL cholesterol concentration in men except for a very weak ($r = 0.08$) one with dietary cholesterol; all correlation coefficients were less than 0.1. In women they found a weak but significant correlation with percentage of energy from saturated fat and serum LDL cholesterol concentration, i.e. only 2% (r^2) of the difference in women's serum cholesterol could be explained by variation in their percentage of dietary energy from saturated fat.

Dietary differences in individual fat consumption do not appear to be an important factor in determining the position of any individual within the population distribution of serum cholesterol concentrations. As already stated in Chapter 3 this may be because a host of other factors affect an individual's serum cholesterol concentration, such as:

• genetic variability in serum cholesterol concentration, including variation in genetic susceptibility to dietary fats
• other dietary influences upon serum cholesterol
• other lifestyle influences on serum cholesterol, e.g. exercise, age, smoking, alcohol, Body Mass Index.

This lack of significant association is thus not incompatible with the proposal that the adoption of a cholesterol-lowering diet by the population will lead to a downward shift in the distribution for serum cholesterol of the population and to a reduction in average serum cholesterol concentration. This general concept was discussed more fully in Chapter 3 using data in Figure 3.10 to illustrate it.

The long term holistic benefits of cholesterol-lowering have not yet been directly demonstrated in intervention trials. Numerous trials of a variety of cholesterol-lowering interventions have been undertaken over the last two or three decades, but none has produced a significant reduction in total mortality in the test group, and many have not even produced significant reductions in cardiovascular mortality. Several have reported that reducing hypercholesteraemia does reduce the overall incidence of coronary heart disease mainly by reductions in the number of non-fatal myocardial infarctions (McCormick and Skrabanek, 1988; Oliver, 1981 and 1991). Some interventions involving use of cholesterol-lowering drugs have actually increased mortality in the test group.

The diet-heart hypothesis, as summarised in Figure 9.5, can be broken up into two key propositions:

1 that a high serum cholesterol concentration is causally associated with increased risk of coronary heart disease

2 that the level of dietary fat consumption, and particularly of saturated fat is an important factor in determining a population's average serum cholesterol concentration and thus the population risk of coronary heart disease.

The evidence for the first of these propositions is very substantial, perhaps overwhelming, although it should also be made clear that serum cholesterol is but one of a number of risk factors and associations. Some of the risk factors are alterable (e.g. diet, smoking, inactivity) but others are unalterable (e.g. genetic propensity and sex). It must also be added that this relationship is most convincing in middle-aged men. Several authors have concluded that this association is much weaker in premenopausal women (Crouse, 1989) and the elderly. In recent editorials in *The Lancet* (Dunnigan, 1993) and *Circulation* (Hulley *et al.*, 1992) doubts have been expressed about extrapolating results derived from middle-aged men, who are at relatively high risk of premature coronary heart disease, to the female population who are at relatively low risk.

It would probably be fair to say that the evidence in favour of the second proposal is strong but not quite as overwhelming as for proposition 1. The absence of association between serum cholesterol and dietary saturated fat intake within populations is a major barrier to universal acceptance of the theory. There is a good explanation for this as discussed above and in Chapter 3 but this explanation is conceptually difficult for non-epidemiologists to understand.

The lack of demonstrated holistic benefit in cholesterol-lowering intervention trials is the other major barrier to universal acceptance of this theory. Despite these apparent "missing links" in the evidence, numerous expert committees in many industrialised countries have evaluated the evidence for the diet-heart hypothesis and in almost all cases the majority view has been to accept the hypothesis. Even some of those who are critical of population measures aimed at reducing coronary heart disease by dietary intervention would accept the great strength of the scientific evidence supporting the diet-heart hypothesis.

Other issues raised by cholesterol-lowering interventions

There are some criticisms of cholesterol-lowering interventions that would not be solved even by absolute scientific proof of the diet-heart hypothesis; some of these are discussed below.

1 How much population reduction in dietary fat and dietary saturated fat intake is realistically achievable? Both NACNE (1983) and NRC (1989b) have suggested target figures of 30% of calories from fat and 10% of calories from saturated fat (see Chapter 4). Considerable doubts were raised in Chapters 1 and 4 as to whether the 30% target for total fat is a realistic one, particularly if sugar intake is also to be substantially reduced. Many consumers probably lack the knowledge and skill to implement these changes even if they wished to. There could well be an inverse relationship between likeliness to implement these changes and likeliness to benefit from them. Young and middle-aged, working class men are at much greater risk of premature coronary heart disease than young and middle-aged, middle class women but seem much less likely to implement change. In 1987, fat still made up more than 38% of calories in the adult UK diet and saturated fat almost 17%. Only 6% of UK men and 8% of women met even the more modest targets of 35% of calories from fat and 15% from saturated fat (Gregory et al., 1990). In the light of these findings, the 30% figure for total fat seems improbable in the UK especially in view of the lack of any measurable change in the propor-

tion of UK energy deri_____ since the 1960s. This d_____ that some reduction in_____ intake cannot be achieve__ perhaps substantial, resultant be__

A little progress has been made in reducing the proportion of saturated fat in the UK diet and in raising the P:S ratio; this has been achieved largely by replacing saturated fat with unsaturated fat. The wisdom of recommending very large increases in intakes of ω-6 polyunsaturates has already been seriously questioned. Monounsaturates and ω-3 polyunsaturates are currently the most favourably viewed of the fatty acids but this is largely on the basis of short term experiments and short duration intervention trials with high risk subjects. It would seem imprudent, on the basis of current evidence, to give advice designed to bring about large increases in the proportions of any particular group of fatty acids. Nutrition education must not create good or bad images of particular fats that later prove to be unjustified. Perhaps the safest option would be to encourage moderation of fat intake and diversity of sources of fat – there is no guarantee that the currently fashionable types of fat will remain fashionable.

2 Dietary fat intake is clearly only one factor in determining serum cholesterol concentration and serum cholesterol is only one risk factor for coronary heart disease. Perhaps undue emphasis placed upon changing these may deflect attention away from other more obvious beneficial changes in lifestyle and may even be inappropriate in some cases. How significant is a high fat diet or perhaps even moderately elevated serum cholesterol concentration in lean, active, non-smoking, moderate drinking men? This question may be even more pertinent in similar women. How significant are reductions in saturated fat intakes for men who remain overweight, inactive and

who smoke and drink heavily?

In an 8.5-year cohort study of male British civil servants, Morris *et al.* (1980) found very low levels of fatal first coronaries in men who did not smoke and who participated in vigorous leisure-time activity; the rates were more than six times higher in cigarette smokers who did not participate in vigorous leisure-time activity. This study took no account of diet or serum cholesterol and the data was collected before the current nutrition education campaigns aimed at lowering dietary fat intakes had gained much momentum in the UK. It suggests that altering these two risk factors offers very great scope for reducing risk of coronary heart disease. Replacing butter with margarine or frying in oil rather than lard are relatively painless changes that may offer reassurance or salve the conscience but are unlikely to compensate for failure to alter other more significant risk factors like cigarette smoking, inactivity, alcohol abuse and obesity.

3 Coronary heart disease has been the primary focus of nutrition education for health promotion in the UK. Coronary heart disease is the single biggest cause of death in the UK, it accounts for over a quarter of all deaths (31% of male and 23% of female deaths). Most of these deaths from coronary heart disease occur in the elderly (median age for death from coronary heart disease in the UK is 74 years) but it also accounts for 30 000 deaths per year in men under the age of 65 years, making it the single biggest cause of premature death in British men. Circulatory diseases (mainly coronary heart disease and stroke) have increased from being the cause of 26% of all deaths in 1931 to 46% of all deaths in 1991 (DH, 1992). Table 9.5 shows a comparison of standardised death rates from coronary heart disease in people under 65 years across the countries of the EC.

There are huge differences in the mortality rates for this disease in these 12 industrialised European countries with rates 3–4 times higher in the British Isles than in the Mediterranean countries.

Statistics such as these, make it entirely understandable that so much of the attention of UK health educators has been focused upon coronary heart disease; but perhaps they give an exaggerated impression of an epidemic of coronary heart disease leading to premature death in a high proportion of Britons however. Circulatory diseases certainly account for a much higher proportion of deaths in the UK than they did 60 years ago, but how much of this is due to decline in death rates from other competing causes? Assuming that human beings are not immortal, if one reduces or eliminates some causes of death, then it is inevitable that other causes must account for an increased proportion of the total; infectious diseases accounted for 13% of deaths in 1931, genito urinary diseases 5% and "other causes" 31% whereas in 1991 "other causes", now including both infectious diseases and genito urinary diseases, accounted for only 17% of the total. In Chapter 3 the very large, post war rises in Japanese death rates from the diseases of industrialisation were highlighted. It was nonetheless argued that over this same period, total life expectancy of the Japanese had increased sharply and that most of the increase in these diseases of industrialisation could be accounted for by increased numbers of elderly people; age-specific death rates from these diseases had changed rather little (Fujita, 1992).

In Table 9.5 life expectancies across the countries of the EC in 1988 are listed. These figures show much less variation in life expectancy across the countries of the community than might be expected given the huge variation in

Table 9.5 Life expectancy at birth in the countries of the EC in 1988. Data source: Echo, a Department of Health newsletter, January 1993

Country	Life expectancy (years)
Spain	76.7
Greece	76.5
Netherlands	76.5
Italy	76.0
France	75.9
West Germany	75.4
United Kingdom	74.9
Denmark	74.9
Belgium (1986)	74.8
Luxembourg	74.4
Portugal	73.7
Republic of Ireland	73.5

Table 9.6 Standardised death rates from coronary heart disease per 100 000 population in persons under 65 years in the EC in 1988. Data source: Echo, a Department of Health newsletter, February 1993

Death rate range	Countries within range
15–29	Portugal, Spain, France, Italy
30–44	Greece, Luxembourg, West Germany, Netherlands, Belgium
45–59	Denmark
60–75	United Kingdom, Republic of Ireland

coronary heart disease mortality rates shown in Table 9.6. The total range is only about 3 years (4%) from 73.5 years in the Republic of Ireland to 76.7 years in Spain with the UK lying close to the mid-point in this range. This means that death rates from causes other than coronary heart disease must compensate or partially compensate for the very large differences in death rates from coronary heart disease, for example: Portugal has the highest death rate from stroke within the EC whereas Denmark has one of the lowest; there are about three times as many deaths from suicide or self-inflicted injury in France than there are in the UK; death rates from cirrhosis of the liver in France and Spain are several times higher than those in the UK; the UK has one of the lowest rates of deaths in road accidents in Europe.

4 Is lowering of serum cholesterol universally beneficial, or at least neutral? Several recent papers have suggested that in people with low serum cholesterol levels (i.e. below 4.1 mmol/l) there is increased total mortality as compared to those in the optimal category (i.e. 4.1–5.2 mmol/l) (e.g. Jacobs *et al.*, 1992; Neaton *et al.*, 1992). This excess mortality is substantial and is accounted for by increased rates of cancer and other non cardiovascular causes. It is estimated that in the US, 6% of middle-aged men are in this low category. Jacobs *et al.* (1992) concluded that this excess mortality was not removed by excluding deaths within the first five years, i.e. reducing the likelihood that the low serum cholesterol was merely an indicator of existing malignant disease; correcting for confounding variables did not remove the association either.

There is thus the very real possibility that the relationship between total mortality and serum cholesterol follows a U curve; at the optimal range (say 4.1–5.2 mmol/l) total mortality is lowest but on either side of that optimum total mortality increases – in the right hand arm due to increasing mortality from atherosclerotic diseases like coronary heart disease but in the left hand arm due to increased numbers of deaths from other causes. Cholesterol-lowering measures directed at the whole population will tend to push more people from the optimal range into the low range and those already in the low range may be pushed still lower. This possibility may be particularly significant for those groups such as premenopausal women and the elderly where the expected benefits from cholesterol-lowering are less secure or at least smaller. Jacobs *et al.* (1992) failed to find any association between high serum cholesterol and increased total mortality in women, perhaps even more surprisingly neither did they find any association between cardiovascular deaths and serum cholesterol. They suggested that the cardiovascular deaths may have remained unaltered with increasing serum cholesterol because increases in mortality from stroke balanced out any decreases in mortality from coronary heart disease. In a 12-year follow-up of a cohort of 15 000 men and women living in the west of Scotland, all cause mortality was found to be not related to serum cholesterol concentration. Although there was a highly significant positive correlation between serum cholesterol and mortality from coronary heart disease, this was counterbalanced by an inverse relationship between cholesterol concentration and other causes of death, including cancer. In the men in this study, the inverse relation between serum cholesterol and risk of developing or dying from cancer was statistically highly significant and remained so even when those developing cancer in the first four years of follow-up were excluded. These authors concluded that it may be a mistake to assume that general advice to lower saturated fat intake will necessarily reduce overall mortality; coronary heart disease may well decrease but other risks may increase (Isles *et al.*, 1989).

If these concerns are substantiated, then it would be difficult to justify population measures, the sole aim of which was cholesterol-lowering, even if one could show that more people were likely to benefit than be harmed by them. This would be particularly so if the intervention has most impact upon those least at risk of premature coronary disease. Premature death from coronary heart disease is relatively uncommon in women and so cholesterol-lowering advice may be particularly dubious for them.

In a recent combined analysis of 35 randomised, controlled trials of cholesterol-lowering interventions, Smith *et al.* (1993) concluded that net benefit (i.e. reduced total mortality) from cholesterol-lowering intervention was confined to those at very high risk of coronary heart disease, i.e. at greater risk than even asymptomatic patients under 65 years with hypercholesteraemia. More than two-thirds of the trials surveyed by these authors involved the use of cholesterol-lowering drugs, and the authors concluded that these drugs should be reserved for the small proportion of people at very high risk of death from coronary heart disease, perhaps only those with both existing coronary heart disease and hypercholesteraemia.

Committed advocates of cholesterol-lowering intervention respond to the lack of any demonstrable effect on overall mortality in primary intervention trials by suggesting quite rightly that the sample sizes in these trials are too small to get statistically significant reductions in overall mortality. In a recent editorial in *The Lancet* (Dunnigan, 1993), it was estimated that a trial involving 80 000 people over a five-year period would be necessary to demonstrate whether there was any beneficial effect of cholesterol-lowering on all cause mortality even in patients with asymptomatic hypercholesteraemia under the age of 65 years. This is, of course, another way of saying that, at least within the timescale of an intervention trial, the difference in risk of dying is only minutely affected by being in the intervention or control group. Of course, the hope is that cholesterol-lowering for the whole population over the whole lifespan will shift the age distribution of deaths from coronary heart disease and eventually from all causes upwards.

One rather bizarre finding that has attracted much attention in the last couple of years has been an apparent increase in suicide and other violent deaths associated with cholesterol-lowering interventions (see Engelberg, 1992). This is not an isolated finding and has been noted by several authors. Engelberg has suggested that cholesterol-lowering drugs, in particular, might increase aggression by altering brain neurotransmission involving the important brain neurotransmitter 5-HT (serotonin). It is ironic that, in my imaginary paper to the centenary meeting of the Nutrition Society in 2041 (see Chapter 1), I also suggested that there were a "freakishly high number of violent deaths" in the test (cholesterol-lowered) group; I made this suggestion because at the time I considered it amusingly improbable – perhaps fact may turn out to be as strange as fiction.

5 Does cholesterol screening have any detrimental effects? Is knowledge that their cholesterol level is above optimal likely to cast an unnecessary and gloomy shadow over the lives of otherwise healthy people? Is it not bound to cause fear and anxiety if it is implied to two thirds of the population that they are "suffering" from some hidden asymptomatic condition that increases the probability that they will be disabled or die prematurely from heart disease? Can this fear and anxiety be justified by the benefits then made available by intervention, particularly as most of the "sufferers" will survive into ripe old age even without taking any corrective measures? Health promotion is a very positive-sounding objective, but its implementation may focus attention upon risk of death and disease which can negatively affect quality of life.

6 Dietary change, as a result of health promotion, has already had significant impact upon national diets; it has been responsible for much of the switch from butter to margarine and low-fat spreads and much of the switch from animal-based cooking fats to vegetable oils. Such changes will inevitably have great social, economic and cultural consequences. Such changes may blight the livelihood of some although equally provide economic opportunity for others. They may produce changes far removed from the dinner-table, kitchen or even supermarket – increasing numbers of fields devoted to growing rapeseed or sunflowers or olive trees and less used as pasture for beef and dairy cattle. What will be the long term economic consequences of promoting skimmed milk as a healthy, calcium-rich food whilst encouraging avoidance of dairy fat? In wealthy countries, people are advised to discard many of the fat calories in animal carcasses whilst millions of people in other countries suffer undernutrition – will health promotion in wealthy nations be at the cost of still greater deprivation in poorer ones? Has the increased growth of rapeseed contributed to increased levels of asthma and hay fever reported in the UK?

One would not wish to start a sterile debate about whether any particular change is good or bad but these are consequences of health promotion that should be considered; the ethical case for such induced changes would be very dependent upon the magnitude of the benefits that they produce.

Diet-heart hypothesis – concluding remarks

These uncertainties emphasise the need for a continuing critical debate about current nutrition education aims and strategies. They underline the need for a readiness to modify strategies as the precise relationship between dietary fats, coronary heart disease and other diseases is clarified. Some might argue that such a debate blurs simple nutrition education messages to the public and thus is likely to hinder their implementation. However, to attempt to hide the uncertainties in the guidelines in order to facilitate their implementation is surely unethical. In most other areas of medical and surgical treatment, the informed consent of the patient is the rule; surely such informed consent should be even more critical if subjects are asymptomatic. Several authors have questioned the ethics of universal cholesterol-lowering advice if there is a real possibility that this may have harmful effects for some (e.g. Oliver, 1991; Hulley *et al.*, 1992).

On a more positive note, it should be said that some of those who remain unconvinced by the diet-heart hypothesis or have reservations about some of the interventions directed towards cholesterol-lowering would still conclude that a moderate reduction in the proportion of calories derived from fat would be desirable. In the COMA (1984) report it was said that each of the ten committee members felt that the evidence supporting the diet-heart hypothesis fell short of actual proof but nine felt that the evidence was sufficient to make it probable that moderating intakes of fat and saturated fat would reduce the incidence or delay the onset of coronary heart disease. Even the one dissenting member felt that the majority recommendations might produce benefit by reducing the incidence of obesity.

It seems highly probable that certain behaviours, identified throughout this book as being likely to promote healthfulness will also reduce or delay an individual's risk of coronary heart disease and reduce serum cholesterol concentrations, e.g. regular exercise, maintenance of ideal body weight, no smoking, moderate use of alcohol, and diets that are closer to nutrition education guidelines than those eaten at present. Serum cholesterol measurements are a useful epidemiological and experimental tool and may also be useful in identifying the relatively small numbers of people with pathological irregularities in their lipoprotein metabolism. (Note that in many cases of pathological hyperlipidaemias there are external clinical indications of the abnormality, e.g. fatty lumps or xanthomas in the skin, tendons and eyelids and fatty deposits in the cornea, corneal arcus.) However, perhaps the current preoccupation with such a narrow and imperfect indicator of wellness as serum cholesterol is unhelpful and unsound as a sole justification for prescribing drugs and restrictive therapeutic diets at the individual level or indiscriminate cholesterol-lowering interventions at the population level.

Fish oils

Overview

A series of papers published in the 1970s by Bang, Dyerberg and their colleagues reported that Greenland Eskimos, who ate the traditional diet high in seal meat, whale meat and fish, had low rates of coronary heart disease and low rates of inflammatory joint disease even when compared to their nearest geographical neighbours, the Danes (e.g. Dyerberg and Bang, 1979). This low rate of coronary heart disease in the Eskimos is despite a diet similar in total fat content to the Danes and despite the fact that most of the fat originates from the animal kingdom. The lipid of the Eskimo diet differs from the Danish diet in two major respects, firstly it is much lower in saturated fatty acids and secondly it has higher levels of ω-3 polyunsaturates (reviewed by Kromhout, 1990).

Fish oils and other marine oils (e.g. from seals and whales) contain large amounts of long chain ω-3 polyunsaturates (i.e. of the linolenic acid series). The three longest chain members of this series, eicosapentaenoic acid, EPA $(20:5_{\omega 3})$, docosapentaenoic acid DPA $(22:5_{\omega 3})$ and docosahexaenoic acid DHA $(22:6_{\omega 3})$

account for around 20% of the fatty acids in many marine fish oils. The ω-3 fatty acids, because of their extra double bond, have greater fluidity at low environmental temperatures than the corresponding ω-6 fatty acid – this may explain their prominence in the fat of cold water mammals and fish. These acids enter the marine food chain via their synthesis by marine plants and plankton which then serve as food for higher marine organisms.

These long chain ω-3 polyunsaturates are widely believed to be the active agents that reduce risk of coronary heart disease and inflammatory joint diseases. It should be noted that many of the fish liver oil products currently available contain high levels of vitamins A and D. Consumption of some of these fish liver oil products in amounts necessary to produce intakes of EPA and DHA equivalent to two fatty fish portions per week (as generally recommended, e.g. in Groom and Ashwell, 1993) might lead to consumption of undesirably large amounts of these vitamins; both vitamin A and D have well documented toxic effects when taken in large excess.

The reports on the health and mortality of Eskimos served to focus scientific attention upon the protective and therapeutic potential of fish oils and the ω-3 polyunsaturates. The increased scientific interest in fish oils may be gauged by the output of research papers on fish oils; less than ten per year in the 1970s but rising sharply during the 1980s to a current level of several hundred per year (see Simopoulos, 1991). Fish oils can now be made available on prescription in the UK for the treatment of certain hyperlipidaemias and for patients with a history of coronary heart disease. The public perception of fish oils as health-promoting is illustrated by the dramatic increase in sales of fish oil preparations. In the UK in 1992, fish oils accounted for over a quarter of the UK market for natural food supplements and fish oils and oil of evening primrose together accounted for 42% of this market. A 1992 UK survey conducted by one of the companies involved in the marketing of fish oils (see Health and Fitness, 1993) suggested a high public awareness of their possible protective effects against coronary heart disease. Around 70% of people were apparently aware of the possible protective effects of fish oil. This awareness has not, however, resulted in any major, sustained increase in sales of oily fish in the UK, although there was a temporary surge in oily fish sales in 1989 following publication of a successful and highly publicised secondary intervention trial (Burr *et al.*, 1989) using fish oils.

Groom and Ashwell (1993) give a wide ranging, referenced review of the nutritional aspects of fish and Simopoulos (1991) has reviewed the ω-3 fatty acids.

Possible protective mechanisms

There are a number of mechanisms by which long chain ω-3 fatty acids have been suggested to reduce the risk of coronary heart disease and inflammatory joint diseases, such as:

1 *Effects on the production of the local regulatory eicosanoid family of compounds* – Long chain ω-3 fatty acids inhibit the conversion of linoleic acid to arachidonic acid by an effect on the rate limiting enzyme that converts linoleic acid ($18:2_{ω6}$) to gamma linolenic acid ($18:3_{ω6}$) – see scheme for essential fatty acid metabolism in Figure 9.2. The ω-3 equivalent of arachidonic acid, EPA, then partially replaces arachidonic acid as a substrate for the enzyme systems that convert arachidonic acid into active eicosanoids, thus producing eicosanoids with different activities to those produced from arachidonic acid (summarised in Figure 9.6).

The thromboxane TXA-2 is produced from arachidonic acid and this increases blood platelet aggregation and the tendency for blood to clot; the ω-3 equivalent is TXA-3 which has much less activity than TXA-2. The overall effect of partially replacing TXA-2 with TXA-3 is a reduction in the tendency of platelets to aggregate and blood to clot. The prostacyclin PGI-2 is produced in vascular endothelial cells from arachidonic acid and it has an anti-aggregating effect on platelets. The ω-3 equivalent in this case, PGI-3, has only marginally lower activity and so partial replacement of PGI-2 with

PGI-3 has little effect on the anti-aggregating system. The overall effect of these changes shown in Figure 9.6 would be predicted to reduce the risk of thromboses forming in blood vessels, reducing in turn the risk of occlusive strokes (due to blockage of cerebral vessels with a clot) and myocardial infarction (heart attacks due to clots lodging in the coronary vessels). Eskimos have extended bleeding times and are prone to frequent and long-lasting

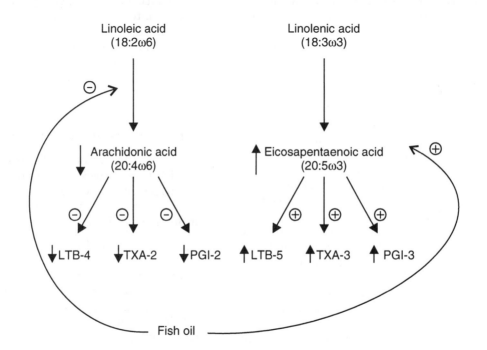

LTB-4 promotes inflammation; LTB-5 has low activity

TXA-2 causes platelet aggregation; TXA-3 has low activity

PGI-2 and PGI-3 both have anti-aggregating effects on platelets

Net effect of fish oil, reduced inflammation and reduced platelet aggregation

Figure 9.6 Possible effects of fish oil consumption on the production of eicosanoids that affect platelet aggregation and inflammation

nosebleeds; they have high stroke mortality (most likely due to increased levels of cerebral haemorrhage). In short term human and animal experiments, high consumption of fish oils has been found to reduce the tendency of blood to clot and to extend the bleeding time (Anon, 1984; Sanders, 1985).

Eicosanoids are also known to be key mediators of inflammation – the leukotriene LTB-4 is produced from arachidonic acid and is a promoter of inflammation. The ω-3 equivalent is LTB-5 which is much less active. The overall effect of fish oil consumption will be the partial replacement of arachidonic acid with EPA as substrate for the leukotriene-producing enzyme system, leading to partial replacement of LTB-4 with LTB-5 and thus a reduced inflammatory response. These changes may reduce the damage caused by the inflammatory response after a myocardial infarction and may also explain the suggested benefits on inflammatory diseases like arthritis and eczema. In a controlled, secondary intervention trial of fish oils in patients who had previously suffered a myocardial infarction, fish oils significantly reduced both cardiovascular and total mortality whereas the other treatments (low-fat diets or increased cereal fibre) did not (Burr et al., 1989). In this trial, the fish oil patients did not have significantly less re-infarcts but these new infarcts were less likely to be fatal – consistent with this suggestion of reduced post-infarct inflammatory damage. In a controlled trial, high intakes of EPA appeared to improve the clinical features of rheumatoid arthritis and the levels of LTB-4 were found to be reduced by the treatment (Kremer et al., 1985).

2 *Effects on blood lipoprotein profiles* – Epidemiological and experimental evidence suggests that fish oils can have marked effects on blood lipoprotein profiles. At high doses both VLDL and LDL levels in blood are reduced in clinical trials and the effect on VLDL (blood triglyceride) is significant even at doses more akin to the amounts likely to be consumed in normal diets (say two portions of fatty fish per week). Some experimental evidence suggests that they may also raise the HDL-cholesterol, and Greenland Eskimos have been reported to have higher HDL levels than those living in Denmark and consuming less marine oils. Sanders (1985) has reviewed the effects of fish oils on blood lipoproteins.

3 *Effects on plasminogen activation* – Clots are broken down by plasmin which is formed when the inactive blood protein plasminogen is activated. Experiments using fish oil supplements in patients with coronary artery disease indicate that they lead to reduced formation of a substance that inhibits the conversion of plasminogen to active plasmin. Clot dissolving drugs like streptokinase are often administered to patients in the immediate period after a myocardial infarction in order to reduce the damage done to the heart; perhaps, fish oils have a similar effect.

Review of the evidence on the possible therapeutic and protective effects of fish oils

There is compelling evidence that in short term, controlled experiments, fish oils affect the blood lipoprotein profile in ways that are currently considered to be beneficial. They also reduce the tendency of blood to clot in such trials and thus would presumably reduce the risk of thromboses forming within the circulation. There is also convincing evidence that in persons with established coronary heart disease that the regular consumption of fatty fish or fish oil supplements produces overall benefits as measured by total mortality in the few years immediately after a first infarction (Burr et al., 1989).

The epidemiological evidence for fatty fish consumption reducing the risk of coronary heart disease or still further, improving overall life expectancy, is rather less convincing (reviewed by Kromhout, 1990). There is no convincing evidence of an independent relationship between fatty fish consumption and reduced risk of coronary heart disease in cross-population studies. Those comparisons that have been made have used total fish consumption as the independent variable (a crude predictor of total ω-3 fatty acid consumption) and the weak negative association with coronary heart disease mortality was very dependent upon the inclusion of the Japanese. In the famous Seven Countries Study there was no significant association between fish consumption and coronary heart disease mortality; some of those populations with negligible fish consumption in inland Yugoslavia had amongst the lowest rates of coronary heart disease whilst some of those with the highest fish consumption in Finland had amongst the highest rates of coronary heart disease. Fish consumption was related to subsequent mortality in a 20-year cohort study of 850 men in Zutphen, Holland. In this cohort, death from coronary heart disease was inversely related to fish consumption; it was 50% lower in men who ate 30 g of fatty fish per day (equivalent to about two servings per week) compared with those who ate no fish at all. The work on Eskimos has, to date been the most positive of the epidemiological evidence in favour of fish oils having protective effects against the development of coronary heart disease (see Kromhout, 1990).

In general, the epidemiological evidence relating fatty fish consumption to reduced coronary heart disease risk is weak or sporadic but this might not be unexpected even if regular consumption of long chain ω-3 fatty acids is protective because:

1 Using total fish consumption as the independent variable is only a very crude indicator of ω-3 fatty acid intake.

2 The cross-population relationship between saturated fat intake and coronary heart disease mortality might well obscure any lesser relationship between fish consumption and coronary heart disease.

The overall evidence at present seems consistent with the recommendation that fish and fatty fish be included in healthful and diverse diets for those who like fish and have no cultural objections to consuming fish. A quantitative recommendation of two portions of fatty fish per week has been suggested. A few years ago fish oil would have been regarded as just another source of fat in our already excessively fatty diets; it now has a much more positive image. There does also seem to be a case for specifically recommending increases in fatty fish consumption or even the use of fish oil supplements in those with established coronary heart disease or those with some types of hyperlipidaemia. This evidence does not yet warrant recommending universal consumption of fish oil supplements or even consumption of fatty fish on purely therapeutic grounds. Some of the favourable epidemiological evidence for fish oils could be interpreted as their being beneficial in preventing coronary heart disease when they replace saturated fat rather than being beneficial *per se*.

Much of the most convincing evidence in the fish oil story comes from very reductionist studies of the effects on particular physiological systems or symptoms or from more holistic studies with high-risk groups. The case has been made in Chapter 1 that extrapolating benefits from high-risk groups to the population as a whole is fraught with danger. It was also argued in Chapter 1 that an apparently beneficial effect on some disease risk marker only becomes a real benefit if it ultimately translates into improved overall life expectancy or reduced morbidity. For persons at high and immediate risk of coronary thrombosis then, reduced tendency for blood to clot may be considered a beneficial effect but would it be necessarily good for everyone, e.g. those with some existing defect in the clotting system or those at high risk of cerebral haemorrhage? In contrast to the reported lower coronary heart disease mortality, stroke mortality is much higher in Greenland Eskimos than in Danes; stroke mortality is also high in some other high fish-consumers like the Japanese and Portuguese. Premenopausal women, in particular, would gain little if a reduction in their risk of death from coronary heart disease was compensated for by an increased risk of cerebral haemorrhage.

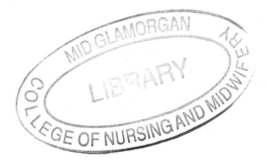

10 The vitamins

Contents

Introduction

Tables 10.1 and 10.2 give a summary of the important factual information about the fat-soluble and water-soluble vitamins respectively: their dietary forms and sources; some indication of human requirements, as indicated by the Dietary Reference Values; their cellular functions; the effects of deficiency; and, likely risk factors for deficiency. Readers with limited biochemical background are urged to refer back to Chapter 5 to facilitate their understanding of the significance of particular biochemical lesions that result from vitamin deficiency. The relevant chapters in Garrow and James (1993) are recommended as a reference source for factual information about the vitamins and the pathological consequences of deficiency. For some of the traditionally important but now uncommon deficiency diseases, more substantial accounts may be found in the previous edition of this book (Passmore and Eastwood, 1986).

Definition, essentiality and roles

Vitamins are a group of organic compounds that are indispensable to body function. Some vitamins cannot be synthesised in the body and others cannot be synthesised in sufficient quantity to meet the metabolic needs; they must therefore be provided in the human diet. Vitamins are only required in small amounts, and they do not serve as sources of dietary

Table 10.1 *The fat soluble vitamins; a summary*

Vitamin names and dietary forms

A: **retinol**; β-carotene and other carotenoids; vitamin A activity is expressed as retinol equivalents.

D: **cholecalciferol** (D_3); **calciferol** (D_2) in supplements and supplemented foods only.

E: **alpha-tocopherol**; other tocopherols have vitamin activity; vitamin E activity   expressed as alpha tocopherol equivalents.

K: **phylloquinone** from plants; menaquinone produced by intestinal bacteria.

Dietary Reference Values

UK RNI adult male/female; (American RDAs)

A: 700/600 µg/day; (1000/800).

D: none, if exposed to sunlight; (5 µg/day).

E: "safe intake" above 4/3 mg/day; (10/8 mg/day).

K: "safe intake" 1 µg/kg/day; (80/65 µg/day).

Dietary sources

A: retinol in dairy fat, eggs, liver, fatty fish and supplemented foods like margarine;   carotene in many dark green, red or yellow fruits and vegetables
  1 cup whole milk – 110 µg retinol equivalents;
  40 g cheddar cheese – 150 µg;
  1 portion (90 g) fried lamb liver – 18 500 µg;
  1 egg – 110 µg;
  1 tomato – 75 µg;
  1 serving (95 g) broccoli – 400 µg;
  1 serving (65 g) carrots – 1300 µg;
  1 banana – 27 µg;
  half cantaloupe melon – 700 µg.

D: dairy fat, eggs, liver, fatty fish and supplemented foods
  1 cup whole milk (UK unsupplemented) – 0.03–0.06 µg;
  1 egg – 1.2 µg;
  40 g cheddar cheese – 0.1 µg;
  5 g cod liver oil – 10.5 µg;
  1 portion (90 g) fried lamb liver – 0.5 µg;
  100 g fatty fish herrings (most), salmon, tuna, pilchards, sardines (least) – 6–22 µg;
  5 g pat of butter/margarine – 0.04/0.4 µg.

E: vegetable oils, wheat germ and whole grain cereals, dark green leaves, seeds and nuts
  1 egg – 1 mg;
  5 g pat of butter/polyunsaturated margarine – 0.1/1.25 mg;
  1 slice wholemeal bread – 0.05 mg;
  5 g sunflower/olive/rapeseed oil – 2.5/0.26/1.2 mg.

K: liver, green leafy vegetables, milk

Biochemical functions

A: precursor of 11-*cis* retinal, a component of visual pigments; maintains integrity of   epithelial tissues; synthesis of glycoproteins containing the sugar, mannose.

D: precursor of 1,25 dihydroxycholecalciferol, hormone produced in the kidney; increases capacity of gut and kidney tubule to transport calcium; regulates deposition of bone mineral.

E: antioxidant in the lipid phase; scavenges free radicals and prevents lipid peroxidation.

K: cofactor in synthesis of clotting factors.

(continued over page)

(Table 10.1 continued)

Effects of deficiency

A: night blindness; xerophthalmia leading to permanent blindness; poor growth; thickening and hardening of epithelial tissue; reduced immunocompetence.

D: rickets/osteomalacia with skeletal abnormalities; low plasma calcium; muscle weakness, possibly tetany; growth failure; increased risk of infection.

E: progressive degenerative neurological syndrome.

K: bleeding, especially brain haemorrhage in the newborn.

Risk factors for deficiency

A: poor diet, based upon starchy staple and unsupplemented with dairy fat, fatty fish or fruits and vegetables; very low fat diet; common in some Third world countries and major factor in child mortality and blindness.

D: inadequate exposure to sunlight, for variety of causes e.g. dress customs, housebound, working indoors for long hours; lack of back-up from limited range of animal foods or supplemented foods; pigmented skin?; high fibre diet?

E: clinical deficiency almost never seen, confined to persons with inherited inability to absorb fat soluble vitamins.

K: normally confined to newborn, especially premature infants; failure of fat soluble vitamin absorption.

---

energy. Many of them, or their derivatives, have clearly defined roles in particular biochemical pathways or physiological processes as illustrated by the following examples:

1 The vitamin A derivative, **11-*cis* retinal**, is the active principle of **rhodopsin,** the light sensitive pigment in the rods of the mammalian retina. Photochemical changes in this pigment are the first steps in converting the light energy reaching the rod into nerve impulses, i.e. vision. All known visual systems, including that of the other light detecting units of the mammalian retina (the cones), are based upon 11-*cis* retinal.

2 Thiamin (vitamin B1) is converted to thiamin pyrophosphate, an essential cofactor for several enzymes including pyruvic oxidase, the enzyme responsible for the conversion of pyruvic acid to acetyl coenzyme A in carbohydrate metabolism. In thiamin deficiency the metabolism of carbohydrates is progressively blocked at this step, leading to the accumulation of pyruvic acid and lactic acid. High carbohydrate intake increases the requirement for thiamin. Thiamin pyrophosphate is also an essential cofactor for a key enzyme of the Krebs cycle (α-oxyglutarate oxidase) and the enzyme transketolase in the pentose phosphate pathway (see Chapter 5).

3 Riboflavin gives rise to **flavin mononucleotide (FMN)** and **flavin adenine dinucleotide (FAD).** These flavin nucleotides are essential components (prosthetic groups) of several key **flavoprotein** enzymes involved in oxidation-reduction reactions. These flavin nucleotides are involved in both the Krebs cycle and oxidative phosphorylation, and so riboflavin deficiency leads to a general depression of oxidative metabolism. Glutathione reductase, an enzyme involved in disposal of free radicals, also has a flavin prosthetic group.

4 Niacin (nicotinic acid) is a component of the important coenzymes nicotinamide adenine dinucleotide (NAD) and the phosphorylated derivative (NADP);

Table 10:2 A summary of the dietetically important water soluble vitamins

Vitamin names and dietary forms

B_1: thiamin
B_2: riboflavin
B_3: niacin/nicotinic acid; may be synthesised from the amino acid tryptophan
B_6: pyridoxine and related compounds
B_1: cyanocobalamin and related compounds
—: Folic acid/folate (folacin)
C: ascorbic acid

Dietary Reference Values

UK RNI adult male/female; (American RDAs)
    Thiamin: 1.0/0.8 mg/day; (1.5/1.1)
    Riboflavin: 1.3/1.1 mg/day; (1.7/1.3)
    Niacin: 17/13 mg/day niacin equivalents; (19/15)
    B_6: 1.4/1.2 mg/day; (2.0/1.6)
    Folate: 200 µg/day; (200/180)
    B_{12}: 1.5 µg/day; (2.0)
    C: 40 mg/day; (60)

Dietary sources

Thiamin: found in all plant and animal tissues but only whole cereals, nuts, seeds and pulses are rich sources
    1 slice wholemeal bread (UK) – 0.12 mg
    1 egg – 0.04 mg
    1 pork chop – 0.7 mg
    1 cup whole milk – 0.06 mg
    30 g peanuts – 0.27 mg
    1 serving (165 g) brown/white rice – 0.23/0.02 mg
    1 serving (75 g) frozen peas – 0.18 mg
    1 serving (200 g) baked beans – 0.14 mg
    1 teaspoon (5 g) yeast extract – 0.16 mg.
Riboflavin: small amounts in many foods, rich sources are liver, milk, cheese and egg.
    1 slice wholemeal bread (UK) – 0.03 mg;
    1 egg – 0.21 mg;
    1 cup whole milk – 0.33 mg;
    40 g cheddar cheese – 0.16 mg;
    1 portion (90 g) fried lamb liver – 4 mg;
    1 teaspoon (5 g) yeast extract – 0.55 mg;
    1 serving (95 g) broccoli – 0.19 mg.
Niacin: distributed in small amounts in many foods but good amounts in meat, offal, fish, wholemeal cereals and pulses; in some cereals, especially maize, much of the niacin may be as unavailable niacytin; the tryptophan in many food proteins is also a source of niacin.
    1 slice wholemeal bread (UK) – 1.4 mg + 0.6 mg from tryptophan;
    1 portion (90 g) lamb liver – 13.7 mg + 4.4 mg;
    1 pork chop – 6.1 mg + 4.9 mg;
    1 serving (95 g) tinned tuna – 12.3 mg + 4.1 mg;
    1 egg – 0.04 mg + 2.2 mg;
    1 cup whole milk – 0.16 mg + 1.5 mg;
    1 portion (75 g) frozen peas – 1.1 mg + 0.7 mg.
B_6: liver is a rich source, cereals, meats, fruits and vegetables all contain moderate amounts.
B_{12}: Flesh foods, milk, eggs and fermented foods.

(continued over page)

(Table 10.2 continued)

Folate: liver, nuts, green vegetables, wholegrain cereals are good sources
    1 portion (90 g) lamb liver – 220 µg;
    1 slice wholemeal bread (UK) – 14 µg;
    peanuts (30 g) – 33 µg;
    1 portion (95 g) broccoli – 100 µg;
    1 banana – 30 µg;
    1 orange – 90 µg;
    1 teaspoon (5 g) yeast extract – 50 µg.
C: fruit, fruit juices, salad and leafy vegetables are good sources.
    1 serving (95 g) broccoli – 30 mg;
    1 serving (75 g) frozen peas – 10 mg;
    1 portion (150 g) boiled potatoes – 14 mg;
    1 portion (45 g) sweet pepper – 45 mg;
    1 tomato – 15 mg;
    1 orange – 95 mg;
    1 banana – 8 mg;
    1 serving (100 g) strawberries – 60 g;
    1 apple – 2 mg;
    1 glass (200 g) orange juice – 70 mg.

Biochemical/physiological roles

Thiamin: gives rise to thiamin pyrophosphate, a coenzyme for pyruvic oxidase (carbohydrate metabolism); transketolase(pentose phosphate pathway); α – oxyglutarate oxidase (Krebs cycle).

Riboflavin: component of flavin nucleotides which are cofactors for several enzymes involved in oxidation-reduction reactions.

Niacin: component of nicotinamide adenine dinucleotide (NAD) and NADP which are coenzymes involved in many oxidation–reduction reactions.

B_6: precursor of pyridoxal phosphate a coenzyme involved in amino acid metabolism.

B_{12}:interacts with folate in DNA synthesis reactions; required for nerve myelination.

Folate: involved with B_{12} in methylation reactions necessary for DNA synthesis.

C: important in synthesis of collagen; promotes iron absorption; functioning of immune system?

Effects of deficiency

Thiamin: beriberi and the neurological disorder Wernicke–Korsakoff syndrome.

Riboflavin: cracking at corners of mouth; raw red lips; enlarged nasal follicles plugged with sebaceous material.

Niacin: pellagra.

B_6: overt deficiency rare, convulsions reported in infants fed on B_6–depleted formula.

B_{12}: megaloblastic anaemia; degeneration of spinal cord leading to progressive paralysis.

Folate: megaloblastic anaemia; see also neural tube defects – Chapter 12.

C: scurvy.

Risk factors associated with deficiency

Thiamin: diet very heavily dependant upon polished rice; alcoholism.

Riboflavin: absence of milk from diet.

Niacin: diet dependent upon maize or sorghum and not supplemented by high protein foods.

B_6: deficiency rare.

B_{12}:vegan diet; failure of absorption in pernicious anaemia.

Folate: poor diet – deficiency common in tropical not developed countries; prolonged heating (e.g. of pulses) destroys folate; poor absorption e.g. in coeliac disease; some drugs (e.g. anti–convulsants) may interfere with folate functioning.

C: living upon preserved foods, absence of fruit and vegetables from the diet.

these serve as hydrogen acceptors and donators in numerous oxidation and reduction reactions in all human biochemical pathways. It is during the re-oxidation of the reduced NAD, produced during the oxidation of foodstuffs, that most of the ATP yielded by aerobic metabolism is produced in the mitochondria of human cells.

5 Vitamin C (ascorbic acid) is necessary for the functioning of the enzyme **proline hydroxylase**. This enzyme hydroxylates residues of the amino acid proline to hydroxyproline once it has been incorporated into the important structural protein **collagen**. Collagen is a major structural protein, it has the capacity to form strong insoluble fibres; it is the most abundant protein in mammals and serves to hold cells together. Collagen is a major structural component of bones, skin, cartilage, blood vessels and fulfils a structural role in most organs. The hydroxylation of proline residues occurs after incorporation of the amino acid into procollagen (the precursor of collagen) and the hydroxylation is necessary for the structural properties of collagen; hydroxyproline is almost exclusively confined to collagen.

6 Vitamin D (cholecalciferol) is the precursor of a hormone produced in the kidney, **1,25-dihydroxy cholecalciferol (1,25-DHCC)**. This 1,25-DHCC acts like a steroid hormone and is classified with the steroid hormones by endocrine physiologists; it stimulates the synthesis of proteins essential for calcium absorption in the gut and kidney and regulates the orderly deposition of calcium and phosphate in bone.

Classification

Vitamins are divided into two broad categories according to their solubility characteristics. Vitamins A, D, E, and K are insoluble in water but soluble in lipid or lipid solvents and they are thus classified as the **fat soluble vitamins**. The B group of vitamins and vitamin C are the **water soluble vitamins**. The term B vitamins actually describes a group of eight different vitamins which were originally grouped together as the B complex because they were found together in, for example, yeast extract. The eight vitamins of the B group are:

- thiamin (B_1)
- riboflavin (B_2)
- niacin (B_3)
- vitamin (B_6 – pyridoxine and related compounds)
- Vitamin (B_{12} – cobalamin)
- folate (folacin)
- pantothenic acid
- biotin.

In general, the fat soluble vitamins are stored in the liver and thus daily consumption is not required provided that average consumption over a period of time is adequate. Excesses of these vitamins are not readily excreted, and so if intakes are very high, toxic overload is possible. Concentrated supplements are the most likely cause of toxic overload but some very rich food sources can also produce symptoms of toxicity, e.g. livers of marine mammals and fish may contain toxic amounts of vitamins A or D and even liver from farm animals may contain enough vitamin A to cause birth defects if eaten by pregnant women. Note that unlike vitamin A itself (retinol) the plant pigment carotene, from which vitamin A can be made, has very low toxicity. As fat soluble vitamins are normally absorbed from the gut along with the fat, then fat malabsorption can increase the risk of fat soluble vitamin deficiency, e.g. in cystic fibrosis, the lack of pancreatic fat digesting enzymes may precipitate fat soluble vitamin deficiencies (see Chapter 13).

The water soluble vitamins, because of their solubility, leach into cooking water and this can result in very substantial losses during food preparation. Stores of these vitamins tend to be smaller than those of the fat soluble vitamins and excesses tend to be excreted in the urine. A more regular supply is usually required than for the fat soluble vitamins, and symptoms of deficiency tend to occur much sooner. Toxicity is much less likely because of their water solubility and urinary excretion and is all but impossible from natural foodstuffs.

The deficiency diseases

Dietary deficiencies of vitamins give rise to clinically recognisable deficiency diseases that may be readily cured by restoration of the vitamin supply. Vitamin discoveries greatly increased the perception of good nutrition as a vital prerequisite for good health; common and frequently fatal diseases could be cured by the administration of small amounts of vitamins or vitamin-containing foods. These cures probably unreasonably raised the expectation of the ability of nutrition to cure or prevent many other diseases. There is evidence that suboptimal intakes of vitamins may predispose to some non-deficiency diseases or impair physiological functioning, there is also some evidence that high intakes of vitamins can ameliorate the impact of some diseases, but vitamins only demonstrably cure or prevent deficiency diseases. In many cases the symptoms of these deficiency diseases, or at least some of them, are readily explicable from a knowledge of the cellular functions of the vitamin.

The diseases that are briefly described here have all represented, and in some cases still represent, major causes of human suffering. These deficiency diseases are rare in industrialised countries and generally confined to alcoholics or precipitated by some other serious medical or social problem. In a survey of British adults it was found that average intakes of all of the vitamins exceeded the then RDA (Gregory *et al.*, 1990). However those 2.5% of the sample with the lowest intakes were in several cases below the current EAR (e.g. thiamin for women, riboflavin and folate for men, and vitamin C for both sexes) in a few cases the recorded intakes of this bottom 2.5% were at or below even the current LRNI (e.g. vitamin A in both sexes and riboflavin and folate in women). Apparently satisfactory overall averages may obscure the fact that a substantial minority may be receiving seriously inadequate intakes of some vitamins. Note that there was some indication of underrecording in this survey particularly amongst women.

Vitamin A deficiency

Mild vitamin A deficiency results in impaired vision at low levels of light intensity, **night blindness**. This night blindness can be readily attributed to the role of retinol in the production of the visual pigments. More serious vitamin A deficiency is also most obvious in its effects on the eyes – the cornea and conjunctiva of the eye become dry, thickened and hard – this may lead on to ulceration and necrosis (cell death) of corneal tissue with the lens ultimately being extruded through the perforated cornea. The general term **xerophthalmia**, which literally means dry eye, is often used as a blanket term to describe all of the ocular manifestations of vitamin A deficiency.

It has been estimated that worldwide as many as a quarter of a million children go blind each year because of vitamin A deficiency; vitamin A deficiency is widespread in southern Asia, large parts of Africa and some parts of South America. Vitamin A deficiency not only affects the epithelial tissues of the eye but results in deleterious changes in epithelial tissue generally, e.g. in the gut, respiratory tract and reproductive tract. Diminished growth and a diminished immune response are also consequences of this deficiency. A combination of impaired immune function and reduced integrity of the epithelial tissues, which normally act as a barrier to pathogen entry, increases the risk of respiratory, gastrointestinal and genitourinary infections. Diarrhoea and respiratory infections are the major determinants of mortality of young children in Third World countries, and epidemiological evidence suggests that vitamin A deficiency is a major factor in the high mortality of young children in southern Asia. In field trials, Vitamin A supplements were associated with 30% reductions in mortality in preschool children in test areas of Indonesia. Reviewed by Rutishauser (1992).

Beriberi

In the first half of this century, **beriberi** was widespread in many countries of the Far East where white (polished) rice is the dietary staple, e.g. in China, Japan, Thailand, the Philippines, Indonesia and Malaysia. Beriberi leads to a progressive loss of sensation in the limbs due to deterioration of peripheral sensory nerves (neuropathy); motor nerves (i.e. those effecting muscle movement) are also affected and this leads to muscle wasting, weakness and in serious, prolonged deficiency, to paralysis (dry beriberi) – severe anorexia and infection may lead to death. Oedema and heart abnormalities may also occur leading to circulatory failure and death (wet beriberi). There may also be neurological manifestations, i.e. Wernicke-Korsakoff syndrome (see under alcoholism later in the chapter).

The clinical manifestations of beriberi can be largely explained by the known biochemical functions of the coenzyme derived from thiamin, thiamin pyrophosphate. Except during starvation, nervous tissue relies upon carbohydrate metabolism for its energy generation. As thiamin deficiency impairs carbohydrate metabolism, it is thus not surprising that many of the symptoms of beriberi are associated with changes in nerve function; heart muscle metabolism also normally relies heavily upon the aerobic metabolism of glucose. Production of the fatty sheath (myelin) covering nerve fibres is dependent upon the enzyme transketolase in the pentose phosphate pathway; this enzyme requires thiamin pyrophosphate as a coenzyme and demyelination of nerves is a feature of beriberi. The oedema of wet beriberi may be due to the accumulation of lactic acid in blood and tissues that results from impaired pyruvic oxidase functioning.

Pellagra

Pellagra is due to niacin deficiency. The specific biochemical role of niacin is as a precursor to the two important coenzymes NAD and NADP; these two coenzymes are involved in a large number of biochemical reactions and processes and it is not easy to directly attribute particular symptoms of the disease to particular biochemical "lesions".

The symptoms of the disease are often referred to as the 3Ds – dermatitis, diarrhoea and dementia. An early sign of pellagra is itching and burning of the skin which becomes roughened and thickened; skin exposed to sunlight is most liable to show dermatitis and a ring of affected skin around the neck (Casal's collar) is a common manifestation. Gastrointestinal symptoms, usually including diarrhoea, are a characteristic manifestation of pellagra. Early neurological symptoms are weakness, tremor anxiety, depression and irritability and, if there is severe prolonged deficiency, eventually dementia. The disease has high mortality and at its peak in the late 1920s and early 1930s caused thousands of deaths in the southern USA. According to Passmore and Eastwood (1986) it was still endemic in parts of southern Africa.

Riboflavin deficiency

According to Miller (1979), manifestations of mild riboflavin deficiency are relatively common even in industrialised countries. No severe deficiency disease has been described for this vitamin. This may be because the wide distribution of small amounts of the vitamin in food prevents mild deficiency progressing to major life-threatening illness or perhaps because riboflavin deficiency is usually associated with concurrent beriberi and the severe symptoms of beriberi mask the symptoms of riboflavin deficiency. In volunteers deliberately made riboflavin deficient, the symptoms were: chapping at the corners of the mouth (angular stomatitis); raw red lips (cheilosis); and, enlarged follicles around the sides of the nose which become plugged with yellow sebaceous material (nasolabial seborrhoea).

Megaloblastic anaemia

This type of anaemia may be caused dietetically either by lack of vitamin B_{12} or lack of folic acid (folacin). In **megaloblastic anaemia**, the red blood cells are large, irregular and fragile; the blood haemoglobin concentration may fall to less than a third of the normal level. Dietetic lack of B_{12} is rare and usually associated with a strict vegetarian diet. Folic acid deficiency is, on the other hand, common in some Third World countries. These two vitamins are necessary for the DNA replication and cell division in the bone marrow which generates red blood cells. High intakes of folic acid can compensate for lack of B_{12} and mask the haematological consequences of B_{12} deficiency. Prolonged B_{12} deficiency also leads to irreversible damage to the spinal cord – **combined sub acute degeneration**. This nerve damage manifests initially as loss of sensation or tingling sensation in the fingers and toes which leads to progressive paralysis. These consequences of B_{12} deficiency upon the nervous system are not corrected by folic acid, and so misdiagnosis and treatment of B_{12} deficiency with folic acid may mask the haematological consequences but allow the insidious progression of the irreversible spinal cord damage.

Scurvy

Scurvy is due to lack of vitamin C (ascorbic acid) and occurs in people deprived of fresh fruits and vegetables for extended periods, typically, in the past, those undertaking long sea voyages or expeditions. Most of the symptoms of scurvy can be attributed to impaired synthesis of the structural protein collagen, i.e. bleeding gums, loose teeth, subdermal haemorrhages due to leaking blood vessels, impaired wound healing and breakdown of old scars. Large areas of spontaneous bruising occur in severe scurvy, and haemorrhages in heart muscle or the brain may cause sudden death. Sudden death from haemorrhage or heart failure may occur even when the outward manifestations of scurvy do not appear particularly severe. Anaemia is usually associated with scurvy almost certainly because vitamin C is an important promoter of iron absorption from the gut. The organic bone matrix is largely collagen, and so osteoporosis may also occur in scurvy.

Rickets and Osteomalacia

Rickets in children and **osteomalacia** in adults are due to lack of vitamin D. During the late 19th century and early 20th century, rickets was extremely prevalent amongst poor children living in the industrial cities of Britain. The symptoms arise from a failure to absorb calcium from the gut which leads to reduced plasma calcium concentration and reduced calcification of bones. Muscle weakness, gastrointestinal and respiratory infections are general symptoms of rickets, and there are a series of skeletal abnormalities that are characteristic of the disease: bowing of the legs or knock knees; swelling of the wrist; beading of the ribs at the normal junction of cartilage and bone (rickety rosary); pelvic deformities which may cause problems in childbirth in later years. Plasma concentrations of calcium may fall low enough to induce tetanic convulsions in severe rickets.

Precursors and endogenous synthesis

Vitamins may be present in food in several different forms, and some substances may act as precursors from which vitamins can be manufactured; some examples are given below:

1 The plant pigment **beta(β)-carotene** can be cleaved by humans to yield two units of vitamin A (**retinol**). Absorption of carotene is less efficient than that of retinol and so 6 mg of carotene is roughly equivalent to 1 mg of retinol when obtained from most dietary sources. Vitamin A content of the diet is expressed in **retinol equivalents, RE** (1 µg RE = 1 µg of retinol). Carotene, and any other similar plant pigments with vitamin A activity, must all be converted to retinol equivalents to give the total vitamin A activity of foods or diets. Cats lack the enzyme necessary for this cleavage of carotene and are thus unable to utilise carotene as a source of vitamin A; most laboratory animals absorb carotene poorly.

2 The amino acid tryptophan can be converted to the vitamin niacin. Niacin can therefore be obtained from the diet either directly as vitamin present in the food or indirectly by the conversion of tryptophan in dietary protein to niacin. Thus, early suggestions that pellagra was due to protein deficiency were partly correct because high protein foods, by providing tryptophan, could permit endogenous niacin synthesis and cure or prevent deficiency. The niacin content of foods and diets is expressed in mg of **niacin equivalents** (1 mg of niacin = 1 mg niacin equivalent). In calculating the niacin equivalents in a food then, 60 mg of tryptophan is usually taken to be equivalent to 1 mg of niacin. In the typical British or American diet tryptophan would make up just over 1% of the total dietary protein.

3 Folic acid (folacin) is present in foods in several different forms, some of them free and some of them conjugated with variable numbers of molecules of the amino acid, glutamic acid. Differential efficiencies of absorption of these different compounds may make it difficult to assess with certainty the amount of biologically available folate in any particular food.

4 The principal source of vitamin D for most people is from endogenous synthesis in the skin. Ultra-violet radiation, from sunlight, acts on the substance 7-dehydrocholesterol which is produced in the skin and converts it to cholecalciferol or vitamin D_3. Dietary vitamin D is widely considered to be a supplement or back-up for this endogenous production. In the UK no Dietary Reference Values are given for vitamin D for the bulk of people between the ages of 4 and 65 years, provided that they have reasonable exposure to summer sunshine; reference values are only given for those groups for whom endogenous production cannot be relied upon to meet physiological needs, i.e. the under 4s, the elderly and pregnant or lactating women. In the USA, an RDA is given for all groups, ranging from 5 µg/day for the over 25s to 10 µg/day for most other groups – in Britain where an RNI is given it is between 7 and 10 µg/day. Average dietary intakes of vitamin D in the UK are around 3 µg/day, and so the reference

values imply the need for supplements in those unable to synthesise their own vitamin D because of lack of sunlight.

5 Most mammals can convert glucose to ascorbic acid (vitamin C) but primates, guinea pigs and a few exotic species lack a key enzyme on this pathway and thus they require a dietary supply of this vitamin. This limits the ability to study the effects of vitamin C deficiency and supplementation in most common laboratory animals. It has also led to speculative estimates of human requirements by extrapolating from calculated rates of synthesis in other mammals (see Chapter 3).

Circumstances that precipitate deficiency

People meeting their energy needs and eating a variety of different types of foods seldom show clinical signs of micronutrient deficiency. Dietary deficiencies arise when either the total food supply is poor, or the variety and nutritional quality of the food eaten is low, or both. Micronutrient deficiencies thus often occur as an added problem of general food shortage and starvation. Vitamin deficiencies may also be associated with diets that are very heavily dependent upon a single staple food that is deficient in a vitamin or are associated with some other very particular dietary circumstance or restriction. A number of circumstances that have been associated with high risk of particular deficiency states are discussed below.

Beriberi

Beriberi (thiamin deficiency) has historically been associated with diets based upon polished rice. Rice is inherently low in thiamin and much of the thiamin is located in the outer layers of the rice grain which are removed by milling; machine milling is much more efficient in this removal than traditional hand milling. Rice is also high in starch which increases thiamin requirements. A diet in which a very high proportion of the total calories are derived from polished rice precipitates beriberi. Beriberi is not a disease of famines and is one of the few deficiency diseases that tended to afflict the more privileged members of society (e.g. the armed forces of Japan and China at the turn of the century) rather than the very poor; the more privileged groups ate the higher prestige white rice, with its thiamin removed, whereas the poor were forced to rely upon the low prestige and cheaper brown rice, with its thiamin still present.

Most parts of India escaped epidemics of beriberi because of different milling practices. The rice was soaked and then steamed or boiled prior to milling (parboiled), and this greatly increases the retention of B vitamins within the rice grain after milling. Introduction of less harsh milling practices, fortification of white rice with thiamin and diversification of the diet have all contributed to the decline in beriberi. Intakes of thiamin are, however, still low in many rice eating countries and offer little margin of safety.

Pellagra

Pellagra (niacin deficiency) has almost always been associated with diets based upon maize. Maize protein (zein) is low in the amino acid tryptophan which can serve as a niacin precursor, and the niacin present in maize is present in a bound form (**niacytin**) that is unavailable to humans. Introduction of maize from the Americas has been associated with major epidemics in those parts of the world where it became established as the dominant staple, e.g. in Southern Europe, North Africa and South Africa. As stated in Chapter 1, in the early decades of this century the disease was so prevalent amongst the poorer residents of southern states of the USA that it was thought to be an infectious disease.

Davies (1964) gives an analysis of the factors that led to the rise and fall of pellagra in the southern United States. At the turn of the century the diets of poor Southerners were based upon corn (maize), pork fat and molasses. The first recorded outbreak of pellagra in the southern USA was in 1907 and Davies attributes this to changes in the way that the corn was milled. At the turn of the century, large scale milling replaced the old inefficient water driven mills and this harsher milling produced a finer and more palatable corn meal, but it also removed the germ of the corn grain and reduced its vitamin content. Paradoxically the disease started to decline at the height of the Great Depression. Davies suggests that this was because demand for cotton, the principal agricultural product of the region, declined very sharply, leading many farmers to cultivate gardens and smallholdings to produce food crops. He thus attributes the decline in pellagra, at a time of great economic deprivation, to departure from the cash-crop monoculture rather than to increased knowledge of the causes of the disease and methods of prevention.

Amongst the people of Central America, where maize originated, its consumption was not associated with pellagra because the traditional method of tortilla preparation resulted in the release of niacin from its bound state; the maize grains were mixed with slaked lime (calcium hydroxide) and subjected to prolonged heating prior to grinding and cooking.

Sorghum consumption is associated with pellagra in some parts of India despite the fact that Sorghum contains reasonable amounts of tryptophan (almost as much as rice which is not pellagragenic). Bender (1983) suggested that this might be because of the high content of another amino acid, leucine, in Sorghum which inhibits key enzymes in the conversion of tryptophan to niacin.

Introduction of harsh machine milling seems to have been a factor in increasing the risk of both beriberi and pellagra. Epidemics of both diseases seem to have been precipitated by the introduction of machine milling. Most of the vitamins in cereal grains are concentrated in the outer layers and in the germ; harsh machine milling processes effectively remove these parts of the grain and thus greatly deplete the nutrient content of the milled product (as well as removing much of the dietary fibre). Traditional milling methods were less efficient in removing these outer layers and left more of the vitamins in the final product.

Scurvy

Scurvy (vitamin C deficiency) is not a disease of famines, it occurred principally among people living for extended periods upon preserved foods, e.g. those undertaking long sea voyages or taking part in expeditions to places where fresh foods were unavailable. The curative and preventative effects of fresh vegetables, fruits and fruit juices were documented almost two centuries before the discovery of vitamin C. In 1795, the regular provision of lime juice (or some suitable alternative) to British naval personnel resulted in the "limey" nickname for British sailors that is still sometimes used to describe the British.

B_{12} deficiency

Vitamin B_{12} is naturally confined to foods of animal origin (flesh foods and dairy produce) and to micro-organisms, although meat substitutes must contain added B_{12} in the UK. This means that strict vegetarians (vegans) may avoid all foods that naturally contain B_{12} and thus be at risk of dietary deficiency of the vitamin unless they eat supplemented foods or take B_{12} supplements. In practice, even amongst those theoretically at risk, dietary deficiency is uncommon because requirements are very small (perhaps only 1 μg/day) and an omnivore might have stores that would represent several years turnover of the vitamin. Contaminants of foods, e.g. mould on nuts, insects on fruit or vegetables, or perhaps synthesis by gut bacteria may contribute significant amounts of B_{12} to the diet of even the strictest vegetarian. Some lactovegetarian Asian women in the UK develop signs of deficiency despite the presence of B_{12} in milk – this is explained by suggesting that the traditional practice of boiling milk with tea may destroy the B_{12} in the milk.

The usual cause of B_{12} deficiency is not dietary lack but an autoimmune disease, **pernicious anaemia,** that results in damage to the parietal cells of the stomach that produce an **intrinsic factor** that is necessary for the absorption of B_{12} from the gut. Until the 1920s, pernicious anaemia was an inevitably fatal condition; nowadays the effects of the resulting B_{12} deficiency can be alleviated by monthly injections of the vitamin.

Rickets

Inadequate exposure of the skin to sunlight is regarded as the primary cause of vitamin D deficiency. Poor dietary supply of the vitamin is usually regarded as an exacerbating factor. The risk of vitamin D deficiency (rickets in children; osteomalacia in adults) is increased by any factors that reduce exposure of the skin to the correct ultra violet wavelengths, e.g. living in northern latitudes, atmospheric pollution, skin pigmentation, customs of dress, being housebound because of illness or immobility, working indoors for very long hours and other cultural or social factors that prevent people getting out of doors during the daytime.

Alcoholism

In affluent countries, alcoholics are a group who are at particular risk of vitamin

deficiencies – most obviously because high alcohol consumption is likely to be associated with low food and nutrient intake. Alcoholic drinks yield substantial numbers of calories but few nutrients and thus substantially reduce the nutrient density of the diet. Poor alcoholics spend their limited money upon alcohol rather than food. High alcohol consumption may also increase the requirement for some nutrients and reduce the efficiency of absorption of others. Several of the deficiency diseases listed earlier do occur in alcoholics in affluent countries, and in many cases there are multiple deficiencies. Some of the harmful effects of very high alcohol intakes may be attributable to dietary deficiency rather than harmful effects of alcohol *per se*.

Alcoholics are particularly prone to thiamin deficiency and some neurological problems caused by thiamin deficiency – Wernicke-Korsakoff Syndrome. This syndrome is characterised by paralysis of eye movements or rapid jerky eye movements (nystagmus), unsteadiness when walking or standing and mental derangements including loss of memory and the ability to learn. Post mortems upon such patients show lesions in various parts of the brain ranging from loss of myelin to complete necrosis. It has been suggested that only a proportion of alcoholics are susceptible to this neurological disorder because of an inherited defect in their transketolase enzyme; it binds thiamin pyrophosphate much less efficiently than normal. The reduction in transketolase activity could explain the demyelination of nerves seen in this syndrome which probably produce the neurological changes (see also Chapter 5).

Low fat diets

Very low fat diets may precipitate fat soluble vitamin deficiencies. These diets contain low amounts of fat soluble vitamins and the absorption of the vitamins may also be impaired by the lack of fat. Children in some Third World countries consume marginally adequate amounts of vitamin A (as carotene in fruits and vegetables) but their extremely low fat intake impairs absorption of the vitamin and may precipitate deficiency. Poor fat absorption (e.g. in cystic fibrosis and coeliac disease) may also be associated with fat soluble vitamin deficiencies (see Chapter 13).

Vitamin K

Vitamin K deficiency leads to a reduced efficiency of the blood clotting system and thus to a tendency to bleed. Primary dietary deficiency of vitamin K is almost never seen but malabsorption for example in coeliac disease can precipitate deficiency and lead to bleeding. Some newborn babies, especially premature babies, may develop intracranial haemorrhages shortly after birth; this tendency to haemorrhage can be prevented by prophylactic administration of vitamin K and the routine administration of vitamin K is common in maternity units (see Chapter 1 for some discussion of this practice). The coumarin group of anticoagulant drugs (e.g. warfarin) exert their effect by blocking the effects of vitamin K and lead to reduced level of prothrombin and other clotting factors in blood. Therapeutic overdosage of these drugs or accidental overdosage due to warfarin-based rodent poisons leads to bleeding and vitamin K acts as an antidote.

Free radicals and antioxidants

What are free radicals?

Free radicals are highly reactive species that have an unpaired electron, e.g. the **hydroxyl** and **superoxide** radicals. Cellular damage caused by these oxygen-derived species has been speculatively implicated in the aetiology of a range of diseases including cancer and cardiovascular disease. It has also been suggested that many of the degenerative changes associated with ageing may be due to the cumulative effects of free radical damage.

These highly reactive species certainly have the potential to cause tissue damage; white blood cells generate superoxide free radicals in order to kill bacteria that they have engulfed. Oxygen free radicals can react with DNA to cause breaks in the DNA chain and alteration of bases (mutation); this could initiate carcinogenesis. Free radicals can react with serum low density lipoprotein (LDL) and the resultant oxidised LDL is much more damaging to arterial walls than LDL. They can also react with membrane lipids leading to peroxidation of polyunsaturated fatty acid residues. Reaction of free radicals with, for example, polyunsaturated fatty acids will generate further unstable compounds (the **lipid peroxyl radical**) and this can lead to a chain of damaging reactions unless antioxidant systems stabilise or quench these chain reactions. Their supposed susceptibility to free radical damage is one of the concerns about diets with very high levels of polyunsaturated fat (COMA, 1991).

Physiological mechanisms to limit free radical damage

Free radicals are normal by-products of the oxidative processes in cells and there are several physiological mechanisms that dispose of free radicals and limit their tissue-damaging effects. There are other mechanisms for the repair of cellular damage induced by free radicals such as the mechanisms to repair damaged segments of DNA.

There are a number of metal containing enzymes, the sole function of which appears to be to scavenge and dispose of free radicals and thus prevent or limit their tissue-damaging effects. Several essential dietary nutrients are components of enzymes that are involved in free radical disposal, for example:

1 Zinc and copper are components of the enzyme **superoxide dismutase** which disposes of the superoxide radical by converting two superoxide radicals to hydrogen peroxide and oxygen.
2 Selenium is a component of the enzyme **glutathione peroxidase** which converts damaging hydrogen peroxide to water and oxygen. It also converts peroxidised lipids into stable and harmless products, thus breaking a damaging chain reaction of free radical production.
3 Iron is a component of the enzyme **catalase** which converts hydrogen peroxide to water and oxygen.
4 The enzyme **glutathione reductase** regenerates glutathione which is oxidised by the glutathione peroxidase reaction mentioned above; this enzyme is a flavoprotein and utilises a riboflavin derivative as a prosthetic group.

In addition to these enzyme systems, some vitamins have innate antioxidant properties and so have the capacity to scavenge free radicals, e.g. vitamin E in the lipid phase and vitamin C in the aqueous phase. These two vitamins are used by food manufacturers as antioxidant food additives. β–carotene and other carotenoids may also function as free radical scavengers.

Figure 10.1 shows some reactions of free radicals and Figure 10.2 some of the mechanisms for their safe disposal – full understanding of these figures requires some understanding of the underlying chemistry; readers without such chemical understanding will probably have to rely upon the descriptive account in the text.

Situations that increase damage by free radicals

Two types of situation are thought to increase the risk of disease due to free radical damage of cellular components:

- increased generation of free radicals beyond the capacity of the mechanisms for their safe disposal and repair of the damage that they induce
- impaired capacity of the disposal mechanisms to handle any free radicals that are generated.

If premature babies are exposed to elevated oxygen concentration in their incubators, then this can cause damage to the retina and lead to blindness – **retinopathy of prematurity**. This is one of the relatively few examples of a disease process being fairly strongly and causally linked to excess free radical production. High oxygen concentration is thought to lead to excessive generation of oxygen free radicals which are responsible for the retinal damage; there is evidence that vitamin E, a free radical scavenger, protects these babies from the damaging effects of oxygen. High oxygen concentration of inspired air also produces lung damage in adults. When water is exposed to ionising radiations, this generates hydroxyl radicals and they are responsible for much of the damage to living cells caused by ionising radiations. There is also evidence that the toxic effects of excess iron may be due to free radical effects; *in vitro*, excess iron in serum stimulates lipid peroxidation and the formation of damaging hydroxyl radicals from hydrogen peroxide. Cigarette smoke and other air pollutants may exert some of their harmful effects by generating free radicals.

In most diseases there is increased formation of oxygen free radicals as a consequence of the disease process. Infiltration of white cells into damaged or diseased tissue will result in excess oxidant load because superoxide generation

The superoxide radical ($O_2^{\bullet-}$) is produced during oxidative phosphorylation, oxygen-haemoglobin dissociation and by phagocytic white cells.

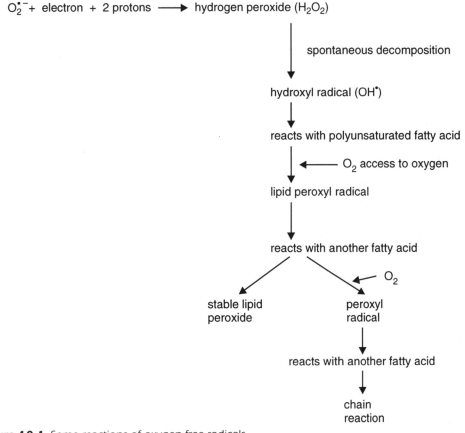

$$O_2^{\bullet-} + \text{electron} + 2 \text{ protons} \longrightarrow \text{hydrogen peroxide } (H_2O_2)$$

spontaneous decomposition

hydroxyl radical (OH$^{\bullet}$)

reacts with polyunsaturated fatty acid

O_2 access to oxygen

lipid peroxyl radical

reacts with another fatty acid

stable lipid peroxide

peroxyl radical

O_2

reacts with another fatty acid

chain reaction

Figure 10.1 Some reactions of oxygen free radicals

is used by these cells to kill pathogenic bacteria. Mechanical injury to tissue also results in increased free radical reactions. This means that injured or diseased tissue generates free radicals much faster than healthy tissue, and so reports that biochemical indices of free radical damage are raised in disease states should be treated with caution. These raised free radical indices may be a reflection of the disease process rather than an indication that free radical "attack" is a key factor in initiating the disease, and they do not necessarily indicate that free radical scavengers like vitamin E will prevent or ameliorate the condition. For example, in experimental deficiency of vitamin E in rats there is a muscular atrophy that resembles that seen in the fatal, inherited human disease, muscular dystrophy. Indices of free radical damage are indeed also raised in the wasting muscles of boys afflicted with muscular dystrophy, but vitamin E does not alter the progress of the disease; the free radical damage is almost certainly a result of the disease rather than its primary cause.

The antioxidant minerals, together with riboflavin, are essential components of enzyme systems involved in the safe disposal of free radicals. Deficiencies of these micronutrients might be expected to

Superoxide dismutase (zinc-containing) converts superoxide radicals to hydrogen peroxide:

$$2H^+ + O_2^{\cdot -} + O_2^{\cdot -} \xrightarrow{\text{superoxide dismutase}} H_2O_2 + O_2$$

Glutathione peroxidase (selenium-containing) converts hydrogen peroxide to water:

$$H_2O_2 + \text{reduced glutathione} \xrightarrow{\text{glutathione peroxidase}} H_2O_2 + \text{oxidised glutathione}$$

Glutathione reductase (riboflavin-containing) regenerates reduced glutathione:

$$\text{oxidised glutathione} \xrightarrow{\text{glutathione reductase}} \text{reduced glutathione}$$

The enzyme catalase (iron-containing) converts hydrogen peroxide to water and oxygen:

$$2H_2O_2 \xrightarrow{\text{catalase}} 2H_2O_2 + O_2$$

Vitamin E can quench free radicals:

$$\text{free radical} + \text{vit E} \longrightarrow \text{water} + \text{oxidised E}$$

$$\text{lipid peroxyl} + \text{vit E} \longrightarrow \text{stable hydroperoxide} + \text{oxidised E}$$

Vitamin E can be regenerated by a mechanism that involves vitamin C:

$$\text{oxidised E} \xrightarrow{\text{regeneration (vit C)}} \text{vit E}$$

Figure 10.2 Some mechanisms for disposal of free radicals

reduce the activity of these disposal mechanisms and thus increase tissue damage by free radicals. However, given this mode of action, it seems unlikely that high intakes would exert any extra protective effects. Selenium or zinc deficiency might be expected to increase free radical damage, but it seems improbable that supplements of these minerals, in well nourished people, would supply any extra protection against free radicals by increasing synthesis of their dependant enzymes. **Keshan disease** may be an example of a deficiency disease due to lack of one of these antioxidant minerals. In this condition there is a potentially fatal degeneration of the heart muscle (cardiomyopathy). This disease has been reported in certain areas of China where the soil is very low in selenium. Activity of the selenium dependant enzyme, glutathione peroxidase, is low and the condition responds to selenium supplements and so the disease has been attributed to lack of dietary selenium with consequent failure of the free radical disposal mechanism.

The other antioxidant vitamins, i.e. vitamin E, vitamin C and carotene have the capacity to react with and quench free radicals without themselves becoming highly reactive. They thus have a free standing antioxidant effect, independent of the enzyme mechanisms. There has, therefore, been considerable speculation as to whether high intakes of these micronutrients might protect against free radical damage and, in particular, reduce the long term risk of cardiovascular disease and cancer. Epidemiological studies consistently report a negative association between high intakes of fruits and vegetables and cancer risk and these foods are the principle dietary sources of carotene and vitamin C. There has also been much speculation about whether high intakes of vitamin E might exert a protective effect against subsequent risk of cardiovascular disease.

Figure 10.3 shows a theoretical scheme that seeks to explain how a free radical mechanism might be involved in the development of atherosclerosis. This scheme could explain the apparent interaction between several risk factors in the development of cardiovascular disease and it might also help to explain why serum LDL cholesterol concentration is such an imperfect predictor of cardiovascular risk. A high fat diet tends to raise the LDL cholesterol concentration; cigarette smoking increases free radical production; and, lack of dietary antioxidants limits the capacity to scavenge free radicals and thus to minimise the damage that they can induce. Any unquenched free radicals can react with LDL to convert it to much more atherogenic oxidised forms. Oxidised cholesterol has been shown to

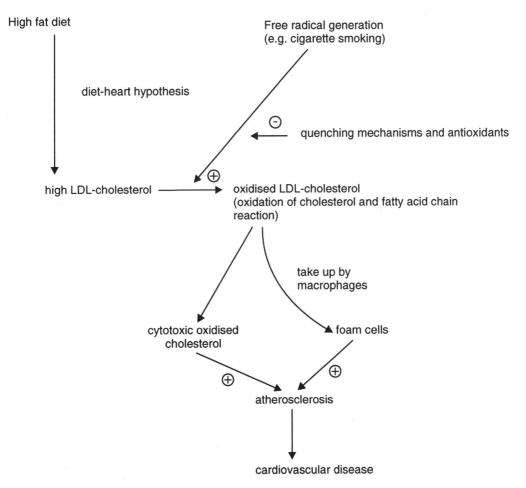

Figure 10.3 A hypothetical scheme to illustrate how free radical generation might contribute to risk of cardiovascular disease

be much more damaging to the arterial wall than cholesterol itself and oxidised LDL is also taken up very readily by macrophages and these LDL-loaded macrophages become foam cells which are characteristically found in atheromatous arterial lesions.

Conning (1991) and Diplock (1991) have written concise referenced reviews of the role of antioxidant nutrients in disease.

Are high intakes of vitamin C beneficial?

The UK panel on Dietary Reference Values (COMA, 1991) listed at least eight benefits that have been suggested for intakes of vitamin C that are well in excess of those needed to prevent or to cure scurvy. They were nevertheless not persuaded to allow any of these suggested benefits to influence their decisions about the reference values for vitamin C. It has been suggested at one time or another that, for example, high intakes might have the following beneficial effects:

1 a serum cholesterol-lowering effect
2 improved physical work capacity
3 improved immune function
4 reduced formation of carcinogenic substances called nitrosamines in the stomach and thus reduced risk of stomach cancer
5 improved male fertility
6 megadoses (several grams daily) might extend life in patients with terminal cancer (a well controlled study found no evidence of such a benefit – Creagan *et al.*, 1979).

Perhaps the most persistent of these claims is that intakes of more than 10 times the RNI/RDA for vitamin C might help prevent the development of the common cold. This view was popularised by a book published in the early 1970s that was written by the double Nobel prize winner Linus Pauling (Pauling, 1972). Since 1970 there have been dozens of controlled trials on the efficacy of vitamin C in preventing colds and/or reducing their duration. Despite this plethora of research effort their remains no convincing evidence that high vitamin C intakes affect either the frequency of colds or their duration (Passmore and Eastwood, 1986). The theoretical basis for advocating very high intakes of vitamin C also seems weak and based largely upon either cross species extrapolations of the amounts synthesised by the rat or upon the amounts consumed by other vitamin C requiring primates like gorillas. More recent recognition that the antioxidant properties of vitamin C may be important in protecting against free radical damage are more persuasive.

One intriguing finding is that there are very high concentrations of vitamin C in the adrenal glands. The adrenal glands are known to be very important in responses to stress. Either stress itself, or mimicking the stress reaction with the pituitary hormone adrenocorticotrophic hormone (ACTH) leads to depletion of the vitamin C content of the adrenals. This has led to the belief that vitamin C requirements may be increased during stress although no clear explanation of the role of vitamin C in the stress reaction has been forthcoming.

Claims for the beneficial effects of vitamin intakes that are orders of magnitude higher than the reference values or usual intake are really the province of the pharmacologist rather than the nutritionist; the vitamin is being used as a potential drug rather than as a nutrient. Vitamin C is one of the antioxidant vitamins and there is a fairly consistent body of epidemiological evidence that diets rich in vitamin C (i.e. high in fruits and vegetables and relatively low in fat) are associated with reduced risk of cancer. There seems to be a good case, based both upon theoretical and observational grounds, for recommending diets rich in vitamin C but there is little convincing evidence that vitamin C supplements *per se* will confer any significant health benefits.

Many thousands of people are unconvinced by arguments against the efficacy of vitamin C supplements and in such individuals the placebo effect may mean that they do in practice derive benefit from these preparations. Such widespread consumption of doses that are far in excess of those that can be obtained from normal human diets means that the potential toxicity of these preparations needs to be considered. The vitamin appears to be non-toxic even at doses many times the RNI/RDA, say 1 g/day, and much of the excess is excreted in the urine. Some concerns about intakes of gram quantities of the vitamin are listed below (after Hamilton *et al.*, 1991).

1 Very large excesses may lead to diarrhoea and gastrointestinal symptoms.
2 Sudden withdrawal of the supplement may precipitate scurvy because of induction of mechanisms for disposal of the excess vitamin.
3 Products of vitamin C metabolism may increase risk of gout and kidney stones in susceptible people.
4 Large doses of vitamin C may interfere with anticoagulant therapy.
5 Large amounts of vitamin C excreted in the urine may make urinary tests for diabetes unreliable.

Doses of up to 1 g/day can probably be tolerated for very long periods with no obvious ill effects in most people.

Do high intakes of vitamin A or β–carotene help prevent cancer?

This topic has been reviewed by Rutishauser (1992) and Peto *et al.* (1981) and many of the uncited references used for this discussion are listed in these reviews.

Early observations of the effects of experimental vitamin A deficiency in animals found a characteristic overgrowth (metaplasia) of the epithelial tissues of the respiratory tract, gut and genito-urinary tract. These epithelial changes, due to vitamin A deficiency, closely resemble precancerous changes in epithelial tissues. These observations led to the suggestion that vitamin A deficiency might predispose individuals to epithelial cancers and that high vitamin A intakes might exert a protective effect against such cancers. Retinol (vitamin A) and related compounds (the retinoids) have been shown to protect against experimentally induced cancers and precancerous changes in studies with experimental animals. Retinol derivatives (e.g. etretinate and isotretinoin) have been successfully used to treat some malignant conditions in humans. Note, however, that retinol itself is far too toxic to be therapeutically useful in cancer treatment and these therapeutic retinoids have little or no vitamin A activity. Indeed, these therapeutic agents have been designed to retain the anti tumour effect of retinoids but to lose the vitamin A activity which is responsible for their toxicity.

Several studies in the 1970s and early 1980s (e.g. Wald *et al.*, 1980) reported that stored blood samples from patients who subsequently developed cancer contained significantly lower plasma retinol concentrations than those who did not go on to develop cancer. There are many reasons why such results from prospective case-control studies might not necessarily indicate a protective effect of dietary vitamin A on cancer risk (see Chapter 3 for fuller discussion of this example). Two very obvious criticisms of such studies are:

1 That one may be simply observing changes in the dietary intake or direct changes in plasma retinol that are a consequence of the early stages of existing disease. It is very difficult to know how long the gap between sample collection and tumour identification needs to be before one can confidently exclude this as a possible explanation.

2 Except at the extremes (i.e. very low or very high intakes) then plasma retinol concentration is not related to vitamin A intake.

In general, studies in which intake of retinol has been related to subsequent cancer risk have not found any association, although a weak association between total vitamin A intake and cancer risk has been reported (Rutishauser, 1992). Peto *et al.* (1981) concluded that even if the relationship between plasma retinol and cancer risk is eventually confirmed then this may be of very limited dietary significance because factors other than dietary vitamin A intake (e.g. hormonal factors) are the primary determinants of plasma retinol concentration. There are overwhelming grounds, unrelated to cancer risk, for measures to ensure adequacy of vitamin A intake in areas of the world where deficiency exists. There is, however, no convincing evidence that supplemental intakes of retinol, well in excess of the RNI/ RDA, are likely to be beneficial; given the known toxicity and teratogenicity of vitamin A, they are undesirable.

Peto *et al.* (1981) raised the possibility that β–carotene, and perhaps other dietary carotenoids, might exert a protective effect against cancer risk that was independent of their role as precursors of vitamin A. Since that time, authors have tended to separate out preformed vitamin A (retinol) and carotenoid precursors when assessing any possible protective effects of vitamin A. There is some evidence that carotenoids protect against experimentally induced cancers in animals but the doses needed are high, perhaps because β–carotene is very poorly absorbed by laboratory animals. A high intake of fruits and vegetables has fairly consistently been associated with reduced cancer risk in both retrospective case-control studies and in more reliable cohort studies. Several studies have also found a negative association between serum β–carotene levels and subsequent risk of lung cancer. The currently favoured mechanism of any cancer preventing effects of the carotenoids in food would be by their free radical scavenging action. This might, for example, explain the apparent protective effect of high carotenoid intake on cancer of the lung induced by cigarette smoking because smoking is known to increase free radical production. β–carotene is, unlike preformed vitamin A, relatively non toxic and so supplements can be taken without apparent risk of poisoning. It must be said, however, that the evidence for a protective effect of carotenoid-rich diet is much stronger than for this effect being wholly or even partly due to the presence of β–carotene within the food.

Are vitamin E supplements beneficial?

Vitamin E is a potent antioxidant and it has been shown to protect against some conditions where the symptoms are confidently thought to be due to free radical-induced tissue damage, e.g. the retinopathy induced by exposure to high oxygen concentrations in premature babies. Riemersma *et al.* (1991) identified around a hundred men suffering from undiagnosed angina pectoris (chest pain due to atherosclerotic narrowing of the coronary blood vessels) by using a self-administered chest pain questionnaire. They matched them with around 400 controls who appeared to be free of angina. They found that plasma concentrations of the three antioxidant vitamins (vitamin C, vitamin E and carotene) were inversely related to risk of angina. Only the relationship for vitamin E remained statistically significant when allowance was made for confounding variables like smoking. This same group of workers (Wood *et al.*, 1987) had previously suggested an inverse relationship between intakes of polyunsaturated fatty acids and risk of angina. Dietary vitamin E comes principally from the same sources as polyunsaturated fatty acids of the linoleate series, i.e. vegetable fats. The analysis of Riemersma *et al.* did not exclude the possibility that the apparent association between vitamin E intake and angina was a secondary consequence of higher intakes of polyunsaturated fatty acids. Riemersma *et al.* (1991) did not apparently record intake of vitamin supplements but at the time this data was collected very few men in the region of Scotland used would have taken supplements of either vitamin E or β–carotene although some may have taken vitamin C or multivitamin supplements.

Two very recent and large cohort studies have suggested that in both women (Stampfer *et al.*, 1993) and men (Rimm *et al.*, 1993) consumption of high levels of vitamin E was associated with reduced risk of coronary heart disease. In neither of these studies was the association removed by correction for expected confounding variables. In neither of these studies was any significant association found between vitamin E intake from food and risk of coronary heart disease and thus the apparent benefit was only observed at doses of vitamin E beyond those consumed in typical US diets. In the women's study, the follow up period was eight years and detailed information was given on other causes of mortality during this period. Neither vitamin E supplements nor multivitamin supplements were associated with any significant reduction in overall mortality, despite a sample size of almost 90 000 women – there was a non significant reduction in those taking vitamin E supplements but equally there was a non significant increase in those taking multivitamins. One should be very wary of advising long term, mass consumption of pharmacological intakes of vitamins (as with any other drug) unless the long term and holistic benefits have been unequivocally demonstrated and the very long term safety of the dosing confirmed for all people (neither group of authors advocate such supplementation yet). COMA (1991) felt that there was still insufficient information about human vitamin E requirements to even offer a full set of UK Dietary Reference Values and only a safe intake was given.

Vitamin E is found in leafy vegetables, whole grain cereals, liver and egg yolks but the richest sources are vegetable oils and the fat fractions of nuts and seeds. Recommending diets specifically aimed at raising vitamin E concentrations could thus conflict with the general advice to reduce total fat intakes although increased intakes of vegetables and whole grain cereals is consistent with other recommendations. It is generally assumed that the requirement for this vitamin is increased by high intakes of polyunsaturated fatty acids because of their susceptibility to peroxidation by oxygen free radicals.

After this section was written, a Finnish group (Group, 1994) reported the results of a randomised, double-blind, placebo-controlled trial of the effects of vitamin E and/or β–carotene supplements in a sample of 30 000, 50–69 year-old, male smokers. Neither supplement appeared to afford any protection against the development of lung cancer during the follow-up period (5–8 years). The rates of lung cancer in the β–carotene supplemented men were, in fact, significantly higher than in those not receiving β–carotene. There was no significant difference in total mortality between those receiving and not receiving vitamin E (2% higher in the vitamin E group supplemented). The total mortality was significantly higher in those receiving β–carotene supplements (8%) due to increased deaths from lung cancer, heart disease and stroke. More detailed breakdowns are given of the comparative incidence and death rates from several cancers and other diseases. The authors conclude that "this trial raises the possibility that these supplements may have harmful as well as beneficial effects".

11 The minerals

Contents

Introduction

In the UK, Dietary Reference Values are offered for 11 minerals and safe intakes listed for a further four (COMA, 1991); these same 15 minerals are also deemed to warrant a recommendation of some type in the American RDAs (NRC, 1989a). There is, therefore, international acceptance that at least 15 dietary minerals are essential.

Several of these essential minerals are required only in trace amounts and in some cases requirements are difficult to establish with confidence. A further 19 minerals were considered by COMA (1991), most they classified as non-essential or of unproven essentiality, a few they regarded as probably essential in trace amounts.

Incidence of clinically-recognisable, dietary deficiency states are extremely rare for most essential minerals. Only two such deficiencies diseases have either historically or currently been generally regarded as anything other than extremely rare or localised, i.e. **goitre** a swelling of the thyroid gland caused by lack of dietary iodine and **iron-deficiency anaemia**, these are both discussed below. This has not prevented very active debate about whether suboptimal intakes and subclinical deficiencies of other minerals are widespread, particularly for calcium, selenium and zinc.

Table 11.1 gives a selective summary of factual information about the dietetically important minerals, their functions, sources, adult reference values and deficiency states.

Table 11.2 on page 241 shows the measured intakes of five minerals in a representative sample of British men and women together with the corresponding RNIs and LRNIs. Several of the mean values are below the RNI, i.e. iron and magnesium in women and potassium in both sexes.

Table 11.1 *Selective summary of the dietetically important minerals*

Dietary Reference Values

UK adult RNI male/female; (American RDAs)

Calcium: 700 mg/day; (800)

Phosphorus: 550 mg/day, equivalent in molar terms to calcium RNI; (800 same as calcium RDA)

Magnesium: 300/270 mg/day; (350/280)

Sodium: 1.6 g/day; (estimated minimum requirement, 500 mg/day)

Potassium: 3.5 g/day (estimated minimum requirement, 2 g/day)

Chloride: 2.5 g/day, equivalent in molar terms to the sodium RNI (estimated minimum requirement, 750 mg/day)

Iron: 8.7/14.8 mg/day; (10/15)

Zinc: 9.5/7 mg/day; (15/12)

Copper: 1.2 mg/day; (safe intake 1.5–3 mg/day)

Selenium: 75/60 µg/day; (70/55)

Iodine: 140 µg/day; (150)

Dietary sources

Calcium: milk and milk products are rich sources with high biological availability; fish, especially if fish bones can be eaten as in tinned fish; green vegetables; pulses; nuts; whole grain cereals (white flour is supplemented in the UK); the calcium in vegetables and in cereals may have relatively low biological availability

1 cup (195 g) whole milk – 225 mg

40 g slice of cheddar cheese – 290 mg

1 serving (20 g) almonds – 50 mg

1 slice wholemeal bread – 19 mg

1 serving (95 g) broccoli – 72 mg

1 serving (75 g) cabbage – 40 mg

1 portion (85 g) tinned sardines – 390 mg

1 serving (80 g) peeled prawns – 120 mg

1 portion (130 g) grilled cod – 13 mg

Magnesium: vegetables; pulses; fruits

Sodium: major sources of dietary salt (sodium chloride) are processed foods; small amounts in natural foods; discretionary salt, added during cooking and at the table

1 slice wholemeal bread – 0.5 g salt

40 g slice cheddar cheese – 0.6 g salt

40 g slice Danish blue type cheese – 1.4 g salt

1 serving (45 g) All-Bran – 1.9 g salt

1 serving (25 g) cornflakes – 0.7 g salt

4 fish fingers – 0.9 g salt

1 portion (85 g) tinned sardines – 1.5 g salt

1 (80 g) portion prawns – 3.2 g salt

1 (120 g) gammon steak – 6.5 g salt

2 slices (60 g) corned beef – 1.5 g salt

2 pork sausages (UK) –1.5 g salt

small packet salted peanuts – 0.3 g salt

1 bowl (145 g) tinned tomato soup – 1.7 g salt

small packet crisps(chips) – 0.4 g salt

1 portion (200 g) baked beans – 2.4 g salt

1 serving (60 g) liver pate – 1.1g salt

Potassium: fruits and vegetables are the best sources; some in milk and flesh foods

1 orange – 490 mg

1 banana – 470 mg

(continued over page)

(Table 11.1 continued)

    1 apple – 145 mg
    1 portion (95 g) broccoli – 210 mg
    1 portion (75 g) frozen peas – 100 mg
    1 tomato – 220 g
    1 portion (265 g) chips (French fries) – 2700 mg
    1 glass (200 g) tinned orange juice – 260 mg

Iodine: richest natural sources are seafood; amounts in fruits, vegetables and meat depend upon soil content of iodine; modern farming and processing methods greatly increase amounts in milk and some bakery products; iodised salt

Zinc: meats; whole grain cereals; pulses; shellfish
    1 slice wholemeal bread – 0.7 mg
    1 pork chop – 2.8 mg
    1 portion (75 g) frozen peas – 0.5 mg
    1 portion (90 g) fried lamb liver – 4 mg
    1 serving (70 mg) tinned crabmeat – 3.5 mg

Copper: green vegetables; many types of fish; liver

Selenium: meat; cereals; fish

Iron: meat (particularly offal); fish; cereals; green vegetables; the biological availability of iron is much higher from meat and fish than from vegetable sources
    1 pork chop – 1 mg
    1 portion (90 g) fried lamb liver – 9 mg
    1 egg – 1.1 mg
    1 serving (80 g) peeled prawns – 0.9 mg
    1 serving (85 g) tinned sardines – 3.9 mg
    1 portion (75 g) frozen peas – 1.1 mg
    1 portion (95 g) broccoli – 1 mg
    1 50 g bar of dark (plain) chocolate – 1.2 mg
    1 serving (130 g) spinach – 5.2 mg
    1 slice wholemeal bread – 1 mg

Biochemical/physiological functions

Calcium: 99% of body calcium is in bone mineral; important in nerve and muscle function; release of hormones and nerve transmitters; blood clotting; intracellular regulator of metabolism

Phosphorus: 80% of body phosphorus is in bone mineral; phosphorylation–dephosphorylation reactions are an important feature of all biochemical pathways (see ATP functioning in Chapter 5); component of phospholipids which are important in membrane function; buffering systems

Magnesium: most of body magnesium is in bone; important role in calcium metabolism; many magnesium–requiring enzymes

Sodium: major cation in extracellular fluid; maintains fluid and electrolyte balance; nerve impulse transmission; acid–base balance

Potassium: major cation in intracellular fluid; nerve impulse transmission; contraction of muscle and heart; acid–base balance

Chloride: major anion in the body; maintains fluid and electrolyte balance

Iron: component of haemoglobin, myoglobin and cytochromes; there are several iron–containing enzymes such as catalase

Zinc: numerous zinc containing enzymes, including superoxide dismutase; insulin is stored as complex with zinc in the pancreas

Copper: there are numerous copper–containing enzymes

Selenium: component of enzyme system glutathione peroxidase, involved in disposal of free radicals; other selenium–containing enzymes

Iodine: a component of thyroid hormones

(Table 11.1 continued)

Effects of deficiency
> Overt deficiency states attributed to lack of an essential mineral are in most cases rarely, if ever, seen

Calcium: overt, primary calcium deficiency is rare; vitamin D deficiency leads to poor absorption of calcium and the disease, rickets; osteoporosis suggested as a long term consequence of calcium insufficiency

Iron: iron deficiency anaemia

Copper: anaemia due to copper deficiency has been reported in premature babies and patients fed by total parenteral nutrition

Selenium: Keshan disease, a progressive and potentially fatal cardiomyopathy seen in parts of China where soil is low in selenium; experimental deficiency in animals has many similarities to vitamin E deficiency presumably because of their common role in disposal of free radicals

Iodine: goitre

Risk factors for deficiency

Iron: chronic blood loss due to e.g. heavy menstrual bleeding, malignancy, intestinal parasites or repeated pregnancies; a vegetarian diet that is low in iron, has low in bioavailability and lacks promotors of absorption like vitamin C

Iodine: living in areas where soil iodine content is low

Calcium: vitamin D deficiency

The median for iron intake of women is substantially below the mean because of skewing of the distribution by supplemental iron and this median intake represents only around two-thirds of the RNI. As with the vitamins, the intakes of the lowest 2.5% is in several cases below the LRNI. Note that there was some suggestion of under recording of habitual intakes in this survey. Note also the very high intakes of iron of the top 2.5%; in the case of men these intakes were over three times the RNI.

The role of salt in the aetiology of hypertension and the significance of dietary calcium in the aetiology of osteoporosis are important mineral-related topics which have been singled out for discussion at the end of this chapter.

The role of dietary fluoride in dental health was discussed in Chapter 7. Fluoride has not been proven to be an essential nutrient, and in both the UK and the US only safe intakes are given; in the UK, even this safe intake is restricted to infants. The roles of zinc, selenium, iron and copper as prosthetic groups for antioxidant enzyme systems were discussed in Chapter 10.

Iodine and Iodine Deficiency Diseases (IDD)

Distribution and physiological function of body iodine

The only known physiological function of iodine is as a component of the thyroid hormones, **thyroxine** and **triiodothyronine**. The thyroid gland traps and concentrates absorbed iodine very efficiently; if radioactively labelled iodine is taken in, then this radioactivity can be shown to be rapidly concentrated within the thyroid gland. The ability of the thyroid to concentrate "labelled" iodine is used diagnostically as a measure of thyroid function, and high doses of radioactive iodine may be used to selectively destroy thyroid tissue as an alternative to its surgical removal in some cases of hyperthyroidism or thyroid carcinoma. Nuclear emissions released after accidents or explosions contain large amounts of relatively short-lived radioactive iodine, and this is accumulated in the thyroid where it can ultimately cause thyroid carcinoma; administration of iodine-containing tablets can be used as a public health measure in such circumstances to compete with and competitively reduce the uptake of the radioactive iodine into the thyroid.

Causes and consequences of iodine deficiency

In goitre, there is a swelling of the thyroid gland. This swelling ranges from that which is only detectable to the trained eye to massive and sometimes nodular overgrowth. The thyroid swells because of excessive stimulation by the pituitary hormone, **thyrotropin**. Thyrotropin output is normally inhibited by circulating thyroid hormones, and so any reduced output of thyroid hormones caused by iodine deficiency leads to compensatory increases in thyrotropin output and con-

sequent thyroid growth (see Figure 11.1). In some cases, the swelling of the thyroid is the only apparent symptom of iodine deficiency.

In severe iodine deficiency, there are symptoms of thyroid hormone deficiency; in places where goitre is endemic, there will be increased rates of spontaneous abortion and stillbirth. Large numbers of children may be born with congenital physical and neurological abnormalities, e.g. deaf-mutism, spasticity and mental deficiency, that are due to iodine deficiency. In children, iodine deficiency can lead to **cretinism**, a condition characterised by impaired mental and physical development; there is evidence of a general impairment of intellectual performance and psychomotor skills in children from iodine deficient areas. In

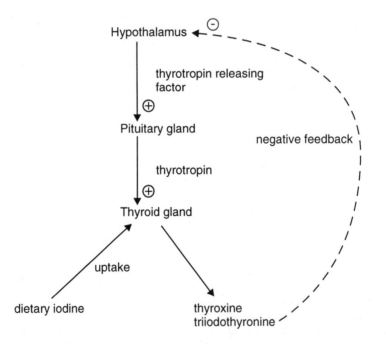

Lack of dietary iodine reduces negative feedback and leads to compensatory overproduction of thyrotropin and this results in overstimulation and swelling of the thyroid – goitre.

Figure 11.1 The regulation of thyroid hormone output and the origins of goitre

adults, iodine deficiency causes not only goitre but can also lead to impaired mental functioning and other symptoms of thyroid hormone deficiency. If a goitre is very large, it may lead to problems with breathing or swallowing that may require surgery and occasionally large nodular goitres may become malignant. Controlled studies by Marine in Ohio in the 1920s showed that iodine supplements were effective in the treatment and prevention of goitre in schoolchildren. Women and girls are more susceptible to goitre than males.

Dietary sources of iodine

The richest sources of dietary iodine are seafoods. The smaller amount of iodine in other foods varies according to the iodine level in the soil. The iodine content of drinking water gives a good indication of the general iodine level in the soil in an area. In many regions of the world, the soil iodine content is low, e.g. mountainous regions, the area around the Great Lakes in America and in Derbyshire and the Cotswold areas of England. In areas where the soil iodine content is low and where seafood is not available or consumed, then the Iodine Deficiency Diseases, manifesting most apparently as goitre (Derbyshire neck), have been, and in many places still are, endemic. There are over a billion people in the Third World at risk of iodine deficiency, with around 200 million suffering from goitre and around 20 million of these suffering from some degree of resultant mental defect; more than a quarter of these suffer from gross cretinism and mental retardation. Iodine deficiency is still endemic in large parts of Central and South America, large parts of India, China and Southeast Asia, some regions of Africa and the Oceanic islands; around 85% of those suffering from overt cretinisn are in Asia (Hetzel, 1993).

Nowadays, few affluent communities rely solely upon food produced in their locality and this reduces the risk of goitre. In both the UK and US, the iodine content of cow milk is high because of iodine-supplementation of feed and the use of iodine disinfectants. In many goitre areas, including Switzerland and the USA, iodised salt has been effectively used as a prophylactic measure to prevent goitre. In some other areas, injections of iodised oil have been used; a single injection gives protection for 2–3 years.

Requirements and intake of iodine

The adult RNI (RDA) for iodine is 140 (150) µg/day and intakes are typically double this in the UK and much more than double in the US. The very high intakes in the US, which reached a peak of 800 µg/day in 1974, have been a cause for concern. Very high intakes (say 5000 µg/day) can cause toxic nodular goitre and hyperthyroidism. COMA (1991) suggested a safe upper limit of 1000 µg/day.

Certain foods of the cabbage (*Brassica*) family and cassava contain goitrogenic substances that either block the uptake of iodine by the thyroid gland or block the synthesis of thyroid hormones. The presence of such goitrogens may precipitate deficiency where intakes of iodine are at the borders of adequacy. Cassava, in particular, may be a significant factor in precipitating iodine deficiency in some tropical areas where it is the principal energy source for around 200 million people. Hetzel (1993) suggests that intakes of iodine should be doubled to 200–300 µg/day where there is high intake of these goitrogens.

Iron and iron deficiency anaemia

Distribution of body iron

A typical well-nourished male body will contain an average of about 4 g of iron. About two-thirds of this total will be present in the respiratory pigments **haemoglobin** in blood and **myoglobin** in muscles. Most of the body's non haem iron will be stored as the iron-protein complex, **ferritin**. Small amounts of iron will also be found in a variety of important iron-containing enzymes and proteins and bound to the protein **transferrin** in plasma; transferrin is responsible for the transport of iron around the body. The first effect of iron deficiency would therefore be expected to be a depletion of iron stored as ferritin followed by reduced levels of the iron-containing, respiratory pigments haemoglobin and myoglobin, i.e. iron deficiency anaemia.

Requirement for dietary iron

Iron is very efficiently conserved by the human body with daily losses of body iron in a typical healthy male amounting to only around 1 mg/day (i.e. only 0.025% of normal body iron content). This tiny net loss of iron compares with around 20 mg of iron in the ageing red blood cells that are removed from the circulation and destroyed each day. This iron released from broken down red cells is recycled, and the small amount of iron lost from the body is that present in lost skin, nails, hair, body fluids and sloughed cells from the alimentary and genito-urinary tracts. In premenopausal women losses in menstrual blood and the losses of iron at parturition also contribute to body iron loss. Average menstrual blood loss represents an additional increment of around 80% to the general iron losses of women, but in some women (say 10%) these extra menstrual losses may represent an addition of 150% or more to the general

iron loss. Any condition which results in chronic blood loss will increase the risk of anaemia, e.g. ulcers, intestinal parasites, intestinal cancer.

Average intakes of iron in the UK are around 14 mg/day in men and 12.3 mg/day in women (see Table 11.2), i.e. around 14 times average daily losses in men and, even in those women with particularly high menstrual losses, still around 5 times estimated losses. The iron RNI (RDA) is 8.7 (10) mg/day for men and 14.8 (15) mg/day for premenopausal women and according to COMA (1991) even this RNI may be insufficient for those women with particularly high menstrual losses. The very large differences in estimated requirements for iron and estimated losses are because only a small and variable proportion of dietary iron is absorbed. The proportion of dietary iron that is absorbed varies with:

- the iron status of the individual
- the form in which the dietary iron is present
- the presence of promoters and inhibitors of iron absorption in the diet.

Haem iron from meat and fish is far better absorbed (10–30%) than the iron in vegetable foods (2–10%). Vitamin C, stomach acid and the presence of meat and fish all promote iron absorption. Vitamin C is a major factor in promoting the absorption of iron from vegetable foods. Fibre, phytate (from unleavened bread) and tannin in tea all tend to hinder iron absorption. Alcohol increases gastric acid secretion and facilitates iron absorption; White *et al.*, (1993) found a positive association between alcohol consumption and level of iron stores in both men and women. In all the examples of iron overload, discussed by Passmore and Eastwood (1986), iron-containing alcoholic drinks were considered to be a major underlying factor.

COMA (1991) assumed an average efficiency of absorption of 15% when making their calculations of Dietary Reference Values.

Regulation of iron balance

The principle physiological mechanism for regulating body iron balance is by controlling the efficiency of absorption; when iron stores are low, then it is absorbed more efficiently than when body iron stores are full. The efficiency of iron absorption may double when iron stores are depleted. This regulatory system is not sufficient to prevent iron toxicity if intake is chronically high. Chronic iron overload leads to cirrhosis of the liver. Single, very high doses of iron can cause diarrhoea, vomiting, gastrointestinal bleeding, circulatory collapse and liver necrosis; iron poisoning resulting from children consuming pharmaceutical preparations of iron has been one of the most common causes of accidental poisoning in the UK. There is no physiological mechanism for excreting excess iron, and so iron overload and toxicity is a major problem for those with certain conditions that require repeated blood transfusions, e.g. the inherited blood disorder, thalassaemia. Drugs which bind or chelate iron and facilitate its excretion can be used to treat or prevent iron overload.

Nature and consequences of iron deficiency anaemia

In iron deficiency, there is impaired ability to synthesise haemoglobin. Anaemia has traditionally been diagnosed by measurement of blood haemoglobin concentration. Iron deficiency anaemia is characterised by reduced blood haemoglobin concentration and reduced red blood cell size – a **microcytic anaemia** (small cell) as compared to the **macrocytic anaemia** (large cell) of vitamin B_{12} or folic acid deficiency. A blood haemoglobin concentration of less than 12 g/100 ml of blood has traditionally been taken as "the level below which anaemia is likely to be present", and the prevalence of anaemia has usually been established by use of a cut-off value like this.

Other measures of iron status have been increasingly used in recent years. The plasma ferritin level indicates the state of body iron stores, and these stores may become depleted without any fall in blood haemoglobin concentration and would be expected to be a more sensitive measure of iron status than blood haemoglobin concentration. Plasma ferritin levels of less than 25 µg/l are said to be indicative of low body iron stores (White *et al.*, 1993) and values of 12 µg/l taken by COMA (1991) to indicate frank depletion. In iron deficiency, the concentration of the iron transport protein, transferrin, in the plasma rises but the amount of iron in plasma drops and so low ratio of iron to transferrin in plasma, the **transferrin saturation**, indicates low iron status.

The symptoms of anaemia result from the low haemoglobin content of blood leading to impaired ability to transport oxygen and they include general fatigue, breathlessness on exertion, pallor, headache and insomnia.

Prevalence of anaemia

A major problem in determining the prevalence of iron deficiency is to decide upon the criteria that are to be used – which measure of iron status should be used and what cut off point used to indicate unsatisfactory iron status? In a series of studies, Elwood and his colleagues found that women with haemoglobin concentrations that would indicate mild to moderate anaemia showed little or no evidence of clinical impairment, even cardiopulmonary function under exercise appeared to be little affected by this degree of apparent anaemia (reviewed by Lock, 1977). More recently it has been suggested by several groups that functional impairment due to iron deficiency (as measured by plasma ferritin) may occur in the absence of anaemia (COMA, 1991). Reduced work capacity and changes in certain brain functions that adversely affect attention, memory and learning in children are some of these suggested adverse consequences of mild iron deficiency.

Miller (1979) listed anaemia as the most common of the diseases due to inadequate nutrient intake. He gave an estimated prevalence of 5% in developed regions and 30% in developing regions – these figures would have been based upon the classical criterion of haemoglobin concentration. More recent WHO figures are not substantially at variance with these figures. The incidence is higher in women than in men because of the extra demands of menstruation and pregnancy upon body iron stores. In the developed countries, the condition is considered to be uncommon in young men. In the UK, it was estimated that in 1991, only 4% of women had haemoglobin levels below 11 g/100 ml but 34% had serum ferritin levels below 25 µg/l and 16% less than 13 µg/l – the level taken by COMA, 1991 to indicate depletion of body stores; the serum ferritin levels of premenopausal women were lower than those of older women with almost half of those under 45 years having serum ferritin levels below 25 µg/l (White *et al.*, 1993). Several studies have found high levels of anaemia in young children in the UK, especially in children of Asian origin where rates of around 25% have been reported (COMA, 1991). Adolescents, pregnant women and the elderly are other groups regarded as being at increased risk of anaemia.

Preventing iron deficiency

In people consuming the same type of diet, iron intake is likely to be directly related to total energy intake. This means that, if the diet provides enough iron for women to meet their dietary standard, then men consuming the same type of diet are likely to take in around double theirs. Any dietary supplementation programme that seeks to eliminate iron deficiency anaemia in those women with particularly

high needs will increase still further the surplus intake of men. Note in Table 11.2 that some British men already take in more than treble their RNI.

In Sweden, the prevalence of iron-deficiency was reduced by three-quarters over a ten-year period from the mid 1960s (Anon, 1980). Increased fortification of flour with iron was considered to be one of the factors that contributed to this decline in anaemia and it had been suggested that more effective iron fortification could help to eliminate the final 7% incidence of anaemia in Swedish women. However, as this *Lancet* editorial (Anon, 1980) points out, any fortification programme designed to eliminate anaemia in women with high iron needs inevitably results in men and even many women receiving iron intakes greatly in excess of their needs. This excess iron intake might cause harm, particularly to subjects inherently sensitive to iron overload.

Widespread use of prophylactic iron was also credited with much of this reduced prevalence of anaemia in Sweden. In 1974 sales of pharmaceutical iron preparations in Sweden amounted to almost 6 mg per head per day. Indiscriminate use of pharmaceutical preparations leads to risk of side-effects, accidental poisoning, and chronic iron overload.

Another factor thought to have contributed to the decline in iron deficiency anaemia in Sweden was increased vitamin C intake; high intakes of vitamin C may account for the relatively low levels of anaemia found in vegetarians. Current advice to increase consumption of fruits and vegetables should increase iron absorption, although increased consumption of cereal fibre might tend to reduce iron availability.

If premenopausal women and other groups at increased risk of anaemia are advised to eat a diet containing more available iron, then such a diet would probably contain more meat (and/or fish). This would probably, but not inevitably, also lead to increased intake of saturated fat and would therefore not be entirely consistent with other nutrition education guidelines. It might also be unacceptable or impractical for many women.

It is still not clear to what extent biochemical measures of low iron status predict impairment. Given the potential problems of measures to "improve" iron status, it would not seem prudent to undertake population measures aimed at eliminating iron deficiency in developed countries. Rather, treatment should be restricted to those identified as needing it and likely to benefit from it.

Calcium, diet and osteoporosis

Rolls (1992) and Halliday and Ashwell (1991) are recent reviews of calcium nutrition that have been used in preparing this section.

Distribution and functions of body calcium

A typical adult human body contains more than 1 kg of calcium and 99% of this calcium is in the skeleton. This skeletal calcium is present as crystals of **hydroxyapatite** (a calcium phosphate hydroxide) which are deposited upon an organic matrix composed of the protein collagen. Hydroxyapatite gives bone its strength and comprises about half its weight. In addition to its role in providing mechanical strength for the skeleton, calcium has a multitude of other vital functions which are fulfilled by the small non-skeletal component of body calcium, for example:

1 Calcium plays a major role in the release of hormones and neurotransmitters
2 It acts as an intracellular regulator
3 It is an essential cofactor for some enzymes and is necessary for blood clotting
4 It is involved in nerve function and in muscle and heart contraction.

This multitude of functions for non-skeletal calcium means that variation in calcium concentration of body fluids can have diverse effects on many systems of the body, and so the extracellular calcium concentration is under very fine hormonal control. The skeletal calcium can be regarded not only as fulfilling a strengthening role, but also as a reservoir of calcium that can donate calcium or soak up excess, thus enabling the concentration in extracellular fluid to be regulated within very narrow limits. A fall in blood calcium concentration, as seen after removal of the parathyroid glands or in extreme vitamin D deficiency, leads to muscle weakness and eventually to tetany and death due to asphyxiation when the muscles of the larynx go into spasm. A rise in plasma calcium is seen in vitamin D poisoning and in hyperparathyroidism. Hypercalcaemia can lead to gastrointestinal symptoms, neurological symptoms, formation of kidney stones and in some cases may lead to death from renal failure.

Hormonal regulation of calcium homeostasis

The hormone **1,25 dihydroxycholecalciferol (1,25DHCC)** which is produced in the kidney from vitamin D is essential for the active absorption of dietary calcium in the intestine. 1,25 DHCC promotes the synthesis of key proteins involved in active transport of calcium in both the gut and kidney. Some passive absorption of calcium occurs independently of 1,25 DHCC, and this passive absorption increases with increasing dietary intake. Parathyroid hormone and calcitonin (from the thyroid gland) regulate deposition and release of calcium from bone and also the rate of excretion of calcium in the urine. Parathyroid hormone also indirectly regulates the intestinal absorption of calcium by activating the renal enzyme that produces 1,25 DHCC. Typical daily fluxes of calcium are illustrated in Figure 11.2, and the hormonal influences upon these calcium fluxes summarised in Figure 11.3.

Requirement and availability of calcium

The adult RNI for calcium in the UK is 700 mg/day for both males and females, slightly less than the American RDA of 800 mg/day; the extra increments allowed for growth and pregnancy are also generally higher in the US than the UK. Almost two-thirds of even non-pregnant women in the US fail to meet the current RDA. Current adult intakes of UK men and women are shown in Table 11.2 and these suggest a very substantial minority of British women also take in much less than the RNI. In the UK, COMA arrived at the RNI by calculating the amount required to replace typical urinary and skin losses (Figure 11.2), assuming that around 30% of the dietary intake is absorbed. In Western countries, 50–70% of dietary calcium is from dairy produce and the calcium in dairy produce tends to be well absorbed.

This predominance of dairy produce as the major source of dietary calcium, makes calcium intake vulnerable to changes in the image of dairy produce induced by health education messages. In the UK, daily calcium intake has fallen by about 15% since 1975 as a result of reduced total food intake and milk consumption; this trend has been most pronounced in young women and teenage girls (Rolls, 1992). Note that lower fat milks contain just as much calcium as whole milk, and so reduced intake of dairy fat does not inevitably lead to reduced

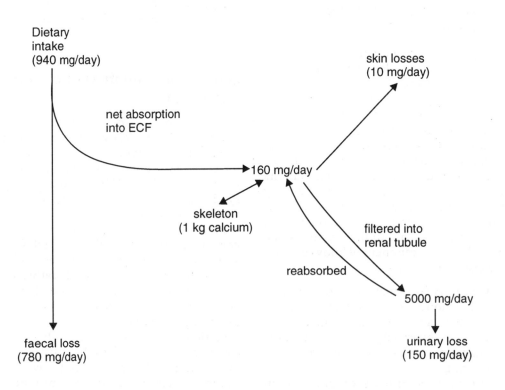

Figure 11.2 Typical daily calcium movements in an adult UK male

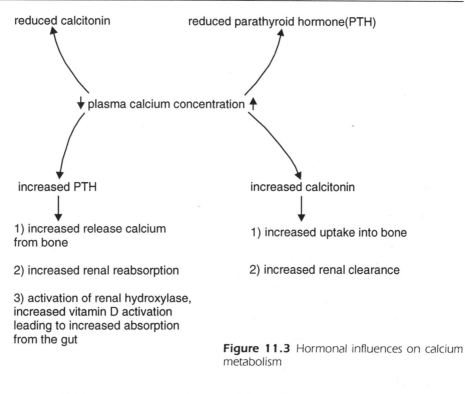

Figure 11.3 Hormonal influences on calcium metabolism

calcium intake. Table 11.1 shows the calcium content of some common foods.

The efficiency of absorption of calcium varies according to the phase of the life-cycle, the dietary source and total dietary intake, for example:

1 The efficiency of calcium absorption increases markedly in pregnancy but is reduced in the elderly
2 Efficiency of absorption from breast milk is very high (66%) but less from infant formula (40%). In general,

Table 11.2 Comparison of measured intakes and Dietary Reference Values for selected minerals in British adults. Data sources: COMA, 1991; Gregory et al., 1990

Mineral		Mean intake	Lower 2.5 percentile	RNI (19–50 years)	LRNI
Iron (mg)	(men)	14.0	6.5 (27.1*)	8.7	4.7
	(women)	12.3 (10.0†)	4.7 (30.7*)	14.8	8.0
Calcium (mg)	(men)	940	410	700	400
	(women)	730	266	700	400
Magnesium (mg)	(men)	323	156	300	190
	(women)	237	105	270	150
Zinc (mg)	(men)	11.4	5.7	9.5	5.5
	(women)	8.4	3.6	7.0	4.0
Potassium (g)	(men)	3.2	1.7	3.5	2.0
	(women)	2.4	1.2	3.5	2.0

EAR is mid way between RNI and LRNI * Upper 2.5 percentile † Median (middle value if arranged in rank order) may be more useful than mean with a skewed distribution.

calcium from vegetable sources is less well absorbed than that from milk and cheese

3 At low calcium intakes the active, vitamin D-dependent absorption process predominates, whereas at high intakes the less efficient passive process predominates. So the proportion of the oral load that is absorbed tends to decline with increasing intake.

Many people who do not consume large amounts of dairy produce as adults, have average calcium intakes that are less than half the current UK RNI and thus below even the current LRNI. Despite this, overt symptoms of acute dietary deficiency are not seen. For example, Prentice *et al.* (1993) reported calcium intakes in pregnant and lactating women in rural Gambia in 1979 of only around 400 mg/day and a follow-up report by Jarjou *et al.* (1994) suggests that this has since fallen still further, to less than a quarter of the current UK RNI for lactating women. Despite this, there is no overt evidence of acute calcium deficiency nor of excessive rates of osteoporotic bone fractures in The Gambia. There is a considerable body of evidence suggesting that during calcium deprivation individuals can adapt to low calcium intakes by increasing efficiency of absorption and by reducing their urinary losses of calcium (Passmore and Eastwood, 1986).

Osteoporosis – definition and incidence

Osteoporosis is a thinning of the bones, involving the loss of both organic bone matrix and bone mineral. This thinning of bones makes them more prone to fracture; fractures of the vertebrae, the wrist and the neck of the femur (hip fracture) are especially likely. Rates of osteoporotic fractures have increased very substantially in many industrialised countries over the last 50 years (e.g. Spector *et al.*, 1990). Fractures of the hip are currently

considered to be the major public health priority. In the UK, there are around 50 000 cases of hip fracture each year, a significant proportion of those affected die within a few months of the initial fracture and many more are permanently disabled or never regain full mobility after the fracture. Up to 20 000 deaths each year in the UK may be consequences of hip fracture or the associated surgery. In the US, there are over a 200 000 hip fractures each year that are attributable to osteoporosis. Cummings *et al.* (1985) and Johnell *et al.* (1992) give substantial detail on comparative rates of osteoporotic fracture in different countries.

Bone mass declines in adults once they get past middle age and thus the increased prevalence of osteoporosis is partly accounted for by the increased numbers of people surviving into old age. Wickham *et al.* (1989) in a prospective study of 1400 elderly British people found that incidence of hip fracture was four times higher in women over 85 years than in women in the 65–74 year age band. There has, however, also been a real increase as demonstrated by the large increases in age-specific incidence of fractures seen in the UK in the last three decades (Spector *et al.*, 1990). Risk of fracture depends upon the ability of bone to withstand trauma and the amount of trauma to which it is subjected. Smith (1987) suggested that thinning of the bones in osteoporosis takes them below a threshold value above which bone is unlikely to fracture unless subjected to severe trauma. Once below this threshold value, bones become liable to fracture when subjected to relatively minor trauma. Although a subthreshold density is a necessary permissive factor for osteoporotic fracture, bone mineral density measurements are imperfect predictors of individual susceptibility to fracture especially for fractures of the hip (Smith, 1987; Cummings *et al.*, 1986). Leichter *et al.* (1982) measured bone density and the shear stress required to fracture the femoral neck using isolated human bones obtained from cadavers. They found a high statistical correlation between shear stress at fracture and both bone density and bone mineral content. Breaking stress, bone density and bone mineral content all declined with the age of the subject. However, they found that breaking stress declined with age much faster than either bone density or bone mineral content. They concluded that changes in bone strength are apparently influenced by factors other than bone density and mineral content.

Fractures of the hip usually occur after a fall, and so susceptibility to falling is the other factor contributing to increased risk of hip fracture in the elderly. Bone density can be readily and non-invasively measured, and so much scientific work has been done looking at the factors that may affect bone density with a view to the prevention of osteoporotic fracture. In contrast, the factors that make people susceptible to falling have been a relatively neglected area of study.

The imperfect association between fracture risk and measured bone density needs to be borne in mind when evaluating reports of weak associations between environmental/lifestyle variables and bone density. Likewise, evidence that interventions can have acute effects on bone density need to be treated with caution – will any short term increase be maintained in the longer term? will small measured increases in bone density significantly reduce fracture risk?

Effects of age, sex and genetics upon bone density

Bones are dynamic structures; the processes of bone deposition and bone resorption continue throughout life. When bone mass is increasing, e.g. during growth, this is because the rate of deposition exceeds the rate of resorption. When bone mass is stable in younger adults this is because of a dynamic equilibrium between the two processes rather than a static state. People reach their **peak bone mass** in their thirties; after this the rate of resorption exceeds the rate of bone formation, and there is a steady decline in bone mass in older adults.

In women, the decade immediately after the menopause is associated with a marked acceleration in the rate of bone loss. This postmenopausal acceleration in the rate of bone loss is due to the decline in oestrogen production and means that women reach the threshold bone density long before men. Osteoporotic fractures are much more common in women than men, e.g. Wickham *et al.* (1989) recorded no fractures in their sample of men under 75 years and the incidence in the over 85s was doubled in females as compared to males. Spector *et al.* (1990) recorded a 4:1 female-to-male ratio in the age specific incidence of hip fracture in the UK. The high female to male ratio in fracture rates is only seen in countries where rates of osteoporosis are high (Cummings *et al.*, 1985).

Many conditions in which there is reduced sex hormone output are associated with reduced bone density, for example:

- early menopause or surgical removal of the ovaries
- a cessation of menstruation due to starvation or Anorexia Nervosa
- amenorrhoea due to extremely high activity and low body fat content in women athletes
- hypogonadism in men.

There is also clear evidence that **Hormone Replacement Therapy (HRT)** in postmenopausal women prevents or reduces the postmenopausal acceleration in rate of bone loss and reduces the risk of osteoporotic fracture. This treatment is widely accepted as being effective in the prevention of osteoporosis. The controversy about HRT is about whether the benefits of the treatment are sufficient to outweigh any possible risks such as increased risk of uterine cancer or perhaps even of breast cancer.

There are clear racial differences in bone density, with persons of European and Asian origin having bones that are less dense than those of African origin. In the United States, white women are much more likely to suffer from osteoporotic fractures than black women. Even within racial groups there is almost certainly a very large inherited variability in bone density and susceptibility to osteoporotic fracture (Cummings et al., 1985).

Lifestyle factors in the aetiology of osteoporosis and osteoporotic fracture

The increasingly sedentary lifestyle of those living in the industrialised countries is widely believed to be a major precipitating factor in the increased age-specific incidence of osteoporotic fracture. Activity is known to increase bone density and immobilisation or extreme inactivity (e.g. confinement to bed or the weightlessness experienced by astronauts) is known to result in loss of bone mass. Increased activity in the early years increases the peak bone mass, and maintaining activity in later years slows down the rate of bone loss (Rolls, 1992).

Children who spent more than two hours daily in weight bearing activity were reported to have greater bone mineral density than those who spent less than one hour daily in such activity (see Cooper and Eastell, 1993). Pocock et al. (1986) found a significant correlation between measured fitness level and bone mineral density in 84 normal women. In the postmenopausal women in this sample, fitness was the only measured variable that correlated significantly with bone mineral density. A randomised, controlled trial of the effects of exercise upon bone density found that it had a significant positive effect in young women (see

Cooper and Eastell, 1993). In the 1400 elderly people sampled by Wickham et al. (1989) risk of hip fracture was reduced in those people with higher levels of outdoor physical activity.

Being underweight is associated with a higher risk of osteoporotic fracture, and in the elderly this is often as a result of low lean body mass caused by inactivity; correcting the association between osteoporotic risk and inactivity for body mass may thus lead to underestimation of the strength of this association. More active and fitter elderly people may also be less prone to osteoporotic fracture because they are better co-ordinated and stronger and therefore less prone to falling or less liable to injury if they do fall. Cummings et al. (1985) suggest that in the already osteoporotic adult, reducing the tendency to fall may offer the greatest potential for reducing the risk of fractures.

Many studies have suggested that cigarette smoking is associated with reduced bone density and with increased fracture risk (Cummings et al., 1985). In their sample of elderly British people, Wickham et al. (1989) reported a strong association between cigarette smoking and risk of hip fracture. Smoking is associated with:

- lower body weight
- reduced physical activity
- early menopause
- reduced blood oestrogen concentration (even in women receiving HRT).

These are all known associates of high fracture risk.

High alcohol consumption has also been widely reported as a risk factor for osteoporosis. Heavy drinking is associated with extensive bone loss even in relatively young adults (Smith, 1987). High alcohol consumption might also be expected to increase the risk of falling.

A vegetarian lifestyle is generally associated with higher bone density and reduced risk of osteoporosis (e.g. Marsh et al., 1988). To what extent, if any, this as a result of meat avoidance *per se* is difficult to establish; see Chapter 14 for discussion of the health aspects of vegetarianism.

Role of dietary calcium in the aetiology of osteoporosis

The extent to which calcium nutrition affects the risk of osteoporosis has been widely investigated and debated but without yet reaching universally accepted conclusions. There is no compelling evidence to suggest that low calcium intake is a major causative factor for the disease – the disease is uncommon in some populations with calcium intakes much lower than those in the US and UK where the prevalence is high. Rolls (1992) quotes the extreme example of rural Bantu women who suffer only ten percent the fracture incidence of Western women despite taking in only half as much calcium and similar findings of Prentice *et al.* (1993) in rural Gambia were discussed earlier. Gatehouse and Webb (unpublished observations) found a significant *positive* association between age standardised hip fracture rates in women and *per capita* consumption of fresh milk products in eight Western European countries; consumption of fresh milk products is a good predictor of calcium intakes in such countries. Hegsted (1986) also found a *positive* correlation between calcium intake and incidence of hip fracture in a genetically and culturally more diverse sample of nine countries in Europe, the Far East, Australasia and North America. International comparisons may be of limited usefulness in proving cause and effect relationships, especially when used rather anecdotally as above, but they are more persuasive when used to argue against such a relationship. If high calcium intake is associated internationally with high rates of osteoporosis, this makes it improbable that calcium deficiency is an important causal factor. It is still possible, of course, that high calcium intakes or calcium supplements might have some role in offsetting an increase in osteoporosis risk, even though it is primarily due to other causes.

It is often argued that high intakes of calcium in childhood together with ensuring good vitamin D status is likely to increase peak bone mass and thus reduce the later risk of osteoporotic fractures. Calcium intakes substantially below the dietary standard during childhood may limit peak bone mass and thus increase the later risk of osteoporosis. A controlled, double-blind study of calcium supplements (1 g/day) conducted over a three-year period in twin children suggested that the supplements could significantly increase bone density (see Cooper and Eastell, 1993). Good intakes of milk and cheese in growing children will, in most cases, be necessary for children to achieve calcium intakes that reach dietary standard values.

There is little evidence that variation in dietary calcium intake has any major effect on bone density in adults (Smith, 1987; Cummings *et al.*, 1986). Wickham *et al.* (1989) found no relationship between dietary calcium intake and risk of osteoporotic fracture in their sample of elderly adults. There is nonetheless a strong case for ensuring adequacy of calcium and vitamin D in the elderly. Elderly housebound people may be at increased risk of osteomalacia (due to vitamin D deficiency).

Conclusions

An active lifestyle, absence of cigarette smoking, moderate alcohol consumption and a diet that meets the standards for essential nutrients is both consistent with general health education guidelines and offers expectation of reducing the risk of osteoporosis and osteoporotic fracture. There seems to be no convincing evidence that calcium supplements in older adults will prevent osteoporosis or be effective in its treatment. Good intakes of calcium in childhood and early adulthood may

Table 11.3 Factors associated with increased risk of osteoporosis

- Old age; risk of osteoporosis increases with age and accelerates in women when they reach the menopause
- Being female; rates are higher in women than men in Western Europe and North America.
- Being white; there are distinct racial differences in bone density and considerable genetic variations within races
- Lack of sex hormones; factors which reduce sex hormone secretion e.g. early menopause or ovarian removal increase risk and Hormone Replacement Therapy reduces risk
- Never having borne a child
- A sedentary lifestyle
- Smoking
- High alcohol consumption
- Being small or underweight
- Inadequate calcium intake in childhood?
- High consumption of carbonated, cola drinks?
- Being an omnivore; vegetarians have lower rates of osteoporosis.

contribute to increased peak bone mass, but other lifestyle factors (e.g. activity level) are probably more significant. There is no case for the use of calcium supplements.

Detailed discussion of the pros and cons of HRT is beyond the scope of this book but, on the narrow question of whether it reduces the risk of osteoporosis, the evidence is compelling. Factors associated with increased risk of osteoporosis are summarised in Table 11.3.

Salt and hypertension

The problems with salt

High salt intake has long been suspected of being involved in the aetiology of essential hypertension. Salt (sodium chloride) is made up of the two mineral elements sodium and chlorine. It is the sodium component that has been generally regarded as significant in causing hypertension; this has been questioned in recent years, and so this discussion generally refers to salt rather than to sodium alone. Despite the fact that salt (sodium) balance is very effectively hormonally regulated, it is argued that prolonged excess salt intake can lead to excess salt

retention and therefore increased fluid retention and hypertension. Evidence from dialysis patients and those with endocrine disorders confirms the latter part of this hypothesis, namely that salt retention does lead to increased blood pressure.

High salt intake has also been implicated in the aetiology of gastric cancer. One theory suggests that salt acts as a gastric irritant and that continued irritation due to high salt intake leads to atrophy of the acid secreting glands in the stomach. Reduced acid secretion in the stomach then allows proliferation of bacteria, and they produce carcinogenic substances (nitrosamines) from some components of food. Again there is considerable support for the latter part of the hypothesis; patients with pernicious anaemia who produce less gastric acid have markedly increased rates of gastric cancer.

Affluent populations have generally been advised to substantially reduce their dietary salt intake – the WHO have suggested a move towards a population average salt intake of 5 g/day. NACNE (1983) suggested a long term aim of reducing current intakes by 25% and in the US, NRC (1989b) suggested that salt intake should be limited to 6 g/day. The principal aim of such recommendations is to reduce the 15% incidence of essential hypertension in the adult population and thus to reduce the morbidity and mortality from diseases precipitated by high blood pressure, namely strokes, myocardial infarction and renal failure. In a recent survey of English adults, 16–17% were classified as hypertensive but only 76% were normotensive and not taking drugs that could affect their blood pressure. The average blood pressure of this sample and therefore the prevalence of hypertension increased with age (White *et al.*, 1993).

There are a wide variety of antihypertensive drugs now available that are very effective in lowering blood pressure. These drugs also seem to be effective in reducing the renal and cerebrovascular complications of hypertension, although they are less effective in reducing the coronary conditions associated with high blood pressure and may even be associated with increased coronary risk. As with any drug, there may be acute side-effects and long-term problems especially as anti-hypertensives may need to be taken for the rest of the patient's life. There have been suggestions that use of antihypertensives can be associated with increased overall mortality (e.g. MRFIT, 1982). The idea that moderation of dietary salt intake might prevent hypertension or be a useful alternative to drugs in the treatment of hypertension is still an attractive proposition. High intakes of potassium and calcium have also been suggested as having possible protective effects against the development of hypertension.

Requirement for salt

Salt is an essential nutrient. Sodium is the principal cation in extracellular fluid; the standard 70 kg male has around 92 g of sodium in his body, equivalent to around 250 g of salt. Around half of total body sodium is in the extracellular fluid, 38% in bone and the remaining 12% in the intracellular fluid; potassium is the dominant cation in intracellular fluid. Despite its undoubted essentiality, the habitual intake of most affluent populations greatly exceeds minimum requirements. Almost all ingested salt is absorbed in the intestine, and the excretion of salt (principally in urine) is homeostatically controlled by the endocrine system enabling individuals to remain in salt balance over a huge range of intakes. Some populations, such as the Kalahari Bushmen and New Guinea Highlanders manage on habitual salt intakes of around 1 g/day, whereas other populations (e.g. some regions of Japan and Korea) habitually take in more than 25 g/day.

NRC (1989a) estimated that minimum requirements for sodium chloride were only around 1.25 g/day. This minimum figure did not provide for large prolonged losses from the skin through sweat. Individuals do adapt to salt restriction during heavy exercise or in a hot environment by producing very dilute sweat. The UK RNIs for sodium and chloride amount to a salt intake of around 4 g/day; the panel felt that this value allowed for losses in sweat during exercise and high temperatures once adaptation had occurred, but that in the short-term extra intake might be required under these circumstances.

Amount and sources of dietary salt

It is generally accepted that **discretionary salt,** used in cooking and, at table makes the traditional methods of dietary analysis using food tables, an unreliable method of assessing salt intake. The accepted method of reliably estimating salt intake is by measurement of sodium excreted over a 24-hour period. This method relies upon the assumption that, whatever the intake, individuals are in salt balance on a day-to-day basis and thus that sodium excretion equals sodium intake. The method usually involves collecting a 24-hour urine specimen from the subjects. Normally well over 90% of total body sodium loss is via the urine, and the figure can be corrected for the normally small losses via the skin and in faeces. If there is severe diarrhoea or unaccustomed heavy sweating due to physical activity, high ambient temperature or fever, then losses by these other routes may be very considerable. Ideally, a marker substance should be used to ensure that the 24-hour urine specimen is complete, i.e. a substance that is consumed by the subject and excreted in the urine; only where there is complete recovery of the marker is the sample considered to be complete.

Gregory *et al.* (1990) found a very poor correlation (r = 0.25) between salt intake as measured by 24-hour urinary sodium excretion or as calculated from the average salt content of foods, recorded during a 7-day weighed inventory, in a large sample of British adults. There are several factors which can be used to explain the poor agreement between the two methods, namely:

- the sodium excretion method used just one day, which was at a different time to the weighed inventory
- no allowance was made for salt added during cooking or at the table in the weighed inventory
- no marker was used to ensure completeness of the 24-hour urine specimen.

However, the lack of agreement between these methods underlines the difficulty of estimating a subject's habitual salt intake in order to correlate this with, for example, blood pressure in epidemiological studies. Both methods have been used as the measure of habitual intake in epidemiological studies. Potassium intake in food and 24-hour excretion of potassium were also both measured in this sample of

people. In this case there is no discretionary intake from table and cooking use. Despite this, the correlation between the two methods for potassium intake were almost as bad as for sodium. This strongly suggests that, even though 24-hour sodium excretion may be an accurate reflection of sodium intake on that day, large day-to-day variation may make it a relatively poor predictor of the habitual salt intake of an individual.

Using the 24-hour sodium excretion method, James *et al.* (1987) concluded that average salt intake in the UK was around 10.7 g/day for men and 8.0 g/day for women. These estimates of average intakes agree well with other recent UK estimates using this method (e.g. Gregory *et al.*, 1990) but were less than some earlier estimates (e.g. those assumed by NACNE, 1983). The authors suggested this was because those using more traditional methods had not recognised that as much as 75% of cooking salt is not actually consumed and most is discarded with cooking water.

James *et al.* provided their subjects with pots of table and cooking salt that had been "labelled" with lithium; recovery of lithium in urine enabled them to estimate what proportion of total excretion was from these sources. By comparing the amount removed from the pot with the amount recovered they were able to make their estimate of the proportion of this salt that is not consumed, e.g. discarded in cooking water or in uneaten food. They concluded that discretionary salt made up only about 15% of total intake; 9% from table salt and 6% from cooking salt. They estimated that a further 10% of total intake was from salt naturally present in foods but that the remaining 75% was derived from salt added by food manufacturers during processing (the salt content of some common foods is shown in Table 11.1). Such figures indicate that there is very limited scope for individuals to reduce their salt intake by restricting their discretionary use of salt. If salt intake is to be substantially reduced, then either the salt content of manufactured foods must be reduced or the contribution of high-salt manufactured foods to the total diet must be reduced.

Encouraging food manufacturers to use less salt may not be without problems. Salt is used by manufacturers not only as a flavouring agent but also as a preservative and processing aid. Reduced salt content of processed foods may have effects other than on their palatability. In particular, shelf life may be adversely affected, thus increasing costs and threatening the micro-biological safety of the food. If salt is replaced by other alternative preservatives, these may be undesirable, too.

Evidence for an aetiological link between salt and hypertension

In some populations (e.g. Kalahari Bushmen and New Guinea Highlanders) with very low salt intakes (1–2 g/day) then hypertension is practically unknown and neither is there any general increase in blood pressure with age as is seen in the UK and US. In countries like Japan and Korea, average salt intake may be 2–3 times that seen in the UK and there is very high incidence of strokes and gastric cancer which have both been aetiologically-linked to high salt intake. These populations, especially the very low salt populations, have diets and life-style that are very different from those of affluent Westerners. Any number of con-founding variables could explain the apparent link between salt and hyperten-sion, e.g. high physical activity, low levels of obesity, low alcohol and tobacco use and high potassium intake of those populations with low salt intake. Tobian (1979) gives a summary of the early work in this area.

The levels of salt in these low-salt populations, such as that in the traditional Bushman diet, is so low as to be a totally unrealistic goal for those living in affluent countries. More extensive cross population studies, like those of Gliebermann (1973), suggested that there was a linear relation-ship between the average salt intake of a population and the average blood pres-sure in middle-aged and elderly people (see Figure 3.7 in Chapter 3). This would mean that even modest reductions in population salt intake could be expected to lead to reduced average blood pressure, reduced incidence of hypertension and thus eventually to reduced morbidity and mortality from those conditions that are precipitated by hypertension. In Gliebermann's paper, the reliability and validity of many of the measures of salt intake were questionable. As in all such cross cultural studies, there was the recur-ring problem of confounding variables. Gliebermann's data also included some black populations who seem to be geneti-cally salt-sensitive, and this could account for some of the most divergent points on her graphs.

In a more recent cross population study, Law *et al.* (1991a) related blood pressure to salt intake from reported data on 24 populations around the world. They overcame some of the criticisms of Gliebermann's earlier work because:

- they restricted their analysis to data in which salt intake was measured by 24-hour sodium excretion
- they excluded African and other black populations from their study
- they analysed data from developed and economically underdeveloped countries separately so as to reduce the problem of confounding lifestyle variables
- their study included people across a wide age range, enabling them to look at the relationship between salt intake and blood pressure in different age groups

They concluded that there was a highly significant relationship between average blood pressure and population salt intake in both developed and economically un-derdeveloped populations. The effect of salt intake on blood pressure increased with age and with initial blood pressure level. They derived an equation that they suggested would predict the average change in blood pressure of a group that would result from a specified change in salt intake; the variables in this equation were, the groups age, current salt intake and initial blood pressure. They predicted, for example, that in a developed country like the UK, a 60% reduction in salt intake in 60–69-year-olds with a systolic pressure of 183 mm/hg might be expected to lead to a 14 mm/hg reduction in systolic pressure.

Studies of migrant populations confirm that much of the international variation in blood pressure and incidence of hypertension-related diseases is due to environmental rather than genetic factors. People of Japanese origin in the USA, where salt intake is much lower than in Japan, have reduced incidence of strokes when compared to Japanese people living in Japan. Samburu tribesmen in Kenya have a traditional low-salt diet in their villages, but if they join the Kenyan army, the high-salt army rations are associated with a rise in their average blood pressure after 2–3 years (see Tobian, 1979).

Reduced reliance upon salting as a means of food preservation during this century has been associated with falling mortality from strokes and gastric cancer in both the US and UK and indeed in most industrialised countries. On an international basis, there is a strong positive correlation between stroke and gastric cancer mortality rates in industrialised countries. This is consistent with their being a common causative factor for the two diseases. Joossens and Geboers (1981) regressed mean death rates for gastric cancer in 12 industrialised countries with those for stroke; they found a very strong linear correlation between 1955 and 1973 (see Figure 3.8 in Chapter 3).

The weak point in the evidential link between salt intake and hypertension has traditionally been the lack of association between salt intake and blood pressure in individuals from within the same community. This lack of association has been a fairly consistent finding in many within population studies (Tobian, 1979; Law *et al.*, 1991b) and may be because of the general tendency for the influence of other factors upon blood pressure to obscure the relationship with salt intake (see Chapter 3). The difficulty of reliably measuring habitual salt intake would also be an important factor. Others have argued that this lack of association is because only a relatively small proportion of the population is salt sensitive. There will inevitably be genetic variation in salt-sensitivity, but if this variation is so great that effectively only a small sub-group of the population is salt-sensitive, then this would greatly weaken the case for population intervention to reduce salt intake.

Frost *et al.* (1991), in a complex re-analysis of 14 published within-population studies of the relationship between salt intake and blood pressure, concluded that the results were consistent with the results predicted from their equation derived from between population analysis (Law *et al.*, 1991). They argued that day-to-day variation in an individual's salt intake tends to obscure the true association between 24-hour sodium intake and blood pressure in within population studies. This is consistent with the poor correlation between 24-hour sodium excretion and salt content of food in weighed inventories reported by Gregory *et al.* (1990) that was discussed earlier in the chapter.

Salt restriction is principally seen by health promoters as a preventative measure, but it has also long been used as a method of treating hypertension. Before the advent of the antihypertensive drugs, extreme salt restriction was one of the few treatments available for severe hypertension. The Kempner rice and fruit diet aimed to restrict salt intake to 1 g/day. This diet was effective in some individuals, but it was associated with very poor compliance, anorexia and side-effects that greatly limited its practical usefulness. These early therapeutic studies of patients with severe (malignant) hypertension generally suggested that, although extreme salt restriction was effective in some hypertensives, more moderate salt restriction (say 2.5+ g/day) was not effective. The advent of antihypertensive drugs heralded a general loss of interest in this method of treating severe hypertension. There is now, however, renewed interest in the use of moderate salt restriction as a therapy for those people with asymptomatic mild to moderate hypertension where the principal aim is to reduce the long-term risk of hypertension-linked diseases. Drug therapy is effective in reducing hypertension in such subjects, but lifelong consumption of antihypertensive drugs is clearly not an ideal solution and may be associated with a new range of hazards.

A large number of trials of the effectiveness of salt restriction in the treatment of hypertension have been conducted in recent decades, e.g. note the rigorous double blind, random crossover study of Macgregor *et al.* (1982) discussed in Chapter 3. Law *et al.* (1991b) analysed the results of 78 controlled salt reduction trials. They concluded that, in those trials where salt restriction was for five weeks or more, the results obtained closely matched those that they had predicted from their cross population analysis (Law *et al.*, 1991a). Effects of salt restriction were less than predicted when shorter periods of salt restriction were used. They concluded that in 50–59-year-olds in industrialised countries, then a reduction in salt intake of 3 g/day could be expected to lead to an average reduction in systolic blood pressure of 5 mm/Hg with greater reductions in those who were hypertensive. They argue that such a level of salt reduction would, if universally adopted, lead to major reductions in stroke and heart disease mortality.

Other factors involved in the aetiology of hypertension

Much of the evidence implicating salt in the aetiology of hypertension could also be used to support the proposition that high potassium intake is protective against hypertension. In acute studies of sodium loading in both salt-sensitive rats and in people, high potassium intake seems to ameliorate the effects of high sodium loads. Some correlation between Na/K ratio and blood pressure may be found in within-population studies where no relationship can be shown between blood pressure and sodium intake alone.

There is some epidemiological evidence that low calcium intake may be associated with increased risk of hypertension. People who suffer from osteoporosis also have higher incidence of hypertension, a finding consistent with common aetiology; in osteoporosis there is certainly depletion of total body calcium even though the relationship with dietary calcium is controversial. Several intervention trials have suggested that calcium supplements may reduce blood pressure, at least in a proportion of hypertensives. Rolls (1982) contains a brief, referenced review of the relationship between calcium nutrition and hypertension.

Overweight and obesity are generally agreed to lead to increases in blood pressure, and weight loss reduces blood pressure in the overweight hypertensive. White *et al.* (1993) reported that in their representative sample of English adults, blood pressure rose with increasing Body Mass Index. Increased physical activity reduces the tendency to gain excessive weight and also contributes directly to a reduction in blood pressure. Excessive alcohol consumption also leads to a rise in blood pressure, while increasing the risk of stroke even in the absence of hypertension. White *et al.* (1993) found that blood pressure was positively associated with alcohol consumption in male drinkers,

Table 11.4 Factors associated with increased risk of hypertension

- Being black: prevalence is higher amongst blacks in the USA and UK than in whites. There are almost certainly also large individual variations in susceptibility within races
- Being overweight
- High alcohol consumption
- A sedentary lifestyle
- High population salt intake
- High dietary fat intake
- Low potassium or calcium intakes?

but they also found that non-drinkers had higher blood pressures than low-and moderate-drinkers.

A list of several of the factors that are associated with an increase in blood pressure and an increased risk of hypertension are shown in Table 11.4.

Conclusions

An active lifestyle, moderate alcohol consumption and good control of body weight are undoubtedly factors that will lessen the risk of hypertension and hypertension-linked diseases. Increased intakes of fruits and vegetables will increase potassium intakes and lower the Na:K ratio in the diet; processing of foods generally involves an increase in this ratio by some loss of K and addition of salt. There are general grounds for assuring that calcium intakes meet dietary standard levels, and this may have some beneficial effect on population blood pressure.

There is clearly some link between dietary salt intake and hypertension. The argument tends to be about how significant and widespread the benefits of salt restriction would be – would salt intake moderation lead to a general fall in average population blood pressure? Or would effects be limited to a relatively small proportion of salt-sensitive people? Moderate salt restriction will almost certainly be of some value to some salt sensitive people and may be of wider benefit. Salt restriction may also be useful in the treatment of mild to moderate hypertension, either as an alternative to drug use or as an adjunct to pharmacotherapy. Processed foods contain most of the salt in Western diets, and so any substantial reduction in salt intake requires either less reliance upon these high-salt foods or reduced use of salt by food manufacturers.

PART III
NUTRITION OF PARTICULAR GROUPS
AND FOR PARTICULAR SITUATIONS

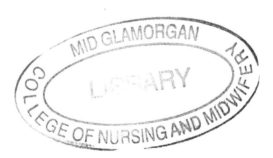

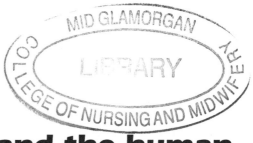

12 Nutrition and the human life-cycle

Contents

Introduction

Nutritional needs and priorities are likely to change during the human life-cycle. One would expect, for example, the relative nutritional needs of an active, rapidly growing adolescent to be markedly different to those of an elderly housebound person. Such differences might well lead to differences in the priority and nature of dietary recommendations for different life-cycle groups. This variation in nutritional needs is well illustrated by a comparison of current dietary recommendations for adults with the composition of breast milk. Adults are currently being advised to limit their fat intake to no more than 35% or even 30% of calories, to particularly reduce their saturated fat intakes, to reduce their intakes of simple sugars and to substantially increase their consumption of starch and non-starch polysaccharide. Yet in breast milk, the ideal food for infants, around 54% of the energy is in the form of fat, and this fat typically has a P:S ratio

substantially below that of the average UK diet. More than 40% of the energy in breast milk is in the form of the simple sugar lactose, and there is no complex carbohydrate in it.

Four phases of the human life-cycle have been identified for discussion in this chapter:

- pregnancy and lactation
- infancy and weaning
- childhood/adolescence
- old age.

Nutritional aspects of pregnancy and lactation

Overview

Nutritional aspects of pregnancy have been reviewed by Morgan (1988).

Healthy, well-fed women have the best chance of having healthy babies and of lactating successfully after the birth. General observation indicates that, although the most obvious manifestations of poor nutrition are specific deficiency diseases, these tend to become clinically recognisable only after severe or prolonged deprivation. Absence of overt deficiency diseases is not a very sensitive indicator of nutritional status and is no guarantee of optimal nutrition. Other less specific manifestations of malnutrition may occur despite absence of clinical cases of deficiency diseases, such as: impaired growth; impaired immune response; slow wound healing and remobilisation after illness or injury; reduced strength and work capacity.

It seems reasonable to assume that those subject to particular nutritional stresses, such as pregnancy or lactation, are likely to be the most sensitive to any marginal deficiencies or suboptimal intakes of nutrients. One would expect pregnancy to be a time of significantly increased nutritional needs for the mother; the phrase "eating for two" has, in the past, been widely used to sum up this expectation. Thus the health and wellbeing of mother or baby might be adversely affected by suboptimal nutrition despite the absence or low frequency of overt malnutrition within the population. Morning sickness affects over half of women in the early part of pregnancy, and this could also compound with other stresses to deplete nutrient stores in some women.

Cross-species comparisons show that human babies are much smaller than would be predicted from the size of the mother and that gestation is also longer than would be predicted. Thus the nutritional burden of pregnancy is likely to be less in women than in other, non-primate species. This difference in the relative burdens of pregnancy in different species is illustrated in Table 12.1. The small size and relatively slow postnatal growth of human babies indicated in Table 12.1 means that similar arguments also apply to lactation. An extreme comparison is between a female mouse and a woman. The mouse produces a litter that represents around 40% of her pre-pregnant weight in 21 days of gestation. She then provides enough nutrients in her milk to enable this litter to double its birth weight within five days. A woman produces a baby that represents 6% of her body weight after nine months of pregnancy and a breastfed baby might then take four to six months to double its birth weight. Extrapolating or predicting the extra nutritional needs of pregnant women from those of non-primate animals may be particularly misleading and would perhaps

Table 12.1 Relationship between maternal weight, offspring weight, gestation length and time to double birth weight in several species; to illustrate variation in the relative burdens of pregnancy and lactation in different species.

Species	Maternal weight (kg)	Litter weight as % maternal weight	Gestation length (d)	Time to double birth weight (d)
Mouse	0.025	40	21	5
Rat	0.200	25	21	6
G-pig	0.560	68	67	14
Rabbit	1.175	19	28	6
Cat	2.75	16	64	7
Woman	56	6	280	120–180

Source: Webb, G.P. (1992b) *Nutrition and the consumer.* ed. Walker, A.F. and Rolls, B.A. London: Elsevier Applied Science.

greatly exaggerate the extra needs of pregnant women.

Behavioural and physiological adaptations to pregnancy also tend to minimise the extra nutritional needs of pregnant women. These extra nutritional needs may thus turn out to be small in comparison to the needs of non-pregnant women. "Eating for two" implies a much greater increase in need than is indicated by measurements of the actual increase in intakes that occur in pregnant women and those indicated by current Dietary Reference Values for pregnant women.

Table 12.2 summarises current UK and US recommendations on the extra nutritional needs of pregnant and lactating women. This table highlights some very substantial differences of opinion about the extra nutritional needs of pregnant and lactating women between the UK and US committees for dietary standards. The American increments for pregnancy and lactation tend to be higher than those in the UK, often substantially higher, e.g. the iron, calcium and B vitamin increments for pregnancy. As noted in Chapter 3, baseline adult values also tend to be higher in the US. This means that for all nutrients, the absolute American RDA for both pregnancy and lactation equals or exceeds the corresponding UK value; in most cases, it substantially exceeds the UK value.

Where the percentage increase in the reference value for a nutrient in Table 12.2 significantly exceeds the percentage increase in the energy value, then this implies the need for increased nutrient density or supplementation in pregnancy/lactation. For example, if a non-pregnant American woman is just meeting her RDA for calcium then, on becoming pregnant, she would need to increase her total food intake by 50% to meet her new calcium RDA if her diet composition did not change. As two-thirds of even non-pregnant women fail to meet the calcium RDA, few pregnant women are likely to meet the now substantially higher RDA. Some values, such as the American RDA for iron in pregnancy and the British RNIs

Table 12.2 *Some daily extra increments for pregnancy (P) and lactation (L) in current UK and US dietary standards (COMA, 1991; NRC, 1989a). Values in parentheses are percentages of the value for other women.*

Nutrient	UK RNI*		US RDA	
	P	L	P	L
Energy (kcal)	200(10)†	520(27)‡	300(14)§	500(23)
(MJ)	0.8	2.18	1.26	2.09
Protein (g)	6(13)	11(24)	10(20)	15(30)
Vitamin A (µg)	100(17)	350(58)	0	500(63)
Vitamin D (µg)	10¶	10¶	5(100)	5(100)
Thiamin (mg)	0.1(13)†	0.2(25)	0.4(36)	0.5(43)
Riboflavin (mg)	0.3(27)	0.5(45)	0.3(23)	0.5(38)
Niacin (mg)	0	2(15)	2(13)	5(33)
Folate (µg)	100(50)	60(30)	220(122)	100(56)
Vitamin C (mg)	10(25)	30(75)	10(17)	35(58)
Calcium (mg)	0	550(79)	400(50)	400(50)
Iron (mg)	0	0	15(100)	0
Zinc (mg)	0	6(86)	3(25)	7(58)

Notes * EAR for energy; † last trimester only; ‡ average for first three months; § last two trimesters; ¶ no RNI for non pregnant/lactating women for vitamin D, require the use of supplements to be realistically achievable. In other cases, average intakes of relatively affluent UK and US women will comfortably exceed the RNI/RDA for many nutrients prior to pregnancy and so, in practice, avoid the need for dietary change that this logic would imply. For example, average intakes of riboflavin in British women are 1.8 mg/day, comfortably in excess of even the raised RNI for riboflavin in pregnancy. Average intakes of all vitamins in British women in 1987 were comfortably in excess of that year's RDAs (Gregory *et al.*, 1990).

There is an inverse correlation between infant mortality rate and birth weight; **low birth weight (LBW)** babies, i.e. less than 2.5 kg, have higher mortality. Thus birth weight of babies is a useful, objective and quantitative measure of pregnancy outcome; this suggests that anything which restricts foetal growth is liable to be detrimental to the chances of the baby's survival and subsequent well-being.

The ideal outcome to pregnancy is not only a healthy baby but also a healthy mother who is nutritionally well-prepared to lactate; lactation is likely to be nutritionally far more demanding for women than is pregnancy. The preparedness of the mother to begin lactation and the general well-being of the mother after parturition are not so readily quantifiable as birth weight but may, nonetheless, be important determinants of successful reproduction. This may be especially true in poorer countries where the presence or absence of a healthy lactating mother may often be a key determinant of the baby's chances of survival.

Maternal weight gain during pregnancy may be one quantifiable measure of the mothers preparedness for lactation. In rats, there is a 50% increase in maternal fat stores during pregnancy, and this fat store is rapidly depleted during the subsequent lactation. This increase in maternal fat stores is a physiological adaptation to enable the female rat to provide enough

milk for her large and rapidly growing litter. The increases in maternal fat typically seen in human pregnancy can also be assumed to be physiological. In women in industrialised countries, who have access to an essentially unlimited supply of palatable, energy-dense and nutrient-rich food, this store of energy to facilitate lactation may not be critical. It may be much more important to women who are subsisting on a marginal diet and who may have limited opportunity to boost intakes to meet the extra needs of lactation.

For those nutrients that accumulate during the pregnancy, either in the mother, or in the products of conception, it is possible to use factorial calculations (see Chapter 3) to predict the likely extra requirements for these nutrients during pregnancy. These are, however, only theoretical predictions, and whilst they may provide a useful basis for discussion or to generate hypotheses, they may not truly indicate extra dietary needs because of behavioural and physiological adaptations to pregnancy.

There has, over the years, been a very considerable amount of discussion about how any extra nutritional requirements of pregnant women are distributed throughout the pregnancy; are they concentrated in the last trimester when foetal growth rate is highest or do adaptive mechanisms ensure that the burden is distributed more evenly throughout the pregnancy? In the first dietary standards (NRC, 1943), the increases in RDAs in pregnancy were even higher than current US values but the increases in 1943 were all confined to the second half of pregnancy, whereas most current increases are for the whole of the pregnancy.

Nutrient needs in pregnancy

Energy needs in pregnancy

A typical British woman gains around 12.5 kg in weight during a typical pregnancy. This weight gain is made up of around 3.5–4 kg of extra maternal fat, around 6 kg as the increased weight of the uterus and contents and the remainder is due to increased body fluid. The total theoretical energy cost of a typical pregnancy has been estimated at about 70 – 80 000 kcal (around 300 MJ), i.e. the energy content of the products of conception and the extra maternal fat stores at the end of the pregnancy. At the end of the first trimester the foetus will only weigh around 5 g and around 500 g at the end of the second trimester – this compares with a typical birth weight of 3.3 kg. Thus foetal growth accelerates throughout pregnancy with most of the foetal weight-gain concentrated in the final trimester. This accelerating foetal growth rate might suggest that the extra energy needs should also be concentrated in the last trimester.

If one simply spreads the theoretical energy cost of pregnancy evenly throughout the pregnancy, then this would point towards an extra daily energy requirement of just under 300 kcal (1.3 MJ). As 85% of the babies total weight gain is concentrated in the final trimester, if the extra energy needs are distributed throughout the pregnancy in proportion to the rate of foetal growth, then this might suggest an extra dietary requirement in excess of 750 kcal/day (3.1 MJ/day) in this last trimester. However, as most of the gain in maternal fat occurs in the first trimester, this should tend to even out any extra energy requirements during the pregnancy. This maternal fat represents not only a reserve to partially offset the high energy costs of lactation but also a potential energy reserve for the last trimester if intake is inadequate.

The current UK Estimated Average Requirement (EAR) for pregnant women is only 200 kcal (0.8 MJ) above that for non-pregnant women and is for the last trimester only (Table 12.2). The UK panel on Dietary Reference Values (COMA, 1991) do suggest, however, that caution needs to be exercised because of the, as yet unresolved, uncertainties;

women who are underweight at the start of pregnancy or who remain active during their pregnancies may need more than suggested by this EAR. The American energy RDA for pregnant women is significantly more generous than the UK equivalent – an extra 300 kcal/day (1.3 MJ) is recommended for the second and third trimesters. Several studies have suggested that pregnant women in Britain only tend to eat more than non-pregnant women in the last few weeks of pregnancy and then less than 100 kcal/day (0.4 MJ/day) extra (COMA, 1991). Such studies, together with similar findings in other industrialised countries, suggest that the spontaneous increases in energy intake during pregnancy, are very small in previously well-fed women (Morgan, 1988). The extra energy needs of pregnant women, in such countries, are thus also likely to be very small because energy balance is physiologically regulated. Clearly, many women reduce their activity levels during pregnancy, and this saves at least some of the anticipated energy costs of the pregnancy – perhaps, more than half of the theoretical predicted cost. Studies on marginally nourished pregnant women, using the doubly-labelled-water method of measuring long-term energy expenditure, further suggest the possibility that physiological energy-sparing mechanisms may operate during pregnancy (Prentice, 1989).

Any reduced energy supply to the foetus during pregnancy is likely to restrict foetal growth and thus increase the risk of low birth weight. There is strong evidence linking maternal weight gain during pregnancy with birth-weight of the baby. According to a survey of 10 000 births in the USA in 1968 (summarised in Morgan, 1988), the chances of having a low birth-weight baby (i.e. below 2.5 kg) was inversely related to maternal weight gain in pregnancy:

- of women who gained less than 7 kg during pregnancy, about 15% had

LBW babies
- with 7–12 kg weight gain, around 8% had LBW babies
- with 12–16 kg weight gain around 4% had LBW babies
- women who gained 16+ kg only around 3% had LBW babies.

To some extent this trend is probably inevitable, i.e. bigger, heavier babies must result in some increase in the maternal weight gain during pregnancy. It does, nonetheless, suggest that attempts to restrict maternal weight gain by dieting during pregnancy may increase the risk of having a low birth-weight baby. Morgan (1988) concludes that, contrary to previous beliefs, **pre-eclampsia** or pregnancy-induced hypertension is not precipitated by high weight gain in pregnancy unless that weight gain is as the result of excessive fluid retention.

The risk of having a LBW baby also seems to be inversely related to maternal weight at the onset of pregnancy. In one study quoted by Morgan (1988) the heaviest 10% of women had only one-third (2.3%) the incidence of LBW babies of the lightest 10%. Energy-restricted diets are probably ill-advised for most women during pregnancy, perhaps even for women who are overweight at the start of pregnancy. In animal studies, even food-restriction of obese mothers during pregnancy reduced foetal weight. Morgan does conclude that obesity prior to becoming pregnant is a significant risk factor for pre-eclampsia. In an ideal world, of course, women intending to become pregnant should ensure that they are at or about their ideal weight prior to conception. Women seeking pre-conception advice can be counselled to normalise their weight before becoming pregnant. At the other end of the scale, if habitual energy intakes and body weights are very low, as seen for example in women suffering from Anorexia Nervosa and endurance athletes, menstruation ceases and they become infertile.

Glucose that has been transferred from maternal blood in the placenta is the primary energy source of the foetus. The concentration of glucose in maternal blood may, under some circumstances, fall to the point where it can limit the availability to the foetus; active transfer of nutrients from maternal blood makes this less likely to restrict supplies of other nutrients to the foetus. Starvation or heavy exercise during pregnancy may restrict foetal growth by reducing glucose concentrations in placental blood. Foetal nutrient supply depends not only upon nutrient concentration in maternal blood but also upon placental blood flow; therefore anything that reduces placental blood flow may also restrict foetal growth and nutrient supply. Smoking may reduce placental blood flow and thus also retard foetal growth. Purely anatomical factors, such as the precise site of implantation and development of the placenta, may affect foetal blood flow and may account for some unexplained incidence of LBW babies.

Poverty is associated with low birth-weight. Babies born in developing countries are, on average, smaller than those born in industrialised countries; proportions of LBW babies are also much higher in many developing countries. Even in industrialised countries, birth weight may be affected by social class and economic status. Nutritional factors seem a likely explanation for some of these differences, which remain even after correction for differences in maternal stature. Studies in Guatemala have shown that women who were marginally nourished, with typical unsupplemented intakes of 1600 kcal/day (6.7 MJ/day), had significantly heavier babies and less LBW babies when they were given food supplements prior to conception and throughout the pregnancy. A similar study in Taiwan, with women whose unsupplemented intake was higher, typically 2000 kcal/day (8.4 MJ/day), showed no significant effect on average birth-weight (both studies reviewed in Naismith, 1980). Analysis of several such intervention studies suggests that at very low baseline levels of intake, energy supplements do favourably affect birth-weight and reduce incidence of LBW babies. However, this favourable effect on birth-weight is not seen at slightly higher baseline levels despite the use of very substantial supplements. This threshold value at which supplements are effective in increasing birth-weight is said to be around 1680 kcal/day (7 MJ/day). Intervention studies also suggest that energy supply is much more likely to limit foetal growth than protein supply (Naismith, 1980; Morgan, 1988).

A lack of measurable effect of supplements on birth weight in the less undernourished women does not necessarily mean that supplementation had no beneficial effects; the supplements may have made mothers better prepared to lactate. In a review of such intervention trials, Morgan (1988) concluded that the supplements probably have a beneficial effect despite their disappointing effect on birth-weight because of increased maternal weight gain and improved lactational performance; these latter outcomes have generally been given relatively little consideration in such studies.

Protein in pregnancy

The current UK RNI for protein is increased by 6 g/day throughout pregnancy. The American RDA is increased by 10 g/day in women who are over 25 years and by 14 g/day in women who are 19–24-years-old. This UK RNI means that, in the first two trimesters (when the energy EAR is unaltered), it represents a rise from 9.3% of energy to 10.7% of energy as protein. In the average UK woman, protein currently makes up 15.2% of total energy intake (Gregory *et al.*, 1990); protein is therefore unlikely to be a limiting nutrient for pregnant women in the UK or in other industrialised countries. In the intervention studies discussed in the previous section, protein-rich sup-

plements appeared to offer no additional benefits over and above their energy value; even in these marginally nourished women, it is energy rather than protein that seems to be the limiting nutrient (Naismith, 1980; Morgan, 1988).

Factorial calculations suggest a total "protein cost" of about 925 g for a typical pregnancy. Theoretical calculations of protein accretion rates during the four quarters of pregnancy suggest rates of 0.6, 1.8, 4.8 and 6.1 g/day respectively (NRC, 1989a). Naismith (1980) provides direct evidence that, in the rat, extra protein is laid down in maternal muscle in early pregnancy, and that this is released in late pregnancy when the demands from the growing foetuses are highest. He argues that limited observations in women are consistent with these observations in the rat and may serve to distribute the extra protein need more evenly throughout the pregnancy. Measurements of nitrogen balance in pregnant women show that a small and fairly constant positive balance occurs throughout the pregnancy. Excretion of the amino acid 3-methyl histidine, is taken as an indicator of muscle protein breakdown, and it increases in the second half of human pregnancy.

Habitual consumption of protein in industrialised countries is almost always in excess of requirements and thus, in practice, it is unlikely that protein supply will be limiting during pregnancy. Pregnant women do not usually need to take specific steps to increase their protein intake despite their increased RNI/RDA. Even in developing countries, energy rather than protein is the likely limiting nutrient in pregnancy.

Minerals in pregnancy

The current RNIs for minerals in the UK indicate no routine extra increment for any mineral in pregnancy. This may initially seem very surprising both in the light of the high priority historically attached to increased mineral intakes during pregnancy and also the high priority that this still attracts in some other countries such as the USA. In the USA, the RDAs for all minerals are increased during pregnancy; details for iron, calcium and zinc are given in Table 12.2.

The estimated "calcium cost" of a pregnancy is around 30 g, i.e. around 30 g of calcium accumulates in the products of conception during pregnancy. This 30 g represents just over 100 mg/day when spread throughout the pregnancy. If one assumes that only a fraction of ingested calcium is retained (say 25–35%), then this factorial approach gives some idea of the origins of the 400 mg increase in the American RDA for calcium in pregnancy. The "calcium cost" of pregnancy represents only around 2–3% of the calcium in the maternal skeleton, and there is clear evidence that the efficiency of calcium absorption in the gut increases during pregnancy. The British panel on DRVs have concluded that in most women the extra calcium cost of the pregnancy can be met by utilisation of maternal stores and by improved efficiency of absorption (COMA,1991). In certain cases (e.g. adolescent pregnancy), they suggest that some extra increment of calcium might be advisable.

Iron supplements have traditionally been given to pregnant women, and the American RDAs clearly suggest that this practice should continue. These iron supplements have been widely reported to cause adverse gastrointestinal symptoms, and it is likely that a high proportion of them are not actually taken; perhaps contributing to the high incidence of accidental iron poisoning in children in the UK. The net iron cost of pregnancy, allowing for the savings due to cessation of menstruation, have been estimated at between 500 and 1000 mg (Morgan, 1988), i.e. 2–4 mg/day throughout the pregnancy. Once again, the UK panel on DRVs have assumed that in most women this extra iron requirement can be met by utilisation of maternal iron stores and by a considerable increase in the efficiency of

iron absorption during pregnancy. There is, therefore, considered to be no need for routine iron supplementation during pregnancy, although targeted supplementation (e.g. to women whose iron status is poor when they enter pregnancy) may be necessary. The American and UK panels have thus come up with very different practical "recommendations" using essentially the same body of factual knowledge.

Vitamins in pregnancy

The increases in vitamin RNIs and RDAs in Britain and the US are summarised in Table 12.2.

The 50% increase in the UK folate RNI and 122% in the American RDA during pregnancy reflects the view of the expert committees, at their respective times of reporting, that folate requirements are increased substantially during pregnancy. The proposal that folate supplements during pregnancy could reduce the risk of **neural tube defects (NTD)** in the offspring of susceptible women has recently been tested in a randomised, double-blind prevention trial using around 2000 women identified as being at high risk because of a previous affected pregnancy (MRC, 1991). There were only six affected babies in the folate supplemented groups but 21 in the same number of women not receiving folate supplements, i.e. a 72% protective effect. This study convincingly demonstrated the benefits of supplements for such high-risk women and suggests that all women should eat a folate rich diet when planning to become pregnant and during pregnancy.

About one in 250 pregnancies are affected; despite screening and termination of affected pregnancies, around one in 4000 babies born in the UK are affected by NTD. The risk is ten times higher in women who have already had an affected pregnancy, but most babies born with NTD are nevertheless first occurrences. The dose of supplements (5 mg/day) used in the intervention trial represent around 25 times the current adult RNI for folate. At this dose some rare but possibly serious and specific side-effects of folate overdose have been predicted; other, unpredicted risks are also possible. An expert advisory group in the UK has recommended that all women in the high risk category should take supplements of 5 mg of folate daily if they plan to become pregnant and during pregnancy. In view of the potential risks of high doses of folate and the relatively low incidence of NTD, all other women were recommended to take a more modest 0.4 mg extra folate if they plan to become pregnant and in the early months of pregnancy; this represents a three-fold increase over the adult RNI. However, as many as half of all pregnancies may be unplanned, and so to have maximum impact on the incidence of NTD, all women of reproductive age would need to increase their current intake by three times. There is currently an active campaign in the UK to increase the range and level of folate fortification of foods, mainly bread and cereals. Such fortified foods are the only realistic way that a high proportion of women will meet this target of 0.6 mg/day (see Halliday, 1993 for a short referenced summary of recent developments).

It seems to be widely assumed that supplementation will result in a similar reduction in general incidence to that seen in the intervention trial with high risk mothers, i.e. almost three-quarters of NTD-affected births will be prevented. However their are several areas of uncertainty that remain, such as:

1 Will the protective effect of folate be as high in the general population as it was in the high risk group selected for the intervention trial?
2 How dose-dependent is the protective effect of folate? If clearly pharmacological doses like those used in the trial are needed to produce significant benefit, then how useful is supplementation

and fortification at lower levels? If lower, physiological doses are effective, then doses even lower than the general level of 0.6 mg/day may well be just as effective.

There is no reason to believe that folate fortification will do any harm at levels commensurate with the 0.6 mg/day intake recommended by the expert committee. However, mass intervention on the basis of extrapolation from secondary intervention trials, using high risk subjects has led to past mistakes and is, as a matter of principle, an insufficient justification for such intervention (see discussion of this issue in Chapter 1). The author would suggest that:

1 the long term effects of chronically high intakes of folate need to be actively investigated
2 levels of any general food supplementation should in the meantime be conservative
3 foods supplemented with folate should be clearly labelled and should contain an indication about the limited population likely to benefit from extra folate and the untested consequences of chronic, high folate consumption
4 unsupplemented versions of all supplemented foods should continue to be readily available for those unlikely to benefit from very high folate intakes, i.e. children, older women and all men; perhaps these groups should be encouraged to use the unsupplemented foods.

This may seem unnecessarily timid with a simple dietary intervention that has been convincingly shown to benefit a section of the population. It is, however, a logical consequence of the criteria for intervention in Chapter 1 and of not assuming that simple changes in diet and lifestyle cannot do any serious harm.

Table 12.2 shows that the UK RNI for vitamin A is increased in pregnancy; there is no extra increment in the US, but the baseline value for women in the US is the same as that for pregnancy in the UK. It is, however, the possible consequences of excessive doses of retinol in pregnancy rather than potential inadequacy that is the current focus of concern about vitamin A in pregnancy in the UK. Very high intakes of retinol during pregnancy are **teratogenic**; they increase the risk of birth defects. Women in the UK are currently advised not to take vitamin A-containing supplements during pregnancy and are advised to avoid eating liver or products containing liver (e.g. paté) because of the high levels of retinol in animal livers (see COMA, 1991).

It is assumed by the UK panel on Dietary Reference Values that most of the adult population obtain their vitamin D principally from endogenous production in the skin via the action of sunlight on 7-dehydrocholesterol; therefore no RNI is offered for these groups. Pregnant women are one of the groups where the panel felt that endogenous production could not be relied upon and, therefore, an RNI was given (Table 12.2). The RNI is over three times average UK intakes and as such supplements are necessary to achieve it.

Alcohol and pregnancy

Foetal alcohol syndrome (FAS) is a recognisable clinical entity that is caused by heavy drinking during pregnancy. Babies with this syndrome:

- are small
- have characteristic facial abnormalities
- are often mentally retarded
- are immunodeficient
- show slow postnatal growth.

This syndrome starts to occur with habitual alcohol intakes in excess of 50 g/day (four glasses of wine) and the frequency increases as alcohol intake rises. The alcohol probably exerts a direct toxic effect on the foetus and may also increase the risk of oxygen or glucose deficit to the foetus.

There are strong indications that moderate amounts of alcohol in pregnancy (habitual intakes of 10–50 g/day) may increase the risk of low birth-weight and congenital malformations (Morgan, 1988). It may be prudent to advise women to limit their alcohol consumption during pregnancy to the occasional small amount, and some suggest that they should avoid alcohol altogether.

Heavy drinking prior to conception not only reduces fertility but also affects foetal growth even if drinking stops after conception. The foetus is also most vulnerable to the harmful effects of alcohol in the early stages of pregnancy. Taken together such observations suggest that moderation of alcohol consumption should ideally begin prior to conception.

Lactation

Lactation is nutritionally far more demanding for the mother than pregnancy. A woman will be producing up to 800 ml of milk containing as much as 9 g of protein and 700 kcal (2.9 MJ) of energy, as well as all the other nutrients necessary to sustain the growing infant.

The amounts by which the British EARs for energy exceed those of other women during the first three months of lactation are:

month 1   450 kcal/day (1.9 MJ)
month 2   530 kcal/day (2.2 MJ)
month 3   570 kcal/day (2.4 MJ).

After three months the EAR depends upon whether the breastfeeding is the primary source of nourishment for the baby or whether the baby is receiving substantial amounts of supplementary feeds. The American RDA for lactating women is increased by a set 500 kcal/day (2.1 MJ/day).

The UK EARs have been estimated by measuring the energy content of milk production and assuming an efficiency of 80% for the conversion of food energy to milk energy. The contribution from the maternal fat stores laid down during pregnancy has been taken as 120 kcal/day (0.5 MJ/day). These increases in the EARs for energy during lactation are said by the panel on DRVs (COMA, 1991) to closely match the extra intakes observed in lactating women in affluent societies.

The RNI for protein is increased by 11 g/day throughout lactation of up to six months duration. When this is expressed as a proportion of the EAR for energy, then it does not rise significantly above that for other women, i.e. 9.3% of calories. As in pregnancy, it seems unlikely that protein will be a limiting nutrient in lactation because habitual intakes are usually well in excess of this, i.e. 15.2% of calories for British women.

The RNIs for eight vitamins and six minerals are also increased during lactation, reflecting the panel's judgement of the extra needs of women at various stages of lactation. Some of these increases are substantial proportions of the standard RNIs for adult women. The increases in the American RDAs are generally even bigger (see Table 12.2).

Infancy

Nutritional aspects of infancy and childhood have been reviewed by Poskitt (1988).

Breastfeeding v bottle feeding

The assumption of most biologists would be that through the process of natural selection, evolution will have produced, in breast milk, a food very close to the optimum for human babies. Only in a few circumstances will breast milk not be the preferred food, such as:

- when babies have some inborn error of metabolism which leaves them unable to tolerate lactose or some amino acid in milk protein

- babies born to women infected with agents that may be transmissible in the milk, such as the Human Immunodeficiency Virus (HIV)
- babies of mothers taking some therapeutic or addictive drugs that may be transmitted in the milk.

Prevalence of breastfeeding

Despite an almost intuitive assumption of the superiority of breast milk as a food for human babies, for many years prior to 1975 the majority of babies born in the UK would not have been breastfed after leaving hospital. During the 1960s perhaps only a quarter of babies born in the USA and parts of Western Europe would have been breastfed for any significant time after delivery. Since then there has been some increase in breastfeeding led by women in the upper socio-economic groups, the same groups that led the earlier trend away from breastfeeding.

Table 12.3 shows the estimated prevalence of breastfeeding in babies of different ages in England and Wales at five-yearly intervals between 1975 and 1990. In 1990, around two-thirds of women made some initial attempt to breastfeed their babies, but less than 40% of babies were still being breastfed six weeks after delivery; by four months, this had dropped to around a quarter of all babies. These low figures nevertheless represent major increases over the figures for 1975, but there have been no significant changes since 1980. The substantial improvement shown

Table 12.3 Prevalence (%) of breast feeding in England and Wales. Data sources: DHSS (1988) and White *et al.* (1992)

Age	Year			
	1975	1980	1985	1990
Birth	51	67	65	64
1 week	42	58	57	54
2 weeks	35	54	53	51
6 weeks	24	42	40	39
4 months	13	27	26	25
6 months	9	23	22	21

between 1975 and 1980 has not been continued, and if anything there may have been a slight drift away from breastfeeding since 1980. These figures in Table 12.3 actually understate the use of bottle feeds because around 40% of breastfed babies received some additional bottle feeds at six weeks of age; thus, by six weeks, only around 24% of babies were being wholly breastfed (White *et al.*, 1992).

Factors influencing choice of infant feeding method

Choice of infant feeding method is very strongly dependent upon social class in Great Britain – in 1990, almost 90% of women in social class 1 attempted to breastfeed their babies and almost 70% were still breastfeeding at six weeks; the corresponding figures for women in social class five were around 40% and 20% respectively. Women with higher levels of education are also more likely to breast feed their children in Britain. The mother's choice of feeding method for her first baby is a major influence on feeding of subsequent children; mothers who had breastfed their first babies usually breastfed subsequent children, whereas women who had bottle fed the first baby usually did not (White *et al.*, 1992).

Many factors will have compounded to decrease the prevalence of breastfeeding, but the availability of a cheap, simple and "modern" alternative was clearly an essential prerequisite. There may have even been a temptation to think that science had improved upon nature if bottle fed babies grew faster than breastfed babies; the high protein content of the early infant feeds may have had a specific growth enhancing effect. Other factors that have contributed to the decline in breastfeeding are:

1 Breastfeeding may be inconvenient to the lifestyle of many women, especially those who wish to resume their careers soon after birth or those women whose income is considered to be a vital part of the family budget. Statutory paid maternity leave should have decreased this influence in more recent years.

2 Breastfeeding prevents fathers and others sharing the burden of feeding, especially night feeds in the early weeks after birth.

3 There are undoubtedly some women (and men) who find the whole idea of breastfeeding distasteful. There is a strong taboo in this country against breastfeeding in public or even amongst close friends or relatives. This coupled with the poor provision of facilities for breastfeeding in many public places can only increase the inconvenience of breastfeeding and restrict the range of activities that women can participate in during lactation.

4 The figures in Table 12.3 clearly indicate that many women who initially try to breastfeed give up after a very short time. Many women experience discomfort in the early stages of lactation, and many women believe that they are unable to produce sufficient milk. Delay in starting suckling (e.g. to allow the woman to rest after delivery) or any prolonged discontinuity of suckling are likely to reduce the likelihood of initiating and maintaining lactation.

5 Breastfeeding is promoted in many Third World countries as the modern, sophisticated, "Western" way of feeding babies – it is thus promoted as the high prestige option. Yet, in many industrialised countries, breastfeeding is more common amongst the higher socioeconomic groups and so in these countries, breastfeeding would appear to be the higher prestige option.

According to a 1990 survey of British women (White *et al.*, 1992), 88% of women chose to breastfeed because this was best for the baby. Other reasons given by 15% or more women were: the convenience of breastfeeding; the bonding it promotes between mother and baby; its cheapness; and, its naturalness. Common reasons given for choosing to bottle feed were: someone else can feed the baby (39%); did not like the idea of breastfeeding or would be too embarrassed to breastfeed (28%); and, around 40% of second or later babies were bottle fed because of the mother's previous experience.

The most common reasons given for early cessation of breastfeeding were lack of milk or failure of the baby to suckle. The discomfort caused by breastfeeding or dislike of breastfeeding were also important causes of early abandonment of breastfeeding. Almost half (44%) of breastfeeding women reported that they had experienced problems in finding somewhere to feed their babies in public places, and almost a quarter of all women with unweaned children, both breastfed and bottle fed, reported that they only went out between feeds (White *et al.*, 1992).

Early feeding experiences in the hospital also strongly influenced the likelihood of early cessation of breastfeeding. Mothers attempting to breastfeed but whose babies were also given some bottle feeds within the first week were almost four times as likely to give up breast feeding within a fortnight as were women whose babies received no bottle feeds. Women were almost twice as likely to continue breastfeeding if feeding on demand rather than at set times was practised in the hospital. Delay in initiating breastfeeding was also strongly associated with early cessation. Early cessation of breastfeeding occurred in 34% of cases where there was a delay of 12 hours or more in putting the baby to the breast but in only 12% of cases where this occurred immediately after birth; even a delay of one hour had a significant effect.

The British statistical data used in this discussion is intended to illustrate principles, patterns and trends that are likely to be common to several industrialised countries. In "Healthy People 2000" (DHHS, 1992) the goal is for 75% of US mothers to be breastfeeding in the immediate post-partum period by the year 2000 and for 50% to continue to breastfeed for 5–6 months. Assumed baseline figures for 1988 were that just 54% of mothers were breastfeeding on discharge from hospital and 21% breastfeeding at five to six months. Only 32% of low income US mothers breastfed their babies at time of hospital discharge, and less than 10% were still breastfeeding at five to six months. These figures are comparable to the 1990 figures for England and Wales. The figures for breastfeeding in Germany, the Netherlands and France are not too dissimilar to those in the UK, and those for Eire rather worse. In contrast, 99% of Norweigian mothers breastfeed their babies at birth and 90% are still at least partially breastfeeding at three to four months (Laurent, 1993).

The benefits of breastfeeding

Table 12.4 illustrates just how different are human milk and cow milk. The latter is an ideal food for rapidly growing calves, but unless substantially modified, is now regarded as an unsuitable food for human babies. Unmodified cow milk is now not recommended for babies until they are at least six months old. This table also demonstrates the scale of changes that are necessary to convert cow milk into a formula that is compositionally similar to human milk. The UK guidelines for formula manufacturers in the table show that even modern "humanised" formula may be quite different from the human milk that it is trying to imitate; they also indicate considerable potential for variation between different brands of infant formula.

Cow milk has around three times the protein content of human milk. This means that babies will need to excrete substantial amounts of urea if fed on cow milk, whereas when breastfed, the bulk of the nitrogen is retained for growth. Around 20% of the nitrogen in cow milk and breast milk is non-protein nitrogen, e.g. urea, creatine and free amino acids; its

Table 12.4 A comparison of the composition of human milk, cow milk and the UK guidelines for infant formulas. All values are per 100 ml as consumed. Data sources: Poskitt (1988) and DHSS (1988).

	Human milk	Cow milk	Formula guidelines Min	Max
Energy (kcal)	70	67	65	75
(kJ)	293	281	272	314
Protein (g)	1.3	3.5	1.5/1.2	2
Lactose (g)	7	4.9	2.5	8
Carb. (g)	7	4.9	4.8	10
Fat (g)	4.2	3.6	2.3	5
Sodium (mg)	15	52	15	35
Calcium (mg)	35	120	30	120
Iron (μg)	76	50	70	700
Vitamin A (μg)	60	40	40	150
Vitamin C (mg)	3.8	1.5	3	
Vitamin D (μg)	0.01	0.02	0.7	

biological significance is unclear, but this fraction will be absent from infant formula. The amino acid **taurine** is added to some infant formula and is thought to be semi-essential for infants. In breastfed infants, the principal bile acid is taurocholic acid, but in infants fed on cow milk it is glycocholic acid and this may adversely affect the emulsification and therefore digestion and absorption of milk fat.

The principal proteins in milk are **casein** and **whey**. The casein:whey ratio is much higher in cow milk than human milk. Casein forms hard clots in the stomach and is also relatively low in cysteine (the usual precursor of taurine). The alternative minimum guideline values for protein content of infant formula depend upon how much the casein:whey ratio has been modified to make it closer to that of human milk. Up to six weeks of age, **casein dominant formula** was used by 51% of a sample of British mothers and **whey dominant formula** by 47% (White *et al.*, 1992). In older infants, use of casein dominant formula became more prevalent, perhaps because of unsubstantiated claims by some manufacturers that a casein dominant formula is more satisfying than a whey dominant formula.

Cow milk fat is poorly digested and absorbed compared to that in breast milk; it is also much lower in essential polyunsaturated fatty acids. Some or all of the butterfat will be replaced by other fats and oils by infant formula manufacturers to give a fatty acid composition closer to that of human milk. Cow milk has only around 1% of energy as linoleic acid, whereas the figure for human milk is up to 16% depending upon the diet of the mother. The infant formula guidelines are for a minimum of 1% of the energy to come from linoleic acid and α-linolenic acid combined with a maximum of 20% from linoleic acid. The differences in digestibility of cow and breast milk fat may be partly due to differences in the nature of the fat itself, partly due to presence of a lipase in breast milk and perhaps also partly due to differences in bile acid secretion.

Breast milk is particularly high in lactose, and this lactose content may increase calcium absorption and act as a substrate for lactobacilli in the lumen of the gut, thus creating an acid environment that will inhibit the growth of pathogens. Breast milk contains a **bifidus factor**, a growth factor for the bacteria *Lactobacillus bifidi*. The stools of healthy breastfed babies have a low pH and contain almost exclusively lactobacilli. Formula manufacturers increase the carbohydrate content so that it corresponds to that of human milk – they may use lactose, sucrose or maltodextrins for this purpose.

Cow milk contains much higher concentrations of the major minerals than human milk. The sodium content is over three times higher; this is a high solute load for the immature kidney to deal with, and it can precipitate **hypernatraemic dehydration**. The risk of dehydration would be exacerbated by fever, diarrhoea or by making the formula too concentrated. High sodium content was the single most important reason why, in the UK in 1976, several formulae, including National Dried Milk, were withdrawn.

The calcium contents of cow milk and breast milk differ by even more than the sodium content, but calcium uptake is homeostatically regulated – calcium absorption from cow milk may be poor despite the high concentration of calcium present.

The vitamin and trace mineral content of formula is generally set so as to match or exceed that in human milk. The iron content of formula is higher than in breast milk to compensate for the much better absorption from breast milk. All formula is fortified with vitamin D.

Even if manufacturers had succeeded in producing a formula that exactly corresponded to breast milk in its nutrient content then there would still be substantial residual benefits to be gained from breast feeding. In many Third World countries, choice of feeding method may greatly affect the chances of survival of the baby. Mortality rates of bottle fed babies are often much higher than those of breastfed babies (Walker, 1990). Even in industrialised countries there are suggestions that deaths from cot death are lower in breastfed babies (see Laurent, 1993). Some additional benefits of breastfeeding are as follows:

1 *Bonding* – Breast feeding is thought to increase bonding between mother and baby.
2 *Anti-infective properties* – Breast milk contains immunoglobulin A which protects the mucosal surfaces of the digestive tract and upper respiratory tract from pathogens. It also contains immune cells which aid in the immunological protection of the infant gut. The iron binding protein lactoferrin has a bacteriostatic effect as well as facilitating iron absorption.

   Colostrum, the secretion produced in the first few days of lactation, is particularly rich in these anti-infective agents. Colostrum is quite different in its composition from mature human milk.

   Anti-infective agents in cow milk will probably be destroyed during processing, and many are in any case likely to be species-specific.
3 *Restoration of maternal prepregnant weight* – It is generally assumed that maternal fat laid down during pregnancy serves as a store to help meet the energy demands of lactation upon the mother. In countries like the UK and USA, where obesity is prevalent, the assumed effect of lactation in reducing this maternal fat after delivery may be an important one.
4 *Cost of formula* – In wealthy industrialised countries, the cost of formula will usually be relatively trivial. In many Third World countries, this cost will be a very substantial proportion of the total household budget. This may seriously reduce resources available to feed the rest of the family, or it may lead to the baby being fed overdiluted formula as an economy measure, thereby effectively starving it.
5 *Hygiene* – It is taken for granted in most industrialised countries, that infant formula will be made up with clean boiled water, in sterile bottles, and the final mixture pasteurised by being made

up with hot water. The risk of contamination in many other countries is a very serious one – the purity of the water, facilities for sterilisation of water and bottles and good storage conditions for pre-mixed feeds may all be poor. This means that bottle fed babies may have greatly increased risk of gastrointestinal infections. Gastroenteritis is the single largest cause of death for babies in developing countries. This is a major reason why breastfeeding should be particularly encouraged in these countries. This is an important cause of the higher mortality of bottle fed babies

6 *Anti-fertility effect* – Although breast feeding cannot be regarded as a reliable method of contraception, it does reduce fertility. In cultures where suckling occurs for extended periods rather than in discreet "meals", then this effect may be increased. In many Third World countries, prolonged breastfeeding will have an important birth spacing effect and will make a contribution to limiting overall population fertility.

7 *Reduced risk of breast cancer* – A large case-control study in the UK has suggested that breastfeeding reduces the risk of developing breast cancer in young women. Breast cancer risk declined both with the duration of breastfeeding undertaken by the woman and with the number of babies that she had breastfed (UK National Case-Control Study Group, 1993).

Weaning

When to wean?

Weaning is the process of transferring an infant from breast milk or infant formula onto solid food. The process begins when the child is first offered food other than breast milk or formula. The process may be very gradual with other foods forming an increasing proportion of total energy intake over several months until breast or formula is eventually phased out completely. During weaning there is ideally gradual transition from a very high fat, high sugar liquid diet to a starchy, moderate fat, low sugar and fibre-containing solid diet. The magnitude of these compositional and textural changes indicates the advisability of a gradual transition to allow babies to adapt to them.

In the report "Present Day Practice in Infant Feeding" (COMA, 1988), it was concluded that very few infants require solid foods before three months of age but that the majority require it by six months of age. It was recommended in this report that weaning should not begin before three months but that infants should be offered a mixed diet by six months of age. After around six months, it is thought that breast milk can no longer supply all of the nutritional needs of the infant; growth is likely to be impaired if the baby receives only breast milk. Breast milk or formula may continue to make a contribution to total food supply after weaning has begun.

The COMA panel considered too-early introduction of solid foods undesirable because:

1 some babies do not properly develop the ability to bite and chew before three to four months
2 the infant gut is very vulnerable to infection and allergy
3 the early introduction of energy-dense weaning foods may increase the likelihood of obesity.

It has been suggested that full production of pancreatic amylase does not occur in human infants until six to nine months of age. As milk contains no starch but most weaning foods are starchy, this may be a physiological indicator that a relatively late introduction of starches into the diet is desirable. Introducing starchy solid foods too early may produce symptoms similar to infectious gastro-enteritis because of poor digestion and absorption due to the lack of pancreatic amylase (COMA, 1988).

In 1975, 18% of British babies had been given some food other than milk in their first month and 97% by the time they were four months old; corresponding figures for 1990 were 3% and 94% respectively (COMA, 1988; White *et al.*, 1992). The practice of introducing solid foods to infants very soon after birth is now much less common. Nevertheless, about two-thirds of British babies do receive solid food before the three months suggested by the COMA panel (White *et al.*, 1992).

What weaning foods?

In the UK, the first foods for most babies are cereals, rusks or commercial weaning foods rather than home-prepared weaning foods (COMA, 1988; White *et al.*, 1992). At six weeks, only 3% of mothers who had offered solid food to their babies had used a home-made food and even at four months, when over 90% had offered some solid food, only a quarter of them had used home-made food (White *et al.*, 1992).

The priorities for weaning foods are as follows:

1 One of the main aims of weaning is to raise the energy density of the infant's diet above that for breast milk. The weaning food should have a suitable texture, but be of high enough energy and nutrient density for the baby to meet its nutritional needs without having to consume an excessive bulk. If very viscous food is introduced too early in the weaning process, then the infant may reject it by spitting it out. A typical Third World weaning food made up to give a suitable viscosity from a starchy staple, such as millet flour, might contain only 0.25 kcal/g (1 kJ/g) compared to around 0.7 kcal/g (3 kJ/g) for breast milk and perhaps 1.5 kcal/g (6 kJ/g) for a typical UK weaning diet (Church, 1979). The child may be incapable of consuming the volume of food required to meet its energy needs

with such a dilute weaning food. This problem may be exacerbated if the child is fed infrequently, has frequent periods of infection and anorexia, and perhaps if the food itself has poor sensory characteristics. In industrialised countries, this could be a problem if parents mistakenly apply the recommendations for low-fat, low-sugar, starchy diets in adults too rigorously to infants.

2 The food should be clean and not contaminated with infective agents. Much malnutrition in the Third World is precipitated by poverty, poor hygiene and contaminated food. Even when dietary intakes are judged sufficient to permit normal growth, infection and diarrhoea may be an indirect cause of dietary deficiency. One survey reported that 41% of traditional weaning foods and 50% of drinking water specimens in rural Bangladesh were contaminated with faecal micro-organisms (see Walker, 1990).

3 In affluent countries, like the UK and US, other aims are also considered important for infant feeds – the food should be low in salt, added sugar and perhaps gluten-free.

High salt foods expose the immature kidney to a high solute load and increase the risk of hypernatraemic dehydration. Sugar is regarded as empty calories and is detrimental to the babies new teeth. Over consumption of sugar in infancy may also create bad preferences for the future. There is very strong evidence that fluoride is protective against dental caries, the UK panel on DRVs suggested a safe fluoride intake for infants of 0.05 mg/kg/day – around 50% of the amount likely to cause fluorosis. To achieve this safe intake most UK infants would need supplements. Swallowing fluoridated toothpaste is one way that many young children receive supplemental fluoride.

Whilst most babies will suffer no harm by early exposure to the wheat protein called gluten, those sensitive to gluten, and thus at risk of coeliac disease (see Chapter 13), cannot be identified in advance. The incidence of coeliac disease has been falling in recent years at the same time as there have been trends towards later introduction of solid foods and towards the use of gluten-free, rice-based weaning cereals.

Childhood and adolescence

The rate of growth of children decelerates steadily from birth until puberty. During adolescence there is a very pronounced and sustained growth spurt; between the ages of 12 and 17 years boys gain an average 26 cm in height and 26 kg in weight, girls gain 23 cm in height and 21 kg in weight between the ages of 10 and 15 years. Adolescence is thus an intensely anabolic period and a time when there is inevitably a relatively high demand for nutrients to sustain this rapid growth. In a proportion of adolescents, high levels of physical activity because of participation in games and sports will still further increase needs for energy and perhaps other nutrients. Adolescence is also a time of major psychological changes brought on by the hormonal changes of puberty, and these may have major effects on children's attitudes to food. Adolescent girls are the most common sufferers from Anorexia Nervosa, and paradoxically, obesity is also a common nutritional problem of adolescence.

As with rapidly growing infants, diets which are too low in energy density (e.g. diets very low in fat and high in fibre) may tend to limit growth during adolescence. Strict vegetarian diets tend to be bulky and have low energy density; this is indeed often cited as one of their advantages. Vegan children tend to be smaller and lighter than other children (Sanders, 1988). The phrase "muesli belt malnutrition" has been widely used in the UK to describe undernutrition in rapidly growing children precipitated by overzealous restriction of calorie dense fatty and sugary foods by health conscious, middle-class parents.

During the five-year period of adolescence, boys accumulate an average of around 200 mg/day of calcium in their skeletons with a peak value of around double this average. They also accumulate an average of 0.5 mg/day of iron and 2 g/day of protein during the five years of adolescence. The onset of menstruation represents a further major stress on the iron status of adolescent girls. Table 12.5 shows some DRVs for 11–14-year-olds, 15–18-year-olds and adults. The energy EAR for 15–18-year-old boys is 8% higher than that for adult men despite the smaller size of the boys. The calcium RNI is 43% higher for both age groups of boys than that for men and clearly reflects the DRV panel's assumptions of the extra calcium needs required for skeletal growth – this RNI would be difficult to meet without drinking good amounts of milk. Similar, relatively high DRVs for girls compared to women are also shown in this table. Similar trends are also seen in the American RDAs; relative allowances (i.e. allowing for size) are higher for adolescents than for adults. American values for all groups tend to be higher than the corresponding British values. Note particularly that the calcium RDAs for both ages of boys and girls are 1200 mg/day (c.f. adult value 800 mg/day); the calcium RDAs for American girls are thus 50% higher than the corresponding UK values.

COMA (1989) published a survey of the diets of a nationally representative sample of British girls and boys at 10–11 years and 14–15 years. They concluded that the main sources of energy in the diets of British children were bread, chips (french fries), milk, biscuits (cookies), meat products (e.g. sausages, burgers, meat pies), cakes and puddings. These foods together accounted for about half

Table 12.5 A comparison of some UK Dietary Reference Values for adolescent boys and girls with those for adults. Data source: COMA (1991)

Nutrient	DRV	Age group		
		11–14 years	15–18 years	Adult
Energy (kcal)	EAR (men)	2200	2755	2550
	(women)	1845	2110	1940
Energy (MJ)	EAR (men)	9.21	11.51	10.60
	(women)	7.92	8.83	8.10
Calcium (mg)	RNI (men)	1000	1000	700
	(women)	800	800	700
Iron (mg)	RNI (men)	11.3	11.3	8.7
	(women)	14.8	14.8	14.8
Zinc (mg)	RNI (men)	9.0	9.5	9.5
	(women)	9.0	7.0	7.0
Niacin (mg)	RNI (men)	15	18	17
	(women)	12	14	13

of the total energy intake. Energy intakes of the two age groups of girls were not significantly different, whereas intakes of the older boys were 20% higher than those of the younger boys. Mean recorded energy intakes were within 5% of the EAR for all groups when these EARs were interpolated from the actual mean body weights of the groups using figures in COMA (1991). Given the tendency for dietary surveys to underestimate total intakes and the satisfactory heights and weights for ages of the population then energy intakes would seem to be adequate to meet the youngsters' needs.

Fat made up about 38% of total energy intake of these British children, very similar to the adult figure recorded by Gregory *et al.* (1990). Three quarters of all children exceeded the 35% target of calories from fat discussed in Chapter 4. Surprisingly, meat and meat products contributed less than 15% of the total fat, marginally less than that contributed by chips (french fries) and crisps (potato chips).

Average intakes of all four groups of children exceeded the current RNIs for most of the nutrients surveyed, i.e. for protein, vitamin A, vitamin C, nicotinic acid, riboflavin, thiamin. Pyridoxine intakes were at or marginally below current RNIs. In the younger children, calcium intakes were well above the RNIs for 10-year-olds but below those of the 11–14-year-old age bands. Calcium intakes of the older children were about 10% below current RNIs. Milk and cheese contributed 40% or more of total calcium intakes for all groups. Milk also contributed about 30% of riboflavin intakes. Iron intakes of the older girls were only 62% of the current RNI; intakes of the younger girls met the RNI for 10-year-olds but represented only 58% of the 11–14-year-old figure which should presumably apply from the start of menstruation.

The overall impression from this survey of British children is that their diets meet most current criteria for adequacy although there are a few areas for concern. In terms of current health education priorities, particularly dietary fats, the diets of children seem to be very similar to those of their parents. These conclusions are as one might expect and the general conclusions would probably apply to most other industrialised countries.

The elderly

Demographic and social trends

The British statistical data is taken from an epidemiological overview of the health of elderly people in Britain (DH, 1992b).

In most industrialised countries, the proportion of elderly people in the population has risen substantially in recent decades, and it is projected to rise still further in the future because of increasing life expectancy. In 1989, around 16% of the population of England and Wales was over 65 years and around 1.6% were over 85 years – the ratio of females to males in the elderly population increases progressively with age. By 2026, the over 65s are expected to represent 19% of the population and the over 85s almost 2.5% of the population. In the USA in 1990, about 13% of the population were over the age of 65 and this proportion is projected to rise to around 22% over the next half-century (Hamilton *et al.*, 1991).

Around 36% of the over 65s in England and Wales lived alone in 1989, and the proportion living by themselves tended to increase markedly with advancing age as a result of the deaths of spouses. In the 85+ age group almost 60% of women and around 45% of men lived alone. The number of elderly people living in residential homes for the elderly has increased by about 60% over the last 15 years, from around 150 000 in 1977 to around 235 000 in 1990. This 1990 figure represents around 3% of all people over the age of 65 years and almost 0.5% of the total population of England and Wales. Catering for the dietary and nutritional needs of the elderly is thus a topic that should warrant an increased educational and research priority.

The household income and expenditure of elderly people in England and Wales tends to be concentrated at the lower end of the range. In both single adult and one man, one woman households, retired persons account for 40–80%
of the three lowest household income groups but they become progressively less well represented in the higher income categories. Retired persons in the upper income groups inevitably receive some income in addition to the state pension. Old age is widely and, for many it would seem, correctly perceived as a time of relative poverty. The increasing ratio of retired to working people in the population and the increasing numbers living in costly, residential homes for the elderly, makes it difficult to foresee any marked improvement in the economic status of the bulk of elderly people in the UK unless this issue acquires a higher political priority.

More than half of all the over 65s report being affected by some long-standing illness and the proportion rises with advancing age. Bone and joint diseases, including arthritis and rheumatism are easily the most common group of long-standing illnesses; other important causes of long-standing illness in the elderly include heart diseases, hypertension, respiratory diseases like bronchitis and emphysema, stroke and diabetes.

Despite this, the majority of elderly people consider themselves to be in good or fairly good general health. In 1985, about 80% of men and women aged over 65 years perceived their own health as good or fairly good and even in the 85+ age group only around 27% of men and 33% of women described their health in the previous year as "not good".

Thus the elderly population in the UK is already a substantial minority of the total population and is growing considerably faster than the population as a whole. The very elderly population (i.e. over 85 years) is expected to almost double over the next 25 years and by the end of the period it will account for one in 40 of the total population. Many people do and will continue to spend a proportion of their later years living alone or in residential homes for the elderly. Many are also required to live upon incomes that are at the extreme low end of the UK range.

Inevitably, the incidence and prevalence of the degenerative diseases and of disabilities will tend to increase with advancing years.

On a more positive note, around 80% of elderly people describe their general health in at least reasonably favourable terms, and this is still true for more than two-thirds of the over 85s. More than 80% of elderly people still report seeing friends or relatives at least once a week, and even in the over 85s this figure is still around 75%. Although the absolute numbers of people living in residential homes for the elderly have increased very substantially, about 95% of people over 65 years still either live in their own homes or with their families. The widespread image of the post-retirement years as being inevitably an extended period of poor health, disability, dependence and social isolation does not seem to be the perceived experience of the majority of older people. As average life expectancy continues to increase and reaches its presumably inevitable plateau, so improving the quality of life of the elderly population will become an increasing priority for health education in industrialised countries.

Nutrition in the elderly

In view of the size of this population and its projected growth, there is a surprising lack of published research data about the nutritional needs, problems, priorities and nutritional status of elderly people. In the preface to a UK report on "The Nutrition of Elderly People" (COMA, 1992) it was noted that the work of the committee was often constrained by lack of available data. Relatively few large scale studies of the nutritional status of elderly people have been undertaken. A survey of 750 elderly people living in the UK in the late 1960s (DHSS, 1972) indicated that only around 3% of the surveyed population were suffering from malnutrition, and that in the great majority of cases,

malnutrition was associated with some precipitating medical condition. Around half of this population were re-assessed in 1972 by which time they were all aged over 70 years (DHSS, 1979). In this second survey the prevalence of malnutrition was found to be around 7%, but twice as high as this in the over 80s. Once again, most of the nutritional deficiencies were related to some underlying disease; certain social factors were also identified as being associated with the risk of malnutrition in the elderly, e.g. being housebound and having a low income. According to this survey the diets of elderly British people were in their general nature very similar to those of other adults.

The general impression created by the results of this survey were that, if elderly people have good general health, are reasonably mobile and affluent, then they tend to have few specific nutritional problems. However, as people get older they are more likely to suffer from a number of medical conditions that may precipitate nutritional problems. The elderly are also more likely to be affected by a range of social factors that were associated with higher risk of nutritional inadequacies, such as:

- to be immobile and housebound
- to be socially isolated
- to have been recently bereaved
- to have a low income
- to live alone.

It is generally accepted that the energy intakes of elderly adults tend to fall with advancing years as a result of reduced energy expenditure. Two factors are thought to be responsible for this decline in energy expenditure:

1 A marked tendency for physical activity to decline with increasing age. This decline may well be accelerated by retirement and is, of course, inevitable in those who are housebound or bedridden.

2 A decline in basal metabolic rate in the elderly. This is probably a function of the decline in lean body mass in the elderly because, when the basal metabolic rate is expressed per kg of lean body mass, there is no decline with age (COMA, 1992). Many elderly people gradually lose lean body mass and body weight in their later years, and this may also be as a result of reduced activity – certainly inactivity increases the rate of decline in lean body mass.

Table 12.6 shows the UK EARs and the American RDAs for energy for different age categories of men and women. These EARs and RDAs represent quite substantial reductions in the estimated energy requirements, and therefore likely total food intake, of elderly people, particularly of elderly men. Longitudinal studies of the food intakes of groups of elderly people in the UK and in Sweden indicate that the average energy intake of these individuals did indeed fall over a five-year period (see COMA, 1992).

There are generally no corresponding decreases in the UK RNIs for other nutrients in the elderly with the exception of small reductions in the male RNIs for protein, thiamin and niacin and a substantial reduction in the female RNI for iron, which reflects the cessation of menstrual blood losses. Similarly, in the American RDAs there are reductions only in the RDAs for the three B vitamins, thiamin, riboflavin and niacin the RDA of which (and RNI in the UK) is based upon the expected energy intake; once again, there is a reduction in the RDA for iron in elderly women. Thus elderly people are perceived as requiring intakes of most nutrients that are similar to those for other adults but requiring average intakes of energy up to 20% lower than those for other adults. This increases the risk that energy needs can be met without fulfilling the requirements for all other nutrients. This risk increases if the nutrient density of the diet is low, i.e. if a substantial proportion of the calories are derived from nutrient-depleted sources such as fatty or sugary foods or from alcohol. According to COMA (1992), in underweight elderly people who are very inactive, the decline in energy expenditure and consequently in food intake is much greater than the average reductions in EAR/RDA seen in Table 12.6. Energy

Table 12.6 A comparison of the energy EARs (UK) and RDAs (US) for elderly adults with those of other adults. Data sources: COMA (1991) and NRC (1989a)

	Age (years)	Men	reduction (%)	Women	reduction (%)
EAR – kcal/day					
(MJ/day)	19–50	2550	—	1940	—
		(10.60)	(8.10)		
65–74		2330	9%	1900	2%
		(9.71)		(8.00)	
75+		2100	18%	1810	7%
		(8.77)		(7.61)	
RDA – kcal/day					
(MJ/day)	25–50	2900	—	2200	—
		(12.14)		(9.21)	
	51+	2300	21%	1900	14%
		(9.63)		(7.96)	

intakes may be so low that it becomes difficult to obtain good intake of the other nutrients without substantial alterations in the nature of the diet. Elderly people, or those responsible for providing meals for the elderly, are advised to ensure that their diet is of high nutrient density so that adequate intakes of the other nutrients can be maintained in the face of a potentially considerable decline in energy and total food intake. COMA (1992) also suggested that the intake of sugars in the elderly tends to be towards the top end of the UK range (i.e. 10–20% of total calories); they concluded that the general dietary guidelines suggesting limiting non milk extrinsic sugars to 10% of calories might be especially appropriate for older people, given their apparent need to ensure a high nutrient density.

Overweight and obesity are also common in elderly adults; this is likely to discourage physical activity and thus lead to an accelerated decline in lean body mass.

There are several specific points raised by COMA (1992) concerning the nutrition of the UK elderly population:

1 *Riboflavin status of the elderly* – 30% of a sample of UK elderly people (DHSS, 1979) had erythrocyte glutathione reductase activation coefficients above the limit taken to indicate satisfactory riboflavin status. Biochemical indications of unsatisfactory riboflavin status in elderly people have been reported in other studies.

2 *B_{12} deficiency* – There may be a high prevalence of vitamin B_{12} deficiency in the elderly because of the increased incidence of diseases that hinder absorption. There may be a case for increased intakes in the elderly.

3 *Vitamin C status* – More than half of a sample of elderly people in the UK had intakes of vitamin C that were below the current RNI of 40 mg/day (DHSS, 1979).

4 *Folate status* – In 1972 red cell folate

levels were marginal or subnormal in around a quarter of a sample of UK elderly people (DHSS, 1979).

5 *Fruit, vegetables and milk* – The panel encouraged increased consumption of fruits and vegetables in elderly people as this would increase intakes of vitamin C, folate, potassium, carotene and of non-starch polysaccharide (fibre). The panel also regarded it as important to maintain reasonable intake of milk in the elderly as it is a good source of most nutrients including riboflavin and calcium.

Nutrition and the elderly – final thoughts

The association between increased serum cholesterol concentration and increased risk of coronary heart disease has been generally assumed to be less convincing in elderly people than in young and middle-aged adults. The benefits of cholesterol lowering have thus been assumed to be reduced or even absent in the elderly. According to COMA (1992), more recent data from both the USA and the UK indicates that the predictive value of a raised serum cholesterol for increased coronary heart disease risk is maintained in later years and thus that the general cholesterol-lowering guidelines should also apply to the elderly. The general nutrition education guidelines for the UK and US populations offer some benefits to the elderly, even if the long-term benefits envisaged for younger adults (e.g. reduced risk of coronary heart disease and cancer) are reduced for them:

1 Increased intakes of non-starch polysaccharides (fibre) are likely to reduce constipation and beneficially affect existing minor bowel problems such as haemorrhoids.

2 Decreased intakes of sugary and fatty foods and their partial replacement by cereals, fruits and vegetables will tend to increase the nutrient density of the diet. It will also increase potassium

intakes and may tend to reduce sodium intakes – this may have beneficial effects in moderating high blood pressure.

3 The reduced energy density of the diet may help to reduce the amount of obesity in the elderly population. Note, however, that the prevalence of underweight increases with age in elderly people and this may be a more serious problem than overweight and obesity. In elderly people, increasing body mass index is associated with increased life expectancy whereas in younger adults high body mass index is a predictor of reduced life expectancy.

Despite this, the nutritional priorities for older people are different to those for younger adults. The maintenance of dietary adequacy re-assumes greater priority in the face of falling calorie consumption. In those elderly people suffering weight loss, loss of taste perception and reduced ability to chew when maintaining high palatability and good food intake may be more important than conforming to current nutritional education guidelines. The nutrition education guidelines discussed in the earlier chapters are directed towards effecting reductions in the long-term risk of degenerative diseases. It seems inevitable that, even if these preventative benefits still occur in the elderly, then they are likely to be considerably reduced. Should healthy elderly people be encouraged to make major changes in their diets if the benefits of change are even less certain for them than for younger people and if the costs of changing practices evolved over a lifetime are likely to be perceived to be higher? Is monitoring of cholesterol levels in the elderly with its attendant anxiety for many and the prescribing of restrictive cholesterol-lowering diets for those with average or even elevated levels really justified, when the holistic benefits of such intervention are difficult to demonstrate even for younger people? Are elderly people sometimes given the standard dietary advice developed primarily for the benefit of younger adults simply because there has not been enough research done to enable guidelines to be developed that are more specifically appropriate for the elderly?

Maintenance of a reasonable level of physical activity would seem to be strongly advisable for the elderly as a complement to sound nutrition in maximising good health and quality of life. In addition to the general beneficial effects upon the cardiovascular system, increased activity will maintain energy expenditure and help to maintain lean body mass. In Chapter 11 it was also noted that fitness and reasonable levels of physical activity were associated with reduced risk of osteoporotic fracture in elderly adults.

13 Nutritional aspects of illness and injury

Contents

- Every careful observer of the sick will agree in this, that thousands of patients are annually starved in the midst of plenty, from want of attention to the ways which alone make it possible for them to take food

    Florence Nightingale (1859)
    Notes on nursing. Reprinted 1980
    Edinburgh: Churchill Livingstone.

- Many people with severe illness are at risk from an unrecognised complication – malnutrition...
    Doctors and nurses frequently fail to recognise under-nourishment because they are not trained to look for it.

    King's Fund Centre report (1992)
    A positive approach to nutrition as treatment. KFC.

Diet as a complete therapy

Overview and general principles

There are a small number of diseases or conditions where dietary change can be a highly effective and complete therapy. Such diseases almost always involve an inherited or acquired intolerance to a specific nutrient or a specific component of food. **Food intolerance** has been defined as "a reproducible, unpleasant (i.e. adverse) reaction to a specific food or ingredient which is not psychologically based". Where there is "evidence of an abnormal immunological reaction to the food" then this is termed a **food allergy**, (Mitchell, 1988).

The therapeutic principles in cases of food intolerance are very simple:

- to identify the nutrient or foodstuff to which the patient is intolerant
- to devise a dietary regimen that provides a healthful and acceptable diet whilst either keeping intakes of the

nutrient within tolerable limits or excluding the offending foodstuff.

In practice, it may prove difficult to pinpoint the food or foods causing the symptoms or even to establish with certainty that the symptoms are really due to food intolerance. For example, a range of symptoms, affecting a variety of physiological systems, have been attributed to food allergy, e.g. abdominal pain and diarrhoea, urticaria (hives), eczema, asthma, allergic rhinitis, migraine and behaviour problems in children (Denman, 1979). Food allergy is not the only cause of such symptoms and is not even a usual cause, and, therefore other, more probable, causes need to be eliminated before a diagnosis of a food allergy can be made.

Once food allergy (or other intolerance) is suspected as a probable cause, then the food or foods responsible need to be identified. Exclusion diets, comprised of foods which infrequently cause allergy, may be used and once symptoms disappear, individual foods added back. If symptoms reappear upon the re-introduction of a particular food, this suggests that this food may be responsible for the allergy. To be confident that symptoms are really due to sensitivity to a particular food, one really needs to **blind challenge** with the suspected allergen. Patients may develop symptoms in response to a placebo if they believe it to contain the suspect food or they may not develop symptoms when they unknowingly consume the suspected food. A procedure analogous to the double blind clinical trials discussed in Chapter 3 is the way to be sure that symptoms are a physiological rather than a psychological response to the suspected allergen. If symptoms do not disappear with the exclusion diet, then an **elemental diet** composed of purified nutrients may need to be used.

Skin sensitivity tests are sometimes used to identify causes of food allergy; small amounts of potential allergens are injected into the skin and the extent of any inflammatory skin reaction is then used to assess sensitivity. It is still unclear how valid these skin reactions are as predictors of response to substances administered by the oral route.

In addition to diseases where exclusion is the primary dietetic aim there are a few diseases that, although they are not of primary dietary origin, can be alleviated by nutrient supplements. **Perncious anaemia** is probably the best known example; autoimmune destruction of the parietal cells of the stomach results in a failure of vitamin B_{12} absorption. Most of the symptoms of this potentially fatal disease can be alleviated by regular injections of B_{12}. **Hartnup disease** is a rare but fatal inherited disorder with symptoms that resemble those of pellagra (niacin deficiency). The symptoms of this disease result from a failure to absorb the amino acid tryptophan (precursor of niacin) which leads to niacin deficiency. The condition responds well to niacin treatment.

Phenylketonuria (PKU) and **coeliac disease** have been selected to illustrate the problems of devising diets that need to severely restrict the intake of an essential nutrient or to exclude a common food ingredient. Coeliac disease also serves as an example of food allergy.

Phenylketonuria

PKU is an inherited disease which affects around 1:10 000 babies in the UK. Since the 1960s, all babies born in the UK have been tested for this condition within the first two weeks of life. Classical PKU is caused by a genetic defect in the enzyme phenylalanine hydroxylase that converts the essential amino acid phenylalanine to the amino acid tyrosine:

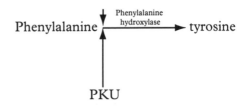

Normally, excess phenylalanine, either from the diet or from endogenous protein breakdown, is metabolised via its conversion to tyrosine. In PKU, this route is blocked and so excess phenylalanine and unusual metabolites of phenylalanine accumulate in the blood where they seriously impair mental development. Untreated children with PKU are severely mentally retarded and prone to epilepsy, but they grow normally and have a normal life expectancy.

The objective of dietary management in PKU is to restrict phenylalanine intake so that mental development is not impaired but to provide enough of this essential amino acid and all other nutrients to allow growth and physical development. This is, in practice, difficult because all foods with good amounts of protein also contain high levels of phenylalanine. The tolerance to phenylalanine depends upon the precise nature of the biochemical lesion and varies from child to child. The amount of phenylalanine that the child can consume whilst keeping blood levels within the acceptable range for age is first determined. The phenylalanine allowance that has been defined in this way, is taken in the form of normal protein-containing foods, e.g. milk, cereals and potatoes. Certainly in young children, meat, fish, eggs, cheese and pulses will be totally excluded and only sugars, fats, fruits and non-leguminous vegetables can be eaten free of restriction. The resultant diet is, by design, very low in protein and is also likely to provide inadequate amounts of energy. Children are therefore given a supplement of free amino acids and may also be given high energy/low protein products originally developed for use by renal patients on low protein diets. Infant formulae that are low in phenylalanine are available prior to weaning.

The prognosis for children with PKU depends upon how strictly the dietary regimen is followed, but even in families where control is poor the children should still be educatable. Prior to the 1960s, and the introduction of universal screening, most PKU children would have been very severely impaired (the average IQ of untreated PKUs is about 50) and many would have spent much of their lives in institutions for the mentally handicapped. Current consensus suggests that some dietary regulation needs to be maintained throughout life. Special care needs to be taken over the diet of PKU women intending to become pregnant because the developing foetus is vulnerable to high phenylalanine levels. The dietary management of PKU has been reviewed by Debenham (1992) and Coutts (1979).

Coeliac disease

Coeliac disease results from a hypersensitivity or allergy to a component of the wheat protein, **gluten**; similar proteins are found in barley, oats and rye and these may also cause symptoms. The disease is classified as a food allergy because it involves an "abnormal immunological response to food", but it differs from classical allergy,, e.g. hay fever, in that it does not involve production of antibodies to gluten of the type (**IgE**) that are usually associated with allergic reactions. In untreated coeliacs, the villi of the small intestine atrophy and there is excessive secretion of mucous. These changes in the small intestine result in severe malabsorption of fat and other nutrients leading to: fatty diarrhoea; distended abdomen; weight loss or growth failure; and, other symptoms that are the result of nutrient deficiencies such as anaemia, rickets/osteomalacia and bleeding due to vitamin K deficiency. In the long term, there may be cancerous changes in the intestine induced by continued exposure to gluten. Coeliac disease may also be present as a chronic skin disorder, **dermatitis herpetiformis.**

The aim of dietary management in coeliac disease is to avoid all gluten-containing foods. The achievement of this goal is complicated because bread and cereals are staple dietary items, and flour is also an ingredient of many prepared foods. Gluten-free flour and bread are available on prescription in the UK and gluten-free cakes and biscuits (cookies) are commercially available. Many food manufacturers use a "crossed grain" symbol to indicate that a particular product is free of gluten. Dietary management of coeliac disease has been reviewed by Debenham (1992).

The symptoms of coeliac disease usually present in early childhood but may first appear at any stage of life. There has been a decline in the number of children developing the disease in recent years but a rise in the number of adult cases. The increased use of rice-based weaning foods, and thus the delayed introduction of wheat into the diet, has probably contributed to the delay in onset of the disease. Before the cause of this disease was identified in the 1950s, around a third of affected children died in childhood, around a third survived into adulthood as chronic invalids and the rest appeared to recover spontaneously (Passmore and Eastwood, 1986).

Diet as a specific component of therapy

There are a number of conditions where diet does not give complete relief from symptoms nor is it the sole treatment but where there is an apparently sound theoretical and empirical basis indicating a specific role for a particular dietary regimen. Three examples, **diabetes mellitus**, **cystic fibrosis**, and **chronic renal failure** are briefly overviewed.

Diabetes mellitus

Diabetes mellitus results from a lack of the pancreatic hormone **insulin** and diet has historically been a key element in its management. In the severe form, **insulin dependent diabetes mellitus (IDDM)**, which usually develops during childhood, there is destruction of the insulin producing cells in the pancreas, which results in an almost total failure of insulin supply. In the more common and milder form of the disease, **non-insulin dependent diabetes mellitus (NIDDM)**, there is a progressive inadequacy of insulin production. This inadequacy seems to stem from a failure of the pancreas to be able to adequately compensate for a progressive decline in sensitivity to insulin in the target tissues.

All diabetes sufferers have high blood glucose concentration, and as a consequence they excrete glucose in their urine which also causes increased water loss, increased thirst and propensity to dehydration. In the untreated, severe form of the disease (IDDM) there is:

- rapid weight loss
- very high blood glucose concentration and severe dehydration
- excessive production and excretion of ketone bodies leading to acidosis, electrolyte imbalance and eventually to coma and death.

NIDDM is treated in some cases by diet alone and in other cases by a combination of diet and oral hypoglycaemic drugs; IDDM is treated by a combination of diet and insulin injections.

The symptoms of the disease suggest that the diabetic is carbohydrate intolerant, and so severe restriction of dietary carbohydrate and almost total exclusion of dietary sugar have been the rule for diabetic diets for most of this century. Prior to the 1970s most diabetic diets would have contained no more than 40% of the calories as carbohydrates and in many cases much less than this; such diets were inevitably high in fat (Keen and Thomas, 1988). According to Leeds (1979), when insulin treatment was first used in the 1920s, diabetic diets typically contained less than 10% of calories as carbohydrate and more than 70% as fat.

The historical aims of diabetic therapy were to alleviate the immediate symptoms of the disease which are at best unpleasant and incapacitating and at worst acutely life threatening. Despite the availability for many years of therapies that are effective in this limited aim, the life expectancy of diabetics was and is considerably less than that of non-diabetics, and diabetics have continued to suffer a high level disability in their later years. A major additional objective of modern diabetic therapy is to increase the life expectancy and to reduce the long-term morbidity of diabetics; so, some discussion of the causes of the high morbidity and mortality of diabetics is necessary. Two major considerations seem to be important in this respect:

1 Diabetics in Western countries have traditionally suffered much higher mortality from cardiovascular diseases than non-diabetics. This high rate of cardiovascular disease is not an inevitable consequence of diabetes because Japanese and black East African diabetics have been relatively free of cardiovascular disease unlike either Japanese American or black American diabetics (Keen and Thomas, 1988). A high fat diet is widely accepted to be a risk factor for cardiovascular diseases, and so the traditional very high fat diet and consequent hyperlipidaemia of diabetics has almost certainly been a factor in their propensity to cardiovascular disease.

2 Diabetics also suffer from a range of conditions that are attributed to degenerative changes in their microvasculature, i.e. capillaries. These changes in the microvasculature are responsible for the **diabetic retinopathy** that causes many diabetics to go blind and also for the high levels of renal disease (**diabetic nephropathy**) seen in diabetics. Changes in the capillaries of diabetics are thought to stem from a chemical change in the proteins of the basement membrane of capillary cells that results from their continued exposure to high glucose levels; the proteins react abnormally with glucose and become **glycosylated**. Glycosylation probably also plays a role in the development of cataract and the degeneration of peripheral nerves and gangrene often seen in older diabetics.

Modern diabetic management seeks to reduce these longer term complications by:

- achieving and maintaining a normal body weight
- minimising hyperlipidaemia and hyperglycaemia.

As a result, the diet recommended for diabetics has changed very considerably over the past 20 years and is almost the opposite of that previously recommended. The modern recommended diabetic diet has more than half of the calories from carbohydrate with the emphasis on unrefined foods high in complex carbohydrate and fibre; it has moderate levels of fat and saturated fat, ideally less than 35% of calories as fat; even the very strict avoidance of sugar has been relaxed, provided it is a component of a meal. The general avoidance of isolated sugary foods except for hypoglycaemic emergency is still recommended. A diet considered ideal for diabetics with NIDDM is very similar to that recommended for the population as a whole; the matching of carbohydrate to insulin dose in IDDM is a specialist topic beyond the scope of this text, but the overall dietary strategy is as outlined here. Note that overdose of insulin causes blood glucose level to fall below normal, hypoglycaemia, and this fall in blood glucose can lead to a variety of symptoms ranging from confusion and disorientation through to coma and even death. Hypoglycaemia is treated by consuming a sugary snack or by infusion of glucose if the patient is unconscious. It occurs, for example, if an IDDM patient misses or unduly delays a meal or takes too much insulin.

There is a strong correlation between obesity and risk of NIDDM, and normalisation of body weight and regulation of caloric intake to match expenditure may in some cases completely alleviate the symptoms of NIDDM. Keen and Thomas (1988) suggest that much of the success of traditional low carbohydrate diabetic diets may be attributed to their regulation of energy intake rather than carbohydrate restriction *per se*. They argue that, provided the diabetic is in energy balance, then short term diabetic control is not really affected by the proportion of calories from fat or carbohydrate. A raised carbohydrate intake increases peripheral sensitivity to insulin and thus does not increase the need for insulin. This adaptation cannot, of course, occur in the absence of insulin, and so carbohydrate does have adverse effects in untreated severe diabetes, thus explaining the past assumption that carbohydrate was inevitably bad for diabetics. The well-documented effects of fibre in improving glucose tolerance were discussed in Chapter 6. Simpson (1981) concluded that an increase in the proportion of energy from carbohydrate, together with an increase in dietary fibre, has a generally favourable effect upon blood glucose control in both IDDM and NIDDM. The reduced levels of fats in diabetic diets would be expected to reduce blood lipid levels and to contribute to a reduction in atherosclerosis.

Cystic fibrosis

Cystic fibrosis (CF) is an inherited disease caused by an autosomal recessive gene, and it affects as many as 1:2000 babies in the UK. There are in excess of 6000 patients with cystic fibrosis in the UK. The genetic lesion results in the production of a sticky mucous which blocks pancreatic ducts and small airways in the lungs. In the pancreas, this blockage leads to formation of cysts and progressive fibrosis and loss of function as these cysts are repaired. Similar changes occur in the lungs; there are repeated chest infections and progressive fibrotic damage to the lungs. In the past, affected children would have been unlikely to survive into adulthood. Improved therapy is steadily increasing the life expectancy of affected patients and the steadily increasing prevalence (in the UK about 130 extra patients per year) is largely accounted for by increased survival of affected patients into early adulthood.

Regular physiotherapy to clear the lungs of the thick secretions and the availability of antibiotics to treat lung infections have been key factors in the improved survival and quality of life of sufferers, but improved dietetic management has also been an important factor. The fibrosis of the pancreas leads to a failure to produce pancreatic juice. As a consequence there is poor digestion and absorption of fat and protein and poor absorption of fat soluble vitamins. Untreated CFs are at high risk of both general malnourishment and fat soluble vitamin deficiencies. Evidence of vitamin A deficiency is frequently found in untreated CF patients and in some cases xerophthalmia (due to vitamin A deficiency) has been the presenting symptom. There is often anorexia in CF patients, especially associated with infection, and there is also increased energy expenditure that is believed to be a primary consequence of the disease.

The principle dietetic objective in this condition is to maintain the nutritional adequacy of the patient. Dietetic management should prevent the wasting, the deficiency diseases and the fatty diarrhoea of untreated CF. There is also very strong evidence of interaction between nutritional status and the pulmonary manifestations of the disease, which ultimately determine survival. Malnourished patients are more prone to respiratory infections whereas well nourished patients suffer fewer episodes of pneumonia; experience of other sick and injured patients suggest that weak, malnourished people have an impaired ability to cough and expectorate (KFC, 1992).

The strategies employed to meet this objective of maintaining dietary adequacy are:

1 pancreatic supplements containing the missing digestive enzymes are given with food; these are now in the form of coated microspheres that are protected from destruction in the stomach but disintegrate in the small intestine (duodenum)
2 a diet that is high in energy and protein and, with the more effective pancreatic supplements, this need not now be low in fat
3 supplements of fat soluble and often of water soluble vitamins are given
4 dietary supplements or artificial feeding are given when patients are unable to take adequate food by mouth.

Dodge (1992) has reviewed the dietary management of cystic fibrosis.

Chronic renal failure

Low protein diets are widely used to give symptomatic relief in chronic renal failure. As the kidney fails, there is reduced excretion of the urea produced by breakdown of excess dietary protein (or body protein in wasting subjects). Increased blood urea (**uraemia**) produces unpleasant symptoms such as headache, drowsiness, nausea, vomiting and anorexia. A diet that minimises urea production should alleviate these symptoms of uraemia.

There is a widespread belief that a low protein diet is not only palliative, but, that if started in the early stages of renal failure, actually slows the pathological degeneration of the kidney. It thus extends the period in which conservative management can be used before either

dialysis or transplantation become essential (Lee, 1988; Debenham, 1992). This latter benefit of low protein diets is still a matter of dispute. Locatelli *et al.* (1991) compared the effects of a low protein diet and a controlled but "normal" protein diet on the progression of chronic renal failure in a large sample of Italian patients with renal disease. Any benefits of the greater protein restriction were at the borderlines of statistical significance, and Locatelli and his colleagues concluded that they did not justify the restrictions imposed upon the patients. They did concede, too, that compliance with the low protein diet was not good with a particular overintake of vegetable protein.

Low protein diets for chronic renal disease aim to restrict protein intake to around 40 g/day (c.f. typical intake of UK male of 84 g/day) and to give a high proportion of this protein in the form of high quality animal protein. Intakes of lower quality cereal proteins with their attendant relatively high nitrogen losses are restricted, and the diet also aims to be high in energy in order to prevent the breakdown of endogenous protein as an energy source. The overall aim is a high energy, low protein but high-quality protein diet. A range of high energy but protein-reduced foods such as protein-reduced flour, bread, pasta and crackers are available not only as direct low sources of low protein calories but also to act as vehicles to carry fats and sugars, e.g. butter and jam (jelly). High energy, low protein supplements may also be used. In advanced renal disease low salt as well as low protein diets may be employed (see Debenham, 1992).

Nutritional support as a non-specific but vital adjunct to therapy in major illness and after surgery or injury

The problem – introduction

In patients for whom diet is a very specific component of their therapy, there is likely to be careful monitoring of their intake and early recognition of nutritional problems. However, less vigilance may be exercised in monitoring the food intake and nutritional status of other hospital or community patients.

Historically, nutrition has been given low priority in medical and nursing education; many doctors and nurses are neither trained to recognise signs of inadequate nutrition nor educated about the key importance of good nutrition in facilitating recovery. The key to improving the nutritional status of hospital patients, and other sick or injured patients, must be a heightened awareness amongst nurses, doctors, and carers in general, of the importance of sound nutrition to prognosis. An increased vigilance in recognising indications of poor or deteriorating nutritional status is also required. A specialist **nutrition team**, no matter how competent and dedicated, can only personally supervise the nutritional care of a small number of patients. The nutrition team must rely upon other medical and nursing staff to identify nutritionally "at risk" patients and to refer them quickly to the team. The general nutritional care of those patients not specifically at risk is also dependent upon non-nutrition-specialist staff. One of the most important roles of the nutrition team is to educate and heighten awareness of other hospital staff to the importance of nutrition in patient care.

In times of economic stringency, there may be strong pressures to economise on the "hotel" component of hospital costs, including the catering costs, and to concentrate resources upon the direct medical aspects of care. Any money saved from the catering budget is, however, likely to be a false economy if it leads to a deterioration in the nutritional status of the hospital population. A worsening of nutritional status will be associated with higher rates of complications, longer durations of stay and thus increased costs in spite of maintained or even improved surgical, medical and nursing care (KFC, 1992). Thus, awareness of the key role of good nutrition in facilitating recovery needs also to permeate through to those with responsibility for budgetary control in hospitals. Some predictions of the financial benefits of nutritional support for undernourished patients and of a specialist nutrition team to supervise parenteral nutrition are given in KFC (1992).

Prevalence of hospital malnutrition

It has been reported that up to 50% of surgical patients in some hospitals in the US (e.g. Bistrian *et al.*, 1974) and the UK (e.g. Hill *et al.*, 1977) show indications of malnutrition, both general protein energy malnutrition and vitamin deficiencies. Since these landmark publications, there have been reports of high prevalence of suboptimal nutrition in children's wards, medical and geriatric wards and in hospitals in other countries (KFC, 1992). For example, almost one in six children admitted to a Birmingham (UK) hospital were stunted or severely wasted – at least a quarter of children admitted with chronic respiratory, cardiac and digestive problems were short for their age (see KFC, 1992 for further examples and references).

Consequences of hospital malnutrition

The practical consequences of hospital malnutrition are likely to be:

1 higher rates of wound infections

2 increased risk of general infections, particularly respiratory infections and pneumonia, because weakening of the respiratory muscles will impair the ability to cough and expectorate

3 increased risk of pressure sores because of wasting and immobility

4 increased risk of thromboembolism because of immobility

5 increased liability to heart failure because of wasting and reduced function of cardiac muscle

6 in the classical studies on the effects of chronic undernutrition in healthy subjects (Keys *et al.*, 1950), apathy and depression were found to be a consequence of starvation, and these will also hinder the recovery of sick and injured people.

Newton *et al.* (1980) and KFC (1992) have reviewed studies on the effects of malnutrition and supplementary feeding in mainly surgical patients. Some specific examples quoted by these sources:

1 malnourished patients undergoing cardiac surgery had extended hospital stays compared to those who were well nourished pre-operatively

2 there were reduced rates of wound infections in patients undergoing surgery for oesophageal and gastric carcinoma who had been given pre-operative supplementary parenteral feeding compared to those who had not

3 more rapid wound healing and reduced wound sepsis was reported in patients given intravenous feeding after surgery for oesophageal carcinoma

4 in patients with fractures to the neck of the femur, malnutrition was associated with slower remobilisation and higher mortality, but artificial feeding decreased the period required to regain mobility and decreased the mortality in malnourished patients

5 mortality was significantly reduced by supplementary feeding in a six-month randomised trial of elderly patients.

The following conclusions were drawn from a recent and general review of the relationship of nutritional status to outcome (KFC, 1992):

1 malnutrition is associated with increased duration of hospital stay and increased hospital charges

2 malnutrition is associated with increased rates of complications and mortality in both medical and surgical patients.

Malnutrition and immune function

It is a general observation that in famine areas, malnutrition is associated with high rates of infectious disease, with increased severity and duration of illness and ultimately with higher mortality. Providing medicines and medical personnel will have limited impact if the underlying problem of malnutrition is not addressed.

Chandra (1993) has recently reviewed the effects of nutritional deficiencies upon the immune system, and he concluded that there were a number of demonstrable changes in immune responses as a consequence of malnutrition, such as:

1 **Delayed-type cutaneous hypersensitivity** (DTH) responses to a variety of injected antigens are markedly depressed, and this depression occurs even in moderate nutritional deficiency. A low plasma albumin concentration predicts a reduced DTH skin response. In this type of test the antigen is injected into the skin and the inflammatory reaction occurs some hours after injection hence, "delayed-type hypersensitivity". The best known of these reactions is the **Mantoux reaction** in which individuals immune to the organism that causes tuberculosis respond to a cutaneous tuberculin injection with a DTH reaction. These DTH reactions are a measure of the cell-mediated immune response which deals with pathogens that have the capacity to live and multiply within

cells, e.g. the bacilli that cause TB and leprosy, some viruses, such as the smallpox virus, and parasites, such as that responsible for the disease toxoplasmosis.

2 Secretion of **immunoglobulin A (IgA)** the antibody fraction that protects epithelial surfaces, e.g. in the gut and respiratory tract, is markedly depressed. Circulating antibody responses (**IgG**) are relatively unaffected in protein energy malnutrition.

3 The ability of phagocytic white cells to kill bacteria after they have ingested them is reduced in malnutrition.

Trauma, whether surgical or accidental, also has an immunosuppressive effect, and the degree of immunosuppression is proportional to the amount of trauma (Lennard and Browell, 1993). This means that, for example, the immune systems of poorly nourished patients undergoing major and traumatic surgery will be doubly depressed. Minimising surgical trauma with modern techniques should lessen the immunosuppressive effect of surgery.

The causes

A combination of depressed intake and increased nutrient requirements compound together to increase the probability of nutritional inadequacy during illness or after injury.

Factors that may depress intake in the sick and injured:

1 physical difficulty in eating, e.g. unconsciousness, facial injury, difficulties in swallowing, oral or throat infection, lack of teeth, arthritis and diseases affecting co-ordination and motor functions

2 malabsorption of nutrients due to disease of the alimentary tract

3 anorexia induced by disease or treatment, most obviously the severe anorexia frequently seen in malignant disease. Anorexia is however, a symptom of many illnesses and a side-effect of

many treatments and is likely in anyone experiencing pain, fever or nausea

4 anorexia resulting from a psychological response to illness, hospitalisation or diagnosis. Starvation itself may lead to depression and apathy and may thus reduce the will to eat in order to assist recovery

5 unacceptability of hospital food. This is most obviously present in patients offered food that is not acceptable on religious or cultural grounds but equally, low prestige, unfamiliar and just plain unappetising food may severely depress intake in people whose appetite may already be impaired

6 unavailability of food. Patients may be starved prior to surgery or for diagnostic purposes, they may be absent from wards at meal times. This may compound with the other factors listed to depress overall nutrient intake.

In general, the more specific and more obvious these influences are, the more likely they are to be addressed. It will be obvious that in someone whose injuries include a broken jaw that particular measures are needed to ensure that they can eat, but a patient who lacks teeth and has a sore mouth and throat is more likely to be overlooked. More allowance is likely to be made for a Jewish patient known to require Kosher food than for a patient who simply finds hospital food strange and unappetising.

Factors that tend to increase the nutrient requirements in the sick and injured:

1 increased nutrient losses, e.g. loss of blood, loss of protein in the exudate from burned surfaces, loss of glucose and ketones in the urine of diabetics and loss of protein in the urine of patients with renal disease

2 increased nutrient turnover – illness and injury lead to hypermetabolism, the **metabolic response to injury**.

In a classical series of studies that began in the 1930s, Cuthbertson demonstrated that in patients with traumatic injury, the initial period of shock after injury was followed by a period of hypermetabolism. He coined the term **ebb** to describe the period of depressed metabolism or shock after injury and the term **flow** to describe the state of hypermetabolism that occurs once the initial period of shock is over. The flow phase is characterised by increased resting metabolism and oxygen consumption and an increased urinary loss of nitrogen associated with increased muscle protein breakdown. Cuthbertson found that the magnitude of this flow response was greater the more severe the injury and the better nourished the patient. He found that the flow response generally reached its peak four to eight days after injury and that the total loss of body protein could exceed 7% of total body protein within the first ten days after injury. He concluded that the increased metabolism was a consequence of the increased rate of body protein turnover and the use of body protein as an energy-yielding substrate. Cuthbertson regarded this catabolic response as an adaptive mechanism to provide a source of energy when incapacitated by injury (traumatic or infective) and a means of supplying amino acids for the synthesis of new tissue and for the functioning of the immune system. This catabolic response is mediated through hormonal responses to the stress of injury or illness, and a patient who is well nourished and able to mount a bigger flow response is enabled to recover more quickly (see Cuthbertson, 1980; Richards, 1980).

The remedies

Aims of dietetic management

The aims of dietetic management of the general hospital population are as follows.

1 The first is to assess and monitor the nutritional status of all patients, and where necessary, to take measures to correct nutritional inadequacy. Where feasible, the nutritional status of poorly nourished patients should be improved prior to elective surgery.

2 After injury, surgery or during illness the input of energy, protein and other nutrients should be maintained to minimise or abolish body depletion during the flow phase. Basal energy requirements can be estimated from the size of the patient. The following additional allowances can then be added to this basal figure:
   - an amount to allow for the hypermetabolism of illness and injury which will depend upon the exact nature of the condition. It might range from + 5–25% in post-operative patients, those with long bone fractures or mild to moderate infections up to as much as + 70–90% in patients with extensive burns
   - an amount to allow for the mobility of the patient ranging from + 20% in the immobile, 30% in the bed bound but mobile to 40% in those able to move around the ward
   - an increment to allow replenishment of stores if the patient is already depleted.

Protein allowances will also need to be increased in line with the extent of the calculated hypermetabolism.

Aids to meeting nutritional needs

The ideal way of satisfying the nutritional requirements of sick and injured persons is to encourage and facilitate the consumption of appetising and nutritious food and drink. In some patients, their needs cannot be met by this route and a variety of additional support measures may be used, such as:

1 *Nutritional supplements* – concentrated energy and nutrient sources that are usually consumed in liquid form and that are readily digested and absorbed.

2 *Enteral feeding* – the introduction of nutrients directly into the stomach or small intestine by use of a tube that is introduced through the nose and into the stomach or intestine via the oesophagus. Tubes introduced directly into the gut by surgical means may also be used on occasion

3 *Parenteral feeding* – the patient may be supplied with nutrients intravenously, either as a supplement to the oral route or as the sole means of nutrition, **total parenteral nutrition (TPN)**. In TPN the nutrients must be infused via an indwelling catheter into a large vein. In some cases of extreme damage to the gut, patients may be fed for years by TPN; observations of deficiency symptoms in TPN patients that respond to nutrient additions have confirmed the essentiality of some nutrients where dietary deficiency rarely occurs. A major factor that has enabled patients to be maintained indefinitely with TPN was the development of a means of safely infusing a source of fat intravenously.

Ideally these artificial feeding methods should be managed by a specialist nutrition team. TPN, in particular, requires specialist management and is usually only used where the enteral route is ruled out, e.g. in patients who have had a large part of the intestine removed or have severe inflammatory disease of the intestine. Infection of the intravenous lines can be a major problem in TPN, but with skilled specialist management it can be largely eliminated (KFC, 1992).

KFC (1992) estimated that around 2% of hospitalised patients in Britain receive some form of artificial feeding, and that in three-quarters of these cases an enteral tube is the method used. Their analysis of the workload of a nutrition team at one general hospital suggested that the number of patients receiving dietary supplements was similar to those being fed artificially.

Measures to ensure sound nutrition of hospital patients

These should include:

1 Active publicity and educational measures to increase the awareness of all nursing and medical staff about the importance of sound nutrition to prognosis and of the potentially high nutrient needs of some immobile patients. Improved training in the recognition of signs of malnutrition is also needed.

2 Provision of appetising, acceptable and nutritious food that reaches patients in good condition. Special provisions for patients with special religious or cultural dietary needs are also necessary.

3 Mandatory inclusion of a nutritional assessment in the standard admission procedure for all hospital patients. This admission assessment should include: information about appetite; recent weight changes; oral and dental health; social characteristics; physical indicators of nutritional status such as body mass index, grip strength or arm circumference (KFC, 1992). Biochemical indicators of nutritional status such as serum albumin concentration are also available and correlate well with functional tests (e.g. Chandra, 1993). Hill *et al.* (1977) in their survey of surgical patients found that only 20% of patients notes contained any reference to their nutritional status and then only a brief note such as "looks wasted". Only around 15% of the patients they surveyed had been weighed at any stage during their hospital stay.

4 Routine monitoring of patients' food consumption and regular weighing (or arm circumference measurement if weighing is not possible) to identify patients whose nutritional status deteriorates significantly after admission. Formal procedures to record absences from wards at meal-times and active measures to provide food for patients who are absent for meals and after a

period of enforced fasting should also be made.

5 Referral of patients identified as "at risk" to a specialist nutrition team with early and active corrective measures for those identified. The management of patients requiring supplementary or artificial feeding is ideally supervised by a specialist nutrition team. Such a team will probably be under the overall control of a senior clinician and will need the support of a nutrition nurse specialist, dietitian, pharmacist (because feeds are dispensed by the pharmacist) and in some cases a speech therapist to assist patients who have swallowing problems. Hill *et al.* (1977) noted that less than 5% of their sample of surgical patients had apparently received any nutritional therapy despite the very frequent indications of malnutrition that they found.

Since writing this section, a new report on the prevalence of hospital malnutrition has been published (McWhirter and Pennington, 1994). This study surveyed the nutritional status of 100 consecutive admissions to each of five areas of a major Scottish acute teaching hospital. They found that many patients (40%) were malnourished at the time of admission and that two-thirds of patients lost weight during their stay. Weight loss was greatest amongst those patients identified as most malnourished on admission. Less than half of the malnourished patients had any nutritional information documented in their notes. Very few patients were given any nutritional support but those who were, showed a substantial mean weight gain. The authors conclude that "malnutrition remains a largely unrecognised problem in hospital and highlights the need for education on clinical nutrition". This conclusion would be essentially the same as that of Bistrian *et al.* (1974) and Hill *et al.* (1977) who drew attention to this problem of hospital malnutrition almost two decades ago.

14 Some other groups and situations

Contents

Vegetarianism

Introduction

Hallas and Walker (1992) and Williams and Qureshi (1988) have reviewed the nutritional aspects of vegetarianism, and they list most of the uncited references used in this discussion.

A strict vegetarian, or **vegan**, avoids consuming any animal products, i.e. meat, fish, eggs, dairy produce and perhaps even honey. Others are less strict in their avoidances, and, although they would not eat meat, they would eat dairy produce, eggs or fish or any combination of these three. The prefixes **lacto, ovo** or **pesco** are used alone or in combination to describe these degrees of vegetarianism, e.g. one who avoids meat and fish but eats eggs and dairy produce is an ovolactovegetarian.

Traditionally, nutritionists have been concerned about the adequacy implications of vegetarian and particularly vegan diets. From an adequacy viewpoint, any major restriction of the categories from which food may be selected cannot be regarded as ideal; the greater the degree of restriction, the greater are the chances of the diet being inadequate and also of any toxicants in food being consumed in hazardous amounts. Paradoxically, most recent interest has been shown in vegetarian diets as a possible means to increasing wellness. There have been numerous reports of low incidence of certain of the diseases of industrialisation amongst vegetarian groups. Indeed, one of the major reasons cited for adopting vegetarianism in the UK has been the belief that it is a healthier option than an omnivorous diet.

Adequacy of vegetarian diets

A recurring theme of the dietary guidance offered in this book has been to encourage diversity of food choice. The avoidance of whole groups of foods runs contrary to that theme, and is therefore regarded by the author as suboptimal. On the other hand, a thoughtfully constructed vegetarian, even vegan, diet is compatible with nutritional adequacy and may well be more diverse and adequate than the current diets of many omnivores. When people decide for cultural, religious, ethical or ecological reasons to adopt some degree of vegetarianism, the role of the nutrition educator should be to facilitate the healthful implementation of that personal choice. The nutrition educator should not seek to dissuade people from adopting particular dietary choices unless they are irrevocably dysfunctional.

Animal-derived foods are the only, or the major, sources of some nutrients in typical UK and US diets. The possibility that supplies of such nutrients might be inadequate in vegan diets needs to be considered and, where necessary, remedial measures identified that are consistent with maintaining the vegan diet. The degree to which less strict vegetarians are also threatened by these potential inadequacies will depend upon the extent of individual restrictions; many vegetarians make liberal use of dairy produce and in some cases also of eggs and fish, and they are no more likely than omnivores to suffer from nutritional inadequacies.

Vegan diets theoretically contain no vitamin B_{12}, no vitamin D and no retinol; they are also likely to contain less total energy, protein, calcium and riboflavin.

Vegan and perhaps other vegetarian diets, are likely to be less energy dense than omnivorous diets because they have less fat and more starch and fibre; total energy intakes are, as a consequence, also likely to be lower than those of omnivores. Indeed, the reduced energy density of vegetarian diets is perceived as one of the major advantages of such a diet for adult populations where there is very high prevalence of overweight and obesity. There is a general consensus that Caucasian vegans have lower energy intakes than omnivores and are lighter and have a lower proportion of body fat.

A less positive view of the low energy density of vegan diets is usually taken when children are the consumers; the low energy density could impair their growth.

Studies in the US, Holland, and UK have found that vegan children tend to be lighter and smaller in stature than omnivorous children. The differences are however, generally small, and the growth patterns and growth curves of vegan children are usually within normal limits. In a sample of British vegan children, Sanders (1988) found that energy intakes were below the RDAs of that time, and that fat intakes were, on average, low but very variable (ranging from only 16% to 39% of calories). Sanders concluded that low fat intake was probably the major determinant of the low energy intakes. In turn, the low energy intakes were probably responsible for the anthropometric differences between vegan and omnivore children rather than any differences in dietary quality.

Vegan diets are likely to be lower in protein than omnivorous or lactovegetarian diets. Individual plant proteins are also generally of lower quality than individual animal proteins. Thus one of the traditional concerns of strict vegetarians has been about the protein adequacy of their diets. The priority attached to protein deficiency as a likely cause of human malnutrition has declined very sharply in recent decades (see Chapter 8). Mutual supplementation also means that the overall protein quality of a good mixed vegan diet is likely to be not substantially different from that of non-vegetarians. This means that, according to current estimates of requirements, vegan diets are likely to be adequate both in terms of their overall protein content and in their ability to supply the essential amino acids.

Vitamin D (cholecalciferol) is naturally present only in foods of animal origin. Vitamin D is added to soya milk, many infant foods, some breakfast cereals and to margarine and other spreading fats in the UK. Average intakes of vitamin D in the UK are generally well below estimated requirements, but intakes of those vegans who consume supplemented foods do not differ substantially from those of omnivores.

Endogenous production (via the action of sunlight upon the skin) rather than dietary intake is regarded as the principal source of vitamin D for most adults and children. For most vegans, even if they avoid supplemented foods, the endogenous production should therefore ensure adequacy. In some groups, current UK DRVs suggest that endogenous production cannot be relied upon, perhaps making supplements of vitamin D necessary. In such groups, the case for supplements in vegans would appear even stronger, especially if they avoid supplemented foods.

Retinol (vitamin A) is only present in animal foods, but ample supplies of carotene in fruits and vegetables will make the total vitamin A content of many vegetarian diets higher than those of typical omnivorous diets.

In strictly vegetarian diets there is no apparent vitamin B_{12}. Symptoms of megaloblastic anaemia and the neurological manifestations of vitamin B_{12} deficiency might thus be expected to be prevalent amongst vegans. However, the human requirement for vitamin B_{12} is extremely small (UK RNI – 1.5 mg/day) and stores of the vitamin in the liver are large and could amount to several years' supply in an omnivore. In the UK, meat substitutes are required to be supplemented with B_{12}, and many vegans take B_{12} supplements. Even in the absence of such alternative dietary sources, cases of clinical B_{12} deficiency amongst Caucasian vegans are rare. There are indirect sources of B_{12} even for those who consume no animal products or supplemented foods, e.g. from micro-organisms and moulds contaminating plant foods; insects or insect remains consumed with plant foods; absorption of vitamin produced endogenously by gut bacteria; from fermented foods or yeast extracts; and, most bizarrely, from faecal contamination of foods like seaweed. A combination of the large stores, extremely low requirement and incidental consumption from the sources listed mean that the practical

hazard of B_{12} deficiency is less than might be expected even for vegans who take no active measures to ensure the adequacy of their B_{12} supply. High intake of folic acid in vegans tends to mask the haematological consequences of B_{12} deficiency, and thus if a deficiency does occur, it is the neurological symptoms that are more likely to be manifested.

Dairy produce and eggs are major sources of riboflavin in UK and US diets and thus intakes of riboflavin are likely to be low in vegan, although not lactovegetarian, diets. Carlson *et al.* (1985) found average intakes of riboflavin in vegans of only 75% of the RDA of the day compared with 140% of the RDA in ovolactovegetarians. There is no evidence of overt riboflavin deficiency amongst strict vegetarians in affluent countries, although Miller (1979) identified it as one of the more prevalent of the diseases of nutritional inadequacy. Plant sources of riboflavin are leafy vegetables, nuts and pulses.

Milk and dairy produce, including soya milk, are major sources of dietary calcium; strict vegetarians who avoid these foods are likely to have lower calcium intakes than omnivores. High fibre and phytate intakes might also be expected to hinder the absorption of calcium from the gut. However, vegans apparently adapt to low calcium intakes and have reduced faecal losses of calcium. Low prevalence of osteoporosis has frequently been reported in vegetarian groups, like Seventh Day Adventists, and even in vegans. This would indicate that low calcium intakes and lack of dietary vitamin D in vegans do not predispose them to low bone density and osteoporosis, further supporting the conclusion reached in Chapter 11 that low calcium intake may, of itself, be of limited significance in the aetiology of osteoporosis.

Haem iron is the most readily absorbed form of dietary iron. Hazell and Southgate (1985) found that between 12–25% of the iron in meat and fish was absorbed compared with 2–7% from a variety of vegetable sources; rice and spinach were at the bottom of the vegetable range and soya at the top. The higher fibre and phytate content of vegetarian diets would also tend to reduce iron absorption, although high levels of vitamin C in vegetarian diets are an important promoter of iron absorption. Several groups have reported lower iron status, as measured by haematological parameters, in vegetarian groups, although there is little evidence of increased clinical symptoms of anaemia.

Vegetarian diets and nutritional guidelines

A vegetarian diet has been reported by a variety of authors using a variety of vegetarian groups as subjects to be associated with reduced incidence of obesity, reduced blood pressure, with reduced prevalence of osteoporosis, reduced incidence of coronary heart disease, and reduced incidence of certain cancers, particularly bowel cancer. It is very difficult to determine whether any of these associations are wholly or partly due to avoiding meat consumption *per se*. Caucasian vegetarians in the UK tend to be from the upper social groups, many of them adopt vegetarianism for health reasons, and thus they are likely to pay particular attention to the healthiness of their diet and their lifestyle in general. Those who are vegetarian for cultural or religious reasons, also tend to adopt other practices that are considered healthful, e.g. avoidance of alcohol and tobacco. American Seventh Day Adventists are a group frequently studied because of their propensity to vegetarianism, and it is generally agreed that they do indeed have lower rates of the diseases listed above. They also tend to avoid alcohol and tobacco, and are, perhaps, different in many other lifestyle characteristics to Americans in general.

Compared to the UK population in general, Caucasian vegetarians in the UK would tend to:

- be more health conscious
- drink less alcohol than other Britons
- make less use of tobacco
- take more exercise
- be lighter and less likely to be obese
- be more likely to come from the upper social groups
- be more likely to be female.

The diets of vegetarians, and vegans in particular tend to be lower in fat, particularly saturated fat and to be higher in complex carbohydrates than the diets of omnivores. Table 14.1 shows a comparison of the sources of dietary energy in a relatively small sample of vegans, lactovegetarians and omnivores along with the corresponding NACNE (1983) guideline values and the values obtained in 1987 from the large scale dietary survey of British adults (Gregory *et al.*, 1990). Several interesting observations can be made from this table:

1 Even the vegans in this sample fail to quite meet the 30% target for proportion of fat calories in the diet. This is despite the fact that they avoid most foods in the two food groups containing most of the "naturally occurring" fat in the diet. They also had the highest intakes of sugars, although the proportion of extracted sugars was not given; this fits in with the idea of a sugar-fat seesaw discussed in Chapter 4.
2 Lactovegetarians are somewhat closer to omnivores than to vegans in these dietary characteristics. In fact, this relatively small sample has a diet composition that appears rather close to that of that found in the recent large dietary survey of British adults (Gregory *et al.*, 1990).
3 The carbohydrate content of both vegetarian diets is higher than that of omnivores, and that of the vegan is much higher than even that of

Table 14.1 A comparison of the major sources of energy (as % of total energy) as recommended in the NACNE (1983) guidelines and as found in the average UK diet and in the diets of a sample of vegans, ovolactovegetarians and omnivores. Data sources: Carlson et al., (1985) and Gregory *et al.* (1990).

Group	Fat	Animal Fat	Carbohydrate (as sugars)	Protein	Alcohol
UK 1987 average	38.5	—	42.4 (18.4)	14.5	4.7
NACNE	30	—	55 (c10)	11.0	4.0
Vegan	32.6	nil	54.4 (20.6)	11.4	2.0
Lactoveg	38.5	15.6	45.1 (15.2)	14.1	2.8
Omnivore	41.0	21.5	38.5 (16.8)	14.0	7.0

lactovegetarians. The starch and non-starch polysaccharide intakes of vegetarians will, almost inevitably, be substantially higher than those of omnivores because they originate only from plant foods. Higher consumption of plant foods will also mean higher intakes of carotene and other antioxidant vitamins in vegetarians.

4 The vegan diet, because of the absence of animal fat will inevitably contain much less saturated fat, almost no cholesterol and will probably have a much higher P:S ratio than the diets of omnivores or even lactovegetarians.

5 The apparent low alcohol content of both the vegetarian diets supports the earlier point that lifestyle variables tend to be interrelated. Although data from a small survey should be treated with caution, vegetarians do probably drink less alcohol than omnivores; those who drink large amounts of alcohol are more likely to make use of tobacco, and those who use tobacco are likely to be less active, and so on...

To assume that any differences in mortality or morbidity patterns of vegetarians are due to the avoidance of meat or animal foods *per se* is clearly a premature assumption. Non-dietary risk factors may be very different in vegetarian and non-vegetarian groups. There are also numerous compositional differences between the diets of vegetarians and omnivores; some of these are almost inevitable, but a thoughtfully constructed omnivorous diet could match the vegan diet in most respects.

The key question is not whether vegetarians are healthier than omnivores but "how would the health records of vegetarians compare with omnivores of similar racial and social backgrounds who have similar smoking, drinking and activity patterns and who take equal care in the selection and preparation of a healthy diet?".

The point of this discussion is to suggest to those reluctantly contemplating vegetarianism on health grounds alone, that giving up meat or "red meat" may well by itself be ineffective, but that adopting some of the lifestyle and dietary practices characteristic of vegetarians will almost certainly be beneficial. This point is even more important for nutrition educators seeking to influence the behaviour of others. The discussion in the next section on the health of British Asians makes the point that vegetarianism and good health statistics are not invariably linked.

Racial minorities

Introduction and overview

Williams and Qureshi (1988) have reviewed nutritional aspects of the dietary practices of racial minorities in the UK. The reader is also referred back to Chapter 2. Several of the topics and issues discussed there are of relevance when considering the nutrition of racial minorities, for example:

- the effects of migration upon food and nutrition
- economic influences upon food choices
- cultural and religious factors that influence food selection and dietary practices.

Those seeking to give dietary or other health education advice to people from a different cultural background need first to identify the particular priorities for that group and the reasons for these priorities. This should then enable them to consider what advice is appropriate from the scientific viewpoint. However, before they attempt to translate those scientific goals into practical advice and recommendations, they need to assure themselves that they have sufficient understanding of the cultural and social influences upon the group's food selection or other behaviour. They can then ensure that their advice is compatible with the beliefs and practices of the group.

There is a general tendency for the health of racial minority groups living in industrialised countries to be inferior to that of the majority population. Indeed, one of the health promotion goals for the American nation is to "reduce the health disparity among Americans" (DHHS, 1992). If improved nutrition is credited with being a major factor in the improving health and longevity of the majority population, then one would have to assume that some of this disparity is due to nutritional improvements lagging behind in minority groups. Racial minorities tend to be economically and socially disadvantaged as compared to the majority population, and this may also be a factor in some of these ethnic disparities in health. One of the most striking inequalities in health of Americans is that between low income groups and all other groups (DHHS, 1992).

The health and nutrition of particular minority groups

The health record of American Indians is particularly poor, with two nutrition-related risk factors, alcohol abuse and obesity, clearly identified as important. Death rates from accident, homicide, suicide and cirrhosis of the liver are all much higher in Indians than in other Americans; all are associated with alcohol abuse. Rates of diabetes are also very high amongst American Indians, with more than 20% of the members of many tribes affected by the disease. The increasing rates of diabetes in American Indians have paralleled increasing rates of obesity; the proportion of overweight adults varies between a third and three-quarters depending upon the tribe. Clearly nutritional factors, including alcohol abuse, are major determinants of the poor health statistics of this minority group (DHHS, 1992).

In 1987, American blacks had a life expectancy of 69.4 years compared with 75 years for the American population as a whole, and this gap has actually widened during recent years. Mortality rates for heart disease are considerably higher for American blacks than whites. The poverty rate amongst blacks is also three times that of whites, and when heart disease rates of blacks and whites are compared within income levels, then the black rates are actually lower than those for whites. A good proportion of the poor health record of some American racial groups seems to result from their generally lower socio-economic status (DHHS, 1992).

In the UK, the two largest racial minority groups are Afro-Caribbeans and British Asians. The Afro-Caribbeans originate from the former British colonies in the West Indies, and large scale immigration of this group started in the 1950s. British Asians are a racially and culturally mixed group, and most of the immigration has occurred since 1960. They originate from the countries of Southern Asia (India, Pakistan, Bangladesh and Sri Lanka) or from the Asian communities of East Africa.

British Asians are made up of three major religious groups – Hindus, Sikhs and Muslims. Rates of vegetarianism are high. Hindus are usually lactovegetarians; they do not usually eat Western cheese. Many from the higher castes are vegans. Sikhs do not eat beef and rarely eat pork, and many are lactovegetarian. Muslims should not eat pork or consume alcohol, and any meat or animal fat should have come from animals slaughtered and prepared according to Islamic ritual.

The potential health problems of vegetarianism, discussed earlier in the chapter, would thus apply to many within this group. For example, Robertson et al. (1982) suggest that nutritional deficiencies of folic acid and vitamin B_{12} are virtually confined to the Asian population in the UK. They suggest that the practice of boiling milk with tea leaves when making tea destroys much of the B_{12} present in the milk, and strict Hindus would have no other apparent source of B_{12} in their lactovegetarian diet. They suggest that prolonged gentle heating of finely cut up foods also destroys much of the folic acid initially present in some Asian diets.

Mini epidemics of rickets and osteomalacia occurred in the 1960s and 1970s amongst Asian children and women in the UK. For example, a five-year-old Asian child living in Glasgow between 1968 and 1978 had a 3.5% chance of being admitted to hospital with rickets before the age of 16 years, whereas the equivalent risk for a white child was negligible (Robertson et al., 1982). Vitamin D deficiency has also been reported as common amongst pregnant Asian women in the UK, and this has serious implications for the health of the baby. Several factors contribute to this high prevalence of vitamin D deficiency:

1 avoidance of those few foods that contain good amounts of vitamin D, e.g. fatty fish, liver, fortified margarine and infant foods and eggs
2 a cultural tendency not to expose the skin to sunlight, perhaps coupled with pigmentation of the skin, would be expected to reduce endogenous vitamin D synthesis. This endogenous synthesis is normally regarded as the primary source of vitamin D
3 high levels of fibre and phytate in chapattis (a traditional unleavened bread), which might impair calcium absorption and perhaps also prevent enterohepatic recycling of vitamin D (Robertson et al., 1982).

The problem appears to be most prevalent amongst recent immigrants, with peaks of rickets cases associated with new waves of immigration. Robertson et al. (1982) suggest that the problem diminishes through acculturation and partial adoption of a Western diet. They concluded that the most practical way of addressing the problem was by increased awareness through health education campaigns and by the provision of vitamin D supplements to those "at risk".

The relative prominence of the different causes of mortality also varies quite considerably between different ethnic groups in the UK. The incidence of hypertension and strokes is high in the Afro-Caribbean population of the UK. It is also high amongst black Americans with stroke mortality amongst black American men almost twice that in the total male population. It is thought that Africans and Afro-Caribbeans have an ethnic predisposition to hypertension due to a hypersensitivity to salt (Law et al., 1991a).

In recent years, the high rates of coronary heart disease amongst the Asian groups in the UK has been an active research area. Age standardised mortality is 40% higher for Asians in England and Wales than for the general population; a similar trend has been reported for Asians living in other industrialised countries. McKeigue *et al.* (1985) compared the dietary and other risk factors for coronary heart disease amongst Asians and non-Asians living in London. They confirmed that rates of coronary heart disease were much higher amongst the Asians, and that the excess morbidity and mortality was common to the three major religious groups despite considerable differences in dietary and lifestyle characteristics between the three. They found that the diets and lifestyles of Asians differed from their white neighbours in the following ways:

- they had lower intakes of saturated fat and cholesterol
- they smoked fewer cigarettes.
- they drank less alcohol
- they had lower serum cholesterol concentrations
- they were much more likely to be vegetarian
- they had low rates of bowel cancer despite the tendency for bowel cancer and coronary heart disease mortality rates to parallel each other on a population basis.

McKeigue *et al.* (1991) reported high levels of insulin resistance amongst British Asians and the prevalence of diabetes was more than four times higher than in the population as a whole. They also reported very high incidence of central obesity in this Asian population (i.e. with a high waist:hip ratio). Vegetarianism amongst the Asian population does not seem to protect against overweight and obesity as it usually does for Caucasian vegetarians. McKeigue *et al.* (1991) suggested that the only known environmental influences associated with insulin resist-

ance are high caloric intake and inactivity. They therefore proposed that these Asian groups are adapted to life in environments where high levels of physical activity and frugal use of food resources have been traditionally required. When these groups migrate to countries where levels of physical activity are low and caloric intakes high, this leads to insulin resistance, central obesity and other associated metabolic disturbances, including maturity onset diabetes; this in turn predisposes them to coronary heart disease.

Nutrition and physical activity

Fitness

It is common experience, not dependent upon scientific measurement, that taking regular exercise contributes to increased levels of physical fitness. Any previously sedentary person, who undertakes a programme of regular vigorous exercise, will notice within a few weeks that he or she can perform everyday activities like garden and household chores, climbing stairs, walking uphill or running for a bus with much less breathlessness and pounding of the heart than previously. Simple personal monitoring would show a reduction in resting heart rate and smaller increases in pulse rate in response to an exercise load.

Scientific appraisal of the benefits of physical activity upon long-term health or the effects of different training schedules upon fitness requires a precise definition of fitness and an objective method of measuring it. This will enable changes in fitness levels within subjects to be monitored as they train, and the fitness levels of different individuals or populations to be compared. The scientific criterion normally used to define fitness is the **aerobic capacity** or the rate of oxygen uptake of the subject when exercising maximally – **the VO_2 max**. This VO_2 max is a measure of the functional capacity of the cardiop-ulmonary system to deliver oxygen to the body muscles and other tissues. Direct measurement of oxygen uptake in maximally exercising subjects is feasible, but it requires relatively sophisticated laboratory equipment and trained personnel. It also requires subjects to perform sustained exercise to the limit of their capacity, which is undesirable and sometimes dangerous in untrained people. For most purposes, therefore, the heart rate measured at several submaximal exercise levels is used to derive a measure of aerobic capacity. In one widely used test, subjects cycle on a static bicycle ergometer at defined work loads. The external work performed by the subject is calculated from the speed of cycling and the resistance applied to the bicycle fly-wheel. In the steady state, work load is assumed to equate with oxygen uptake. Three graded levels of work are performed, and the steady state heart rate is measured at each. The calculated work rate is then plotted against the heart rate on a graph, and the best straight line drawn through the three points (see Figure 14.1). By extending this straight line, the graph can be used either:

- to predict the work rate at the predicted maximum heart rate (220 minus age in years) for the subject, **the maximum physical work capacity, PWC_{max}**
- to predict the work rate at a defined heart rate, e.g. the physical work capacity at 170 beats per minute, the **PWC_{170}**.

Figure 14.1 An idealised plot of work load against heart rate. The straight line drawn through the three measured points can be extrapolated to predict the work load at 170 beats per minuute (the PWC_{170}) or the work load at the estimated maximum heart rate (the maximum physical work capacity, PWC_{max}). These are both used as indices of aerobic fitness

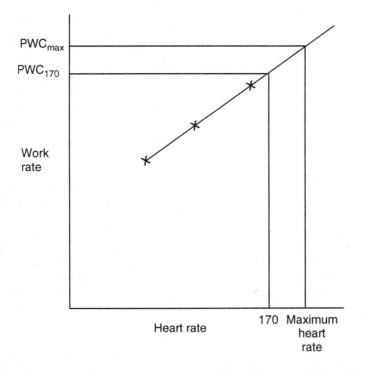

Maximum heart rate = 220 – age in years.

The rate of 170 beats per minute is approximately 85% of the maximum heart rate in young adults, and using this value involves less extrapolation than predicting to maximum heart rate; in older subjects a lower defined heart rate would be used. Similar tests are available that involve walking or running on a treadmill rather than the use of a static bicycle.

Conditioning of the cardiopulmonary system to produce measurable improvements in aerobic capacity requires that the system be significantly exerted for sustained periods. In Healthy People 2000 (DHHS, 1992) it has been assumed that, in order for exercise to increase or maintain aerobic fitness, it must comprise three sessions each week in which heart rate is raised to at least 60% of maximum for at least 20 minutes duration. Sometimes a figure of 70% of maximum heart rate is used.

Regular exercise not only produces measurable increases in aerobic capacity, but also produces other rapid and readily demonstrable benefits in the short term, such as:

1 training increases muscle **strength**
2 training increases **endurance**, i.e. the maximum duration that one is able to sustain a particular activity; both the endurance of individual trained muscle groups and the endurance of the cardiopulmonary system are increased
3 training improves or maintains joint mobility or **flexibility**, i.e. the range of movements that subjects are able to safely and comfortably perform is increased.

These latter benefits accrue at intensities and durations of activity that are considerably below those necessary to produce measurable changes in aerobic capacity. These latter effects of increased strength, endurance and flexibility may be of even greater importance to some subjects than increases in aerobic fitness, e.g. elderly or physically disabled people. There is also a substantial body of evidence suggesting that participation in regular physical activity produces psychological as well as physiological benefits. It improves the general sense of well being and self-confidence, improves the ability to cope with stress and may even reduce the frequency and severity of personality disorders (see Hayden and Allen, 1984). Some of these psychological benefits may be a consequence of the physiological conditioning.

Current levels of physical activity and fitness

The average levels of physical activity of the populations of the wealthy industrialised countries have, by general agreement, declined in recent decades. Car ownership, workplace automation and labour saving aids in the home and garden have drastically reduced the amount of obligatory physical exertion that most people now undertake. Increased voluntary leisure-time activities have not been enough to offset this reduction in obligatory activity. The increased levels of overweight and obesity in the UK and US despite a sharp decline in average energy intakes in recent decades provides compelling evidence of the scale of this reduction in activity (discussed in Chapter 6). Increased levels of overweight in the adult population indicate that energy expenditure (i.e. activity) has been declining faster than caloric intake.

There are estimates of current activity levels of the American population in "Healthy People 2000" (DHHS, 1992), for example it was assumed that in 1985:

1 12% of American over-18s and 66% of 10–17-year-olds engaged in vigorous exercise of sufficient frequency, intensity and duration to promote the development of aerobic fitness. In those over 18s with low incomes this assumed rate was only 7%.
2 22% of over-18s were assumed to engage in light to moderate physical activity (i.e. reaching less than 60% of

maximum heart rate) for at least 30 minutes on at least five occasions each week.

3 24% of over-18s were assumed to engage in no leisure-time physical activity, with figures of 32% for low income people and 43% for the over-65s.

Table 14.2 gives a summary of activity levels determined by interview in a recent health survey of English adults (White *et al.*, 1993). More than half of men and women reported engaging in less than three periods of even moderate level of activity each week. Around 20% had reported engaging in no periods of moderate or vigorous activity in a four-week period. Activity levels of women were on average less than those of men, and there is a marked tendency in both sexes for activity level to decline with age. More than a third of 65–74-year-olds had no period of even moderate activity in a four-week period. Other findings of this survey were:

- Subjects with higher educational qualifications were more likely to be at the highest activity levels (4 and 5).
- Heavy smokers were, as might be expected, less likely to reach the highest activity levels.
- Perhaps more unexpectedly, non drinkers and occasional drinkers were also less likely to reach activity levels 4 and 5.

Also in the UK, the recent Allied Dunbar National Fitness Survey (1992) of a

Table 14.2 Distribution of reported activity levels of a representative sample of English adults. All values are percentages. Data source: White *et al.* (1993)

Activity level		Age group (years)				
		16–34	35–44	45–64	65–74	All
4 and 5	(men)	37	24	9	2	20
	(women)	22	11	8	1	12
3	(men)	23	29	38	31	29
	(women)	28	34	42	21	30
1 and 2	(men)	31	33	33	36	32
	(women)	39	48	34	35	37
0	(men)	8	15	20	31	19
	(women)	10	8	16	43	21

Activity levels:

 4 and 5 – Twelve or more occasions in 4 weeks of vigorous or mixed vigorous/moderate activity;
   3 – Twelve or more occasions of moderate activity in 4 weeks;
 1 and 2 – One to eleven occasions of at least moderate activity in 4 weeks;
   0 – No occasions of moderate or vigorous activity in 4 weeks.

Moderate activity means requiring an energy expenditure of 5+ kcal/min and vigorous activity 7.5+ kcal/min.

Moderate activities: walking a mile at brisk or fast pace; heavy gardening work such as digging or cutting large areas of grass by hand; heavy DIY work such as knocking down walls or breaking up concrete; heavy housework such as walking with heavy loads of shopping or scrubbing/polishing floors by hand.

Vigorous activities: running or jogging; playing squash; several other sporting activities if they caused the subject to breathe heavily or sweat a lot such as aerobics, tennis, weight training or swimming.

representative sample of 4000 adults found very low levels of reported physical activity and low levels of aerobic fitness (short summary by Groom, 1993). This survey report suggested that 70% of men and 80% of women had lower levels of physical activity than would be necessary to achieve aerobic fitness. For around one-third of men and two-thirds of the women, walking at 3 mph up a gradient of 1:20 would be difficult with even higher proportions in the over-65s. A large number of women over 35 years would find even walking at 3 mph on the flat severely exerting and would need to rest or slow down after a few minutes.

Most surveys of physical activity levels in populations use a subjective measure such as an activity questionnaire or diary to assess activity levels. One survey of activity levels of English children (11–16 years) used continuous heart rate monitoring to obtain a more objective measure of activity levels. Armstrong *et al.* (1990) recorded the number of sustained periods in which the heart rate was above 70% of maximum, i.e. over 139 beats per minute. During a period of three weekdays, 5% of boys and 14% of girls recorded no periods when heart rate was above this level for five minutes; around 75% of boys and nearly 90% of girls had no continuous 20-minute periods at or above this rate. Only 4% of boys and 0.6% of girls had three or more 20-minute periods at this rate which the authors took as the appropriate frequency, duration and intensity of activity to maintain aerobic fitness in children of this age group. Levels of inactivity at the week-end were found to be even higher than on weekdays; on Saturdays, 47% of boys and 64% of girls recorded no continuous period of five minutes when the heart rate was above 139 beats per minute. These figures contrast very sharply indeed with the proportions of American children assumed to be taking enough exercise to maintain aerobic fitness in DHHS (1992). There is no indication in this paper of Armstrong *et al.* of how the results would be affected by setting a slightly lower threshold, say the 60% of maximum heart rate (120 beats per minute) used in DHHS (1992).

"Healthy People 2000" also sets a series of very specific targets for increases in the physical activity levels of different sections of the American population for the year 2000, for example:

1 20% of over 18s and 75% of 6–17-year-olds should engage in vigorous physical activity that promotes aerobic fitness, i.e. three or more 20 minutes each week of activity intense enough to raise the heart rate to 60% of maximum

2 at least 30% of those aged six and over should engage in light to moderate physical activity for at least 30 minutes each day (i.e. activities that do not raise heart rate to 60% of maximum, like walking)

3 no more than 15% of people aged over six years, 22% of over-65s and 17% of low-income people should fail to engage in any leisure-time physical activity.

In "The Health of the Nation" (DH, 1992a), the stated intention of the British government is "to develop detailed strategies to increase physical activity" in the light of the activity and fitness levels found in the Allied Dunbar National Fitness Survey (1992).

In "Health People 2000" it is seen as particularly important to encourage children to participate in physical activities that can be carried through into adulthood. Participation in team sports and group games is rarely carried through into adulthood, whereas some other activities are much more likely to be continued, e.g. swimming, cycling, jogging, walking, dancing and games requiring only one or two participants. Increased provision of facilities for participating in such activities is also seen as a necessary component of this encouragement.

Long term health benefits of physical activity

Introduction

In the short-term, increased physical activity improves aerobic capacity, endurance, strength, flexibility and various aspects of psychological well-being. Over a period of weeks or months it also leads to changes in appearance and body composition; increased lean to fat ratio and improved muscle tone. It is inevitable that low levels of physical activity will lead to reduced caloric requirements, and it seems safe to assume that this low-caloric requirement will predispose to overweight and obesity in countries where there is a plentiful supply of energy-dense food. In the longer term, regular exercise contributes to reduced morbidity and mortality from several of the diseases of industrialisation, and therefore increases both life expectancy and years of healthy life.

Activity and body weight control

For those seeking to use exercise as an aid to weight control, then regular, sustained, moderate (aerobic) activity would appear to offer the best possibility of significant weight loss. Inactivity undoubtedly predisposes to overweight and obesity, but regular physical activity is likely to be more effective as a preventative measure rather than as a relatively short-term measure to cure established obesity. An exercise programme is nonetheless an important adjunct to dietary management of overweight or obesity for a number of reasons, such as:

1 it maintains energy expenditure which tends to decline in dieting as in starvation
2 exercise maintains lean body (muscle) mass which tends to fall with weight loss; this is one factor contributing to the fall in energy expenditure during weight reduction
3 exercise increases muscle tone and so "improves" physical appearance as weight is lost

4 as people become fitter and experience the other benefits of exercise, this may encourage them to maintain activity levels after target weight has been reached and help to maintain the weight loss. This maintenance of weight loss is often even more difficult than reaching target weight.

Activity and osteoporosis

Exercise increases and maintains bone density and therefore protects against osteoporosis. For example, Pocock *et al.* (1986) found physical fitness to be a major determinant of bone density in two regions frequently associated with osteoporotic fracture, the neck of the femur and the lumbar spine. Note, however, that extremes of physical exercise in women that are accompanied by very low body weight and amenorrhea almost certainly accelerate bone loss and predispose to osteoporosis (activity in relation to osteoporosis risk is discussed in Chapter 11).

Activity and coronary heart disease/total mortality

Regular physical activity is protective against cardiovascular disease. This may be a direct effect, e.g. by strengthening heart muscles or an indirect consequence of its effects on other risk factors. Physical activity reduces the tendency to overweight, insulin resistance and maturity onset diabetes, it lowers blood pressure, it has beneficial effects on blood lipid profiles (e.g. Blair *et al.*, 1989). In an 8.5-year cohort study of 18 000 middle aged, male, British civil servants, Morris *et al.* (1980) found that those who participated in vigorous leisure-time activity had lower rates of both fatal and non-fatal coronary heart disease than those who did not. This apparent protective effect of exercise was maintained in all age groups and in subgroups classified according to smoking behaviour, family history of coronary heart disease and even in those with existing hypertension and subclinical angina. They concluded that vigorous exercise has "a protective effect in the ageing heart against ischaemia and its consequences".

Several studies have looked at the comparative mortality of different occupational groups with differing levels of work-related activity (reviewed by Leon, 1985). Farmers and farm labourers have been the subject of several such studies because of the perception that their work required considerable activity. Studies in California, North Dakota, Georgia and Iowa have all found lower levels of heart disease amongst farm workers than other inhabitants of these regions (Pomrehn *et al.*, 1982). Less smoking and higher levels of activity were identified as differences between farmers and non-farmers in these studies. Pomrehn *et al.* (1982) analysed all death certificates in the state of Iowa over the period 1964–1978 for men aged 20–64 years. They compared deaths rates of farmers and non-farmers in Iowa over that period. They found that farmers had lower all cause mortality and mortality from heart disease than non-farmers. They also compared the lifestyle and dietary characteristics of a sample of farmers and non-farmers living in Iowa in 1973. They found that the farmers were significantly less likely to smoke (19% v 46% of non-farmers), were more active, were fitter and drank less alcohol. The farmers in their sample also had significantly *higher* total serum cholesterol levels. They concluded that the reduced total and heart disease mortality of farmers could be attributed to a lifestyle that included regular physical activity and much less use of alcohol and tobacco than non-farmers.

In a 16-year cohort study of 17 000 Harvard graduates, ranging in age from 35–74 years, Paffenberger *et al.* (1986) found that reported exercise level was strongly and inversely related to total mortality. They used reported levels of walking, stair climbing and sports play to calculate a relative activity index. The relative risk of death of those with an index of around 3500 kcal per week was around half that of those with an index of less than 500 kcal per week. They found that mortality rates amongst the physically active were lower with or without consideration of other confounding factors, such as: hypertension; cigarette smoking; body weight or weight gain since leaving college; or, early parental death.

In an eight-year cohort study of over 13 000 men and women, Blair *et al.* (1989) found a strong inverse correlation in both sexes between measured fitness level and relative risk of death from all causes. The apparent protective effect of fitness was not affected by correcting for likely confounding variables.

Diet as a means to improving physical performance

An adequate dietary supply of caloric substrates and of micronutrients to enable those substrates to be utilised efficiently are clearly prerequisites for maximum athletic performance. There is no convincing evidence, however, that any particular micronutrient supplement boosts performance in already well-nourished individuals. In recent years, much detailed research has been conducted into dietary means to optimise athletic performance – detailed consideration of this topic is beyond the scope of this book, it has been reviewed by Eastwood and Eastwood (1985); Flynn and Connolly (1989): and, Elliot and Goldberg (1985).

A nutrient-dense diet rich in complex carbohydrate and with a moderate fat content should be suitable for those engaging in sport for leisure or truly amateur competition. Only for those competing at the highest levels, or those participating in endurance events like marathon running is a special diet likely to be considered.

Two important factors do need to be considered by those participating in endurance events like marathons: maintaining adequate body fluid levels during competition and boosting glycogen stores prior to the event.

A marathon runner competing in a warm environment may expect to lose up to six litres of sweat during the run and, even in a more temperate climate, sweat losses will often be in the range three to four litres. Prolonged exercise, particularly in a hot environment, can lead to dehydration, which produces fatigue and reduces work capacity. Profuse sweating and an inability to dissipate excess body heat in a warm, humid environment may lead to a combination of dehydration and hyperthermia, or **heat stroke,** which can have serious, even fatal, consequences. Ideally marathon runners should drink a pint of fluid 15–30 minutes before competition and then take small, regular drinks (say every three miles) although competitive rules may prevent drink stops in the early part of the race.

In sustained physical activity, like marathon running, depletion of muscle glycogen is a factor that potentially limits endurance. One would expect glycogen stores in liver and muscle to be depleted after one-and-a-half to two hours of vigorous exercise, and depletion of muscle glycogen leads to fatigue – the so called **"wall"** that affects marathon runners. Training for endurance events increases muscle glycogen stores. Training also increases the aerobic capacity of muscles enabling them to use fatty acids more effectively. As the duration of exercise increases, so the contribution made by fatty acids to the total energy supply of the muscle increases, although the use of fatty acids as substrates cannot completely stave off fatigue due to carbohydrate depletion. Diets high in carbohydrates (70% of energy) during endurance training also leads to modest increases in endurance.

Many endurance athletes manipulate their diets and exercise schedules prior to competition in an attempt to increase their body glycogen stores – **carbohydrate loading**. There are several theories as to the best way to increase muscle glycogen stores – one regime that is not associated with any obvious side-effects is for the athlete to eat a normal high carbohydrate diet during heavy training up to a week before the event. Then in the week before competition, a very high carbohydrate diet is taken and training intensity wound down with a complete rest on the day before the competition. A high carbohydrate diet should be continued during the week following competition to replenish carbohydrate stores; carbohydrate taken in the first hour or two following the completion of the event seems most effective in replenishing muscle glycogen stores.

PART IV
THE SAFETY AND
QUALITY OF FOOD

15 The safety and quality of food

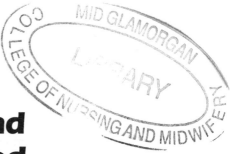

Contents

Scope of the chapter

In this chapter some of the factors that influence the safety and quality of food in an urban industrial society are overviewed, including a short review of the general aims of food safety legislation. The rationale is given for some practical steps that should help the individual consumer to increase the microbiological safety of his or her own food. The theoretical basis of a number of important processing methods is discussed, and their effects on the safety and nutritional value of foods is overviewed. There is a summary of the origins of potentially toxic substances in food and some of the circumstances under which they may represent a real hazard to consumers. The uses and safety of food additives are singled out for particular discussion.

Consumer protection

Food safety legislation

Food safety legislation has traditionally had three major aims:

1 to protect the health of consumers. To ensure that food offered for human consumption is safe and fit for people to eat

2 to prevent the consumer from being cheated. To ensure that verbal descriptions, labels and advertisements for food describe it honestly. When a consumer asks for a particular commodity, he or she should not be dishonestly given some inferior substitute or variant passed off as the requested product

3 to ensure fair competition between traders. Unscrupulous traders should be prevented from gaining a competitive

advantage by dishonestly passing off inferior and cheaper products as more expensive ones or by making dishonest claims about the merits of their product.

A further aim could be added for some current legislation governing the labelling of foods:

4 to provide consumers with enough information on the nutritional content of food to enable them to make informed food choices, and thus to facilitate their adherence to nutrition education guidelines.

In the UK, the first comprehensive food legislation was passed in the middle of the last century, and there have been regular revisions and additions to this legislation ever since. The 1990 Food Safety Act is the latest version. The first food legislation was introduced in an attempt to combat widespread adulteration and misrepresentation of foods designed to cheat the consumer and also to prevent incidences that on occasion resulted in a product that was directly injurious to health. The sweetening of cider with sugar of lead (lead acetate) and addition of red lead to cayenne pepper are examples of practices with serious health repercussions for the consumer. The watering of milk (often with dirty water), addition of alum and bone ash to flour, dilution of pepper with brick dust and the bulking out of tea with floor sweepings are all examples of practices designed to cheat the consumer. The sale of meat from diseased animals slaughtered in knackers' yards, and the passing off of horse flesh as beef also occurred.

Below are some of the main provisions of the UK 1990 Food Safety Act that illustrate a formal legal framework designed to achieve the aims listed above:

1 It is illegal to add anything to food, take any constituent away, subject it to any treatment or process, or use any ingredient that would render the food injurious to health.

2 It is forbidden to sell food not complying with food safety regulations. It fails to comply with food safety regulations if it has been rendered injurious to health by any of the above, if it is unfit for human consumption (e.g. meat from animals slaughtered in a knacker's yard) or if it is so contaminated that it would not be reasonable to expect it to be used for human consumption.

3 It is illegal to sell any food not of the nature, substance or quality demanded by the purchaser, i.e. customers must be given what they ask for.

4 It is an offence to describe, label or advertise a food in a way that is calculated to mislead as to its nature, substance or quality.

Enforcement of this legislation is, in the UK, primarily the responsibility of Trading Standards officers employed by local authorities. A summary of UK food safety legislation may be found in Ryder (1991) or Jacob (1993) and of US legislation in Thompson *et al.* (1991).

Food labelling

Labelling in the UK

Most packaged foods in Britain must contain the following information on the label: the name of the food; a list of ingredients; an indication of its minimum durability; an indication of any special storage conditions or conditions of use that are required (e.g. refrigerate, eat within three days of opening, etc.); and, the name and address of the manufacturer or packer of the food.

If a food is perishable and likely to become microbiologically unsafe after a relatively short storage period, then it carries a **"use by"** date and it is illegal to offer for sale any food that is past its use by date. Such foods usually need to be stored in a refrigerator or chill cabinet, and these foods should not be eaten after their use by date, e.g. cooked meats, ready meals, sandwiches, meat pies, etc. Other foods that are unlikely to become hazardous on storage are labelled with a **"best before"** date; although they are unlikely to represent a hazard after that date, their eating quality may be impaired, e.g. biscuits (cookies), cakes, bread, chocolate. Foods may be legally offered for sale after their best before date provided they have not become unfit for human consumption.

In Britain and the EC, the ingredients of packaged foods must be listed in order of their prominence, by weight, in the final product. All additives must be listed and their function given. Certain foods are exempted from the requirement to carry a list of ingredients such as fresh fruit and vegetables, cheese, butter, alcoholic drinks and any food composed of a single ingredient.

In Britain, the great majority of packaged foods also carry nutritional information on the labels. Most manufacturers voluntarily choose to include some nutritional information on their labels, but from October 1993, such nutrition labelling became compulsory if the manufacturer makes any nutritional claim for the product, e.g. low fat or high fibre. The minimum nutritional information the food must then carry is the energy, protein, carbohydrate and fat content per 100 g together with the amount of any nutrient for which a claim is made.

Labels in the US

American food labelling regulations have just undergone a major revision in the Nutrition Labelling and Education Act of 1990 (NLEA). Many food "activists" would regard this very formal and detailed set of regulations, amounting to 4000 pages, as an ideal model for other countries to follow. This short review is offered to non-US readers as an illustration of the complexity involved when statutory regulation of full nutritional labelling of food is attempted.

The stated aims of the new US legislation are to produce a simple, understandable label that clears up confusion and helps consumers to make healthy choices and also:

> to encourage product innovation, so that companies are more interested in tinkering with the food in the package, not the word on the label.
>
> D.A. Kessler, FDA Commissioner, 1991.

This latter objective would not, as it is stated, be regarded as wholly positive by all consumers or nutritionists; one of the original purposes of food legislation was to stop producers "tinkering with the food in the package". Even the following brief summary of these new regulations illustrates the complexity of trying to frame food labelling rules that cover every eventuality and ensure that all labels contain all the useful information, in a clear, comprehensible and truly informative form, free from misleading information and claims. In 1992, it was suggested in the influential journal, *Nature* (vol. 360, p. 499), that the resulting labels were "all but incomprehensible" and "leaving the consumer in need of a mainframe computer to translate it all into practical terms".

Listed below are a sample of the important changes introduced in NLEA (source FDA, 1992):

1 *Range of foods* – Nutrition labelling is now mandatory on almost all packaged foods. Foodstores are also being asked to display nutrition information on the most frequently consumed raw fruits, vegetables, fish, meat and poultry backed up by the threat of future legislation if there is non-compliance

2 *List of ingredients* – A full list of ingredients is now required on all packaged foods, even those made according to the standard recipes set by the FDA such as mayonnaise, macaroni and bread. The ingredients must be listed in descending order of weight in food and a number of additional specific requirements are listed, e.g. all colours

must be listed by name, caseinate (used in non-dairy coffee whitener) must be identified as being from milk, and the source of any protein hydrolysate must be indicated (e.g. hydrolysed milk protein). One purpose of these specific rules is to assist people with food allergies

3 *Serving sizes* – These have to be stated, and for many products the serving size is laid down so as to properly reflect what an adult actually eats, e.g. the statutory serving size for a soft drink is eight ounces. There are detailed regulations about what happens if packages contain less than two statutory servings, e.g. if the carton also contains less than 200 g/200 ml, then the whole package should be treated as one serving. This measure has been introduced to prevent producers misleading consumers as to, for example, the fat, sugar or calorie content of their product by using unrealistically small portion sizes.

4 *Nutritional information* – The label must contain the amounts of the following per serving: calories; calories from fat; total fat; saturated fat; cholesterol; sodium; total carbohydrate; dietary fibre; sugars; protein; vitamins A and C; calcium; and, iron. Other nutritional information that can be voluntarily listed (e.g. B vitamins) is also specified. The label must not only give the amount of the nutrient in absolute terms but must also put it into the context of an average ideal diet, e.g. if a serving contains 13 g of fat this is equivalent to 20% of the total fat in the ideal 2000 kcal diet. Not only the content of the label but also its format are laid down. A nutrition information panel from a sample label is shown in Figure 15.1.

5 *Descriptive terms* – Ten of the descriptive terms that are frequently used on food labels are formally defined, and the food must comply with this statutory definition, e.g. "free" as in say "fat free" or "sugar free", "low" as in "low calorie" or "low sodium", and "less" as in

"less fat". It is even suggested that there will be a formal definition of "healthy" as applied to food!

Low-fat versions of products like butter, sour cream and cheese need no longer be called imitation or substitute, but may be called simply low fat, provided they comply with certain specified criteria. This is aimed at improving the image of low-fat foods.

6 *Health claims* – Seven relationships between nutrients and disease are regarded as well enough established to be allowed to be used in health claims on food labels, they are:
- calcium and osteoporosis
- sodium and hypertension
- saturated fat and cholesterol and coronary heart disease
- fat and cancer
- fibre containing foods and cancer
- fruits and vegetables and cancer
- fibre containing foods and coronary heart disease.

Other claims are not yet permitted, and only foods that meet the compositional criteria specified for each claim can carry the claim.

The US Food and Drug Administration (FDA) estimate the cost of these labelling changes at $1.4–2.3 billion (£1–1.5 billion) over 20 years. They assume that these costs will be more than compensated for by the improvements in the diet that they facilitate and the resultant reduction in health care costs!

The microbiological safety of food

Introduction

There cannot be many readers of this book who have not experienced several bouts of microbial food poisoning. There seems to be a general acceptance that the incidence of microbial food poisoning has risen sharply in recent decades in many industrialised countries. For example, the number of officially recorded cases of food poisoning in England and Wales rose throughout the 1980s from about 15 000 in 1982 to more than 50 000 now. Such apparently large and rapid increases in the recorded incidence of foodborne diseases does not, however, necessarily mean that our food is becoming less safe. For example, in the 1940s, prior to the introduction of general pasteurisation of milk, 1500 people died in the UK each year from bovine tuberculosis contracted from drinking contaminated milk; this disease has now been all but eradicated in the UK.

The number of recorded cases of food poisoning will, almost inevitably, only represent the "tip of the iceberg"; only a

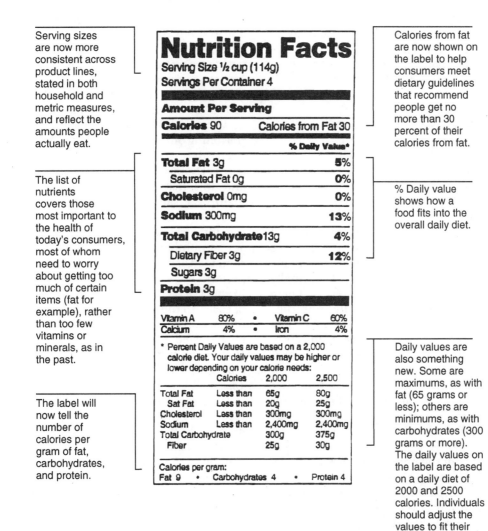

Serving sizes are now more consistent across product lines, stated in both household and metric measures, and reflect the amounts people actually eat.

The list of nutrients covers those most important to the health of today's consumers, most of whom need to worry about getting too much of certain items (fat for example), rather than too few vitamins or minerals, as in the past.

The label will now tell the number of calories per gram of fat, carbohydrates, and protein.

Calories from fat are now shown on the label to help consumers meet dietary guidelines that recommend people get no more than 30 percent of their calories from fat.

% Daily value shows how a food fits into the overall daily diet.

Daily values are also something new. Some are maximums, as with fat (65 grams or less); others are minimums, as with carbohydrates (300 grams or more). The daily values on the label are based on a daily diet of 2000 and 2500 calories. Individuals should adjust the values to fit their own calorie intake.

Nutrition Facts

Serving Size ½ cup (114g)
Servings Per Container 4

Amount Per Serving

Calories 90   Calories from Fat 30

% Daily Value*

Total Fat 3g	**5%**
Saturated Fat 0g	**0%**
Cholesterol 0mg	**0%**
Sodium 300mg	**13%**
Total Carbohydrate 13g	**4%**
Dietary Fiber 3g	**12%**
Sugars 3g	
Protein 3g	

Vitamin A	80%	•	Vitamin C	60%
Calcium	4%	•	Iron	4%

* Percent Daily Values are based on a 2,000 calorie diet. Your daily values may be higher or lower depending on your calorie needs:

		Calories	2,000	2,500
Total Fat	Less than		65g	80g
Sat Fat	Less than		20g	25g
Cholesterol	Less than		300mg	300mg
Sodium	Less than		2,400mg	2,400mg
Total Carbohydrate			300g	375g
Fiber			25g	30g

Calories per gram:
Fat 9 • Carbohydrates 4 • Protein 4

Source: Food and Drug Administration 1992

Figure 15.1 *A typical nutrition information section from a new American food label*

minority of sufferers will even consult a physician. Any attempt to estimate real numbers of cases is going to involve a considerable element of guesswork; reported cases have been variously estimated at representing between 1% and 10% of all cases. As recorded cases represent such a small and indeterminate fraction of all cases, then caution needs to be exercised when interpreting these figures. For example, small changes in the proportion of cases that are recorded may falsely indicate changes in overall incidence; a more serious and long-lasting illness is more likely to be recorded and so may erroneously appear to be more frequent than a shorter or milder one.

The causes of foodborne diseases

The causative organisms

Textbooks of food microbiology usually list more than ten organisms or groups of organisms as significant causative agents for **food poisoning**. In classical food poisoning, large numbers of organisms actively growing in the food are generally required to cause illness which normally presents as acute gastro-enteritis. There are a number of other **foodborne diseases**, e.g. typhoid and cholera which usually require relatively few organisms to cause illness, and in these cases there is usually no need for the organism to grow in food as there is in food poisoning.

The relative importance of the various organisms in causing food poisoning varies in different countries and communities and depends upon the diet and food practices of the population. For example, food poisoning caused by the organism *Vibrio (V.) parahaemolyticus* is associated with consumption of undercooked fish. In Japan, where consumption of raw fish (sushi) is widespread, food poisoning due to this organism is the most common cause of food poisoning. It is, however, a relatively uncommon causative agent in

the UK and US where sushi bars and Japanese restaurants are frequently the source of infection. The cool climate is another factor reducing the incidence of disease due to this organism in the UK and northern parts of the USA.

Roberts (1982) analysed over 1000 outbreaks of food poisoning that occurred in England and Wales, and she found that four organisms or groups of organisms accounted for almost all of these outbreaks; *Salmonellae, Clostridium (C.) perfringens, Staphylococcus (S.) aureus* and *Bacillus (B.) cereus*. Similar analyses of US outbreaks had also identified the first three on this list as the most common causative agents (Bryan, 1978). More recent figures in Hobbs and Roberts (1993) show that Salmonella infections now account for around 95% of all food poisoning outbreaks in the UK. There has been a dramatic increase in the number of cases of Salmonella infections since 1985, and this has reduced the other three major causative organisms listed by Roberts (1982) to a very small fraction of the total cases. For example, although actual numbers of cases of *C. perfringens* remained at a fairly constant level over the period 1985–1991, they nonetheless fell from 11% of all cases to only around 4% of cases. In the late 1970s and early 1980s this organism represented up to a third of all reported cases of food poisoning in some years in the UK. In 1991, *B. cereus* and *S. aureus* each represented less than 1% of all UK food poisoning cases.

Campylobacter jejuni was only recognised as a general cause of food poisoning in the late 1970s when techniques for the isolation and identification of the organism became available; it is difficult to grow on standard laboratory media. The *Campylobacter* are now the organisms most frequently causing acute bacterial gastro-enteritis in the UK (Cooke, 1991). The organism does not grow in food, requires only a few organisms to cause illness and can be spread from person to person, and thus it should probably not be classified as a food poisoning organism but with the other group of foodborne diseases like typhoid and cholera. *Campylobacter* infections are not included in official food poisoning statistics in the UK but are listed separately.

Listeriosis was not mentioned in the earlier report of Roberts (1982); neither is it mentioned in textbooks of food microbiology published well into the 1980s. It has, however, been a cause of great public concern in the UK and US in recent years, with the demonstration of the causative agent (*Listeria monocytogenes*) in many supermarket chilled foods. It has been of particular concern because it may cause miscarriage, birth defects and death of newborn infants if pregnant women are infected.

How bacteria make us ill

Food poisoning organisms produce their ill-effects in one of three ways:

1 Some organims cause illness by colonising the gut when they are ingested, e.g. the *Salmonellae, Escherichia (E.) coli*, the *Campylobacter* and *V. parahaemolyticus*.
2 Some organisms produce a toxin when they grow in the food, and it is the ingestion of this toxin that is responsible for the illness associated with the organism, e.g. *S. aureus, B. cereus* and *Clostridium (C.) botulinum*.
3 *C. perfringens* infects the gut and produces a toxin when it sporulates within the gut, and that toxin evokes the food poisoning symptoms.

Some cases of gastro-enteritis cannot be attributed to bacteria or bacterial toxins, and many are thought to be caused by viruses which may be, in some cases, foodborne.

Circumstances that lead to foodborne illness

In order for foodborne disease to occur then the food must have been contaminated with the causative organism at some stage prior to ingestion. There are many possible means by which the food can be contaminated with microorganisms, such as:

- the organism may be widespread in the environment, e.g. in the soil, water, dust or air
- the organism may be present in the animal carcass at slaughter
- eggs and meat may become contaminated with animal faeces
- fish and shellfish may become contaminated by sewage in sea water – particularly important in filter feeding molluscs like mussels
- fruits and vegetables may become contaminated by being washed or watered with dirty water
- any food may be contaminated by the food handler.
- insects, like flies, may be a source of contamination
- food may be cross-contaminated from contact with another food – particularly important if cooked food that is to undergo no further heat treatment is contaminated by raw meat or poultry.

With some bacteria (e.g. those causing foodborne diseases like *Shigella* dysentery, typhoid, paratyphoid and cholera), illness can result from the consumption of small numbers of organisms (say 10–10 000) and thus contamination of any food with these organisms may in itself be sufficient to cause illness. Such organism are said to have a low **infective dose,** and in these cases infection may well result from drinking contaminated water or in some cases spread from person to person.

Foreign travel and gastro-enteritis, **travellers diarrhoea,** seems to be very frequently associated. Some of these cases may be due to the food poisoning organisms listed earlier, but a high proportion are probably due to strains of *E. coli* to which the traveller has not acquired any immunity. Faecal contamination of drinking water, bathing water or perhaps contamination of water used to irrigate fruits or vegetables are the likely source of the organisms. The lack of immunity means that foreigners may have a much lower infective dose than the indigenous population, and so foreigners become ill but the local population is untouched. Low infective doses from water, ice in drinks, or raw fruit and salad vegetables washed in contaminated water may trigger the infection. Those on short visits to foreign countries, especially where the water supply may be suspect, would be well-advised to consume only drinks made with boiled or purified water, to avoid ice in drinks, to peel, or wash in purified water, any fruits or vegetables that are to be eaten raw. The *Campylobacter* may also be a cause of traveller's diarrhoea.

The common food poisoning organisms need to be ingested in higher numbers (often in excess of 100 000) to cause illness in a healthy adult. These organisms have a high infective dose, and they do not usually cause illness as a result of the consumption of contaminated water because of dilution and because water does not have the nutrients to support bacterial proliferation. Similarly, with those organisms that cause illness by producing a toxin in the food, a large bacterial population usually needs to have accumulated before sufficient toxin is produced to cause illness. For food poisoning to occur in healthy adults then, not only must food be contaminated with the causative organism, but usually the following conditions also need to be met:

1 the food must support growth of the bacteria (and allow production of toxin if relevant)
2 the food must at some stage have been stored under conditions that permit the bacteria to grow (and produce toxin).

Note that even within a group of healthy young adults there will be variation in the susceptibility to any particular infective organism. Infective doses are likely to be at least an order of magnitude smaller and perhaps less in highly vulnerable groups.

Babies are vulnerable because their immune systems are not fully developed; and immunocompetence also declines in the elderly. Others who are at increased risk of food poisoning are those whose immunocompetence has been compromised by illness, starvation, immunosuppressive drugs or radiotherapy. Not only is the infective dose lower in such groups, but the severity of the illness is likely to be greater, perhaps even life-threatening, and the speed of recovery slower.

Prevention of foodborne disease

The safe preparation of food involves measures and practices that involve attempts to do some or all of the following:

1 minimise the chances of contamination of food with bacteria
2 kill any contaminating bacteria, e.g. by heat or irradiation
3 ensure that food is stored under conditions, or in a form that, prevents bacterial proliferation.

Some bacteria produce changes in the flavour, appearance and smell of the food that reduces its palatability, i.e. they cause **spoilage**. The growth of spoilage organisms serves as a warning that the food is stale or has been the subject of poor handling procedures, inadequate processing or poor storage conditions. Food poisoning organisms, on the other hand, can grow in a food without producing changes in palatability. Thus, the absence of spoilage is no guarantee that the food is safe to eat. Otherwise food poisoning would be a rather rare occurrence.

Requirements for bacterial growth

1 *Nutrients* – Many foods are ideal culture media for the growth of microorganisms. The same nutrients that people obtain from them can also be used to support bacterial growth.

2 *A suitable temperature* – Bacterial growth slows at low temperatures and growth of most pathogens ceases at temperatures of less than 5°C. At the temperatures maintained in domestic freezers (–18°C) all bacterial growth will be arrested even though organisms can survive extended periods at such freezing temperatures. Growth of food poisoning organisms will also not occur at temperatures of over 60°C, and most will be slowly killed. At temperatures of over 73°C non-spore-forming bacteria will be very rapidly killed, although those capable of forming spores may survive considerable periods even at boiling point. Note also that, for example, *S. aureus* produces a heat stable toxin, and so foods heavily contaminated with this organism remain capable of causing food poisoning even if heat treatment or irradiation kills all of the bacteria.

3 *Moisture* – Bacteria require moisture for growth. Drying has been a traditional method of extending the storage life of many foods. High concentrations of salt and sugar preserve foods by increasing the osmotic pressure in foods, making the water unavailable to bacteria, i.e. they reduce the **water activity** of the food. Moulds generally tolerate much lower water activities than bacteria and grow, for example, on the surface of bread, cheese and jam (jelly).

4 *Favourable chemical environment* – A number of chemical agents (preservatives), by a variety of means, inhibit bacterial growth. They create a chemical environment unfavourable to bacterial growth. Many pathogenic and spoilage organisms only grow within a relatively narrow pH range; they will not, for example, grow in a very acid environment. Acidifying foods with acetic acid (pickling with vinegar) is one traditional preservation method. Fermentation of food using acid producing bacteria (e.g. the *Lactobacilli*) has also been traditionally used to preserve and flavour foods such as yoghurt, cheese and sauerkraut.

5 *Time* – The contaminated food needs to be kept under conditions that favour bacterial growth for long enough to allow the bacteria to multiply to the point where they represent a potentially infective dose. Note that under favourable conditions, bacteria may double their numbers in less than 20 minutes. A thousand organisms could become a million in three hours.

Roberts (1982) identified the factors that most often contributed to outbreaks of food poisoning in England and Wales (see Table 15.1). Bryan (1978) had earlier concluded that the factors contributing to food poisoning outbreaks in the US and UK were similar. Hobbs and Roberts

Table 15.1 Factors most often associated with 1000 outbreaks of food poisoning in England and Wales (after Roberts, 1982)

Factor	% of outbreaks with factor
Preparation of food in advance of needs	61
Storage at room temperature	40
Inadequate cooling	32
Inadequate heating	29
Contaminated processed food (not tinned)	19
Undercooking	15

* Other factors identified as contributing to 4–6% of cases were: inadequate thawing; cross contamination; improper warm holding; infected food handler; use of leftovers; and, the consumption of raw food.

(1993) suggest that factors contributing to outbreaks of food poisoning are unlikely to have changed significantly since that time. Such analyses give a useful indication of practices that are likely to increase the risk of food poisoning and so indicate some of the practical measures that can be taken to reduce risk.

Some guidelines to avoid food poisoning

These can be summarised as four general aims:

1　to minimise bacterial load of purchased food
2　to minimise risk of contamination during home processing
3　to maximise killing of bacteria during home preparation
4　to minimise the time that food is stored under conditions that permit bacterial multiplication.

Some specific recommendations that should help to achieve these aims are discussed below.

Buy food from retailers and caterers where food is apparently stored and prepared hygienically and under the correct conditions, e.g. maintained cool or hot (as appropriate), protected from insect contamination.

Purchase only foods (especially animal foods) that appear to be fresh and in good condition. Avoid foods with damaged packaging. Reject or discard food that shows evidence of the growth of spoilage organisms, i.e. that is discoloured or that smells or tastes "off". Do not consume foods that have exceeded their "use by" date or have been stored after opening for more than the time recommended on the packaging.

When preparing food ensure that you are not a source of contamination for the food, e.g. wash hands thoroughly before preparing food. If you use the toilet or blow your nose during food preparation then wash your hands before continuing to prepare food. Any infected lesions on the hands represent a potential source of contamination; they should be properly covered when preparing food.

Keep all utensils and surfaces that come into contact with food clean. Always wash any surfaces or utensils that have been used on raw food before they are re-used on cooked food. Separate raw food, especially raw meat, and cooked food. Ensure that cloths used to clean or dry dishes, and those used to wipe down surfaces are clean and changed regularly.

Care should be taken when cooking poultry, meat and probably eggs that they cook right through. To this end, any frozen meat or poultry should be thoroughly defrosted prior to cooking, either in a cool place or in a microwave oven. Meat that is eaten "rare" will not have undergone sufficient heat treatment to kill all bacteria, and thus it represents a potential hazard if contaminated prior to cooking; poultry should always be well-cooked.

The time between food preparation and consumption should be as short as is practically reasonable. Where food is prepared well in advance of serving, then it should be protected from contamination and should not be stored at room temperature. Buffets, where prepared food may be left uncovered at room temperature for some hours before consumption, are particularly hazardous.

Food that is to kept hot should be kept above 65°C, and any food that is to be re-heated should be thoroughly re-heated so that all parts of it reach 75°C. Food that is to be kept cool should be kept below 5°C. Food that has been cooked but is to be stored cool should be cooled rapidly so that it spends the minimum time within the growth range of bacteria. Leftovers, or other prepared foods, that are stored in a refrigerator should be covered and used promptly; care should be taken to ensure that they do not come into contact with raw food, especially flesh foods.

In her analysis of food poisoning outbreaks, Roberts (1982) found that two-thirds of outbreaks could be traced to foods prepared in restaurants, hotels, clubs, institutions, hospitals, schools and canteens; less than 20% of outbreaks were linked to food prepared in the home. These figures are, however distorted due to the low rate of inclusion of home-related incidents because epidemiological data on these outbreaks was often incomplete; Hobbs and Roberts (1993) indicate that 60% of food poisoning incidents occur in the home. It should nonetheless be borne in mind that outbreaks of food poisoning that originate from home-prepared food will tend to generate fewer individual cases than outbreaks associated with commercial and institutional catering:

> Situations where food is prepared in quantity for a large number of people are most likely to give rise to most food poisoning
>
> Hobbs and Roberts (1993)

For example, a flaw in the pasteurisation process of a major US dairy resulted in over 16 000 confirmed cases and around 200 000 suspected cases of food poisoning in Illinois in 1985 (Todd, 1991). The principal aim of this chapter has been to encourage greater care and awareness in the home preparation of food. In order to effect reductions in the rates of food poisoning produced outside the home, there needs to be improved training of catering workers and regulatory changes that lead to improvements to commercial and institutional catering practices. Food hygiene laws and regulations are complex, often extremely detailed, and vary from nation to nation (recent attempts to harmonise food hygiene laws within the EC have highlighted this latter point). Food hygiene laws must remain the province of specialist texts of food microbiology and food technology (e.g. see Jacob, 1993). Note, however, that in principle food hygiene laws represent attempts by governments to enshrine the safety principles and practices outlined for home food preparation into a formal legal framework so as to ensure that they are carried through into mass-catering situations.

In the vast majority of the outbreaks investigated by Roberts (1982), meat and poultry were identified as the source of the infection. Eggs, as well as poultry, are now also recognised as a source of the organism causing the most common type of Salmonella food poisoning (*S. enteritidis*). Certain foods are associated with a low risk of food poisoning:

1 dry foods like bread and biscuits or dried foods – the low water activity prevents bacterial growth
2 high sugar (or salted) foods like jam (jelly) – again because of the low water activity
3 fats and fatty foods like vegetable oil lack nutrients and provide an unfavourable environment for bacterial growth
4 commercially tinned foods because they have been subjected to vigorous heat treatment and maintained in air-tight containers
5 pasteurised foods like milk because they have been subjected to heat treatment designed to kill likely pathogens
6 high acid foods like pickles
7 vegetables generally do not support bacterial growth. They can, however, be a source of contamination for other foods, e.g. if used in prepared salads containing meat, eggs or mayonnaise. Fruit and vegetables contaminated by dirty water may be a direct source of infection if the infecting organism has a low infective dose.

Once opened, tinned or pasteurised foods cannot be assumed to be safe, as they may have been contaminated after processing, or, in the case of dried foods, after rehydration.

This information may be particularly useful if one is obliged to select food in places where food hygiene seems less than satisfactory.

Pinpointing the cause of a food poisoning outbreak

Identifying the cause of food poisoning outbreaks should highlight high risk practices and thus may be useful for improving food handling. If a single event (e.g. serving a contaminated dish at a buffet) is the cause of an outbreak, then a time distribution of cases like that shown in Figure 15.2 would be expected. Each food poisoning organism has a characteristic average incubation period from time of ingestion to the onset of symptoms. Incubation times in individuals will vary around this average; a few people develop symptoms early, most towards the middle of the range, and a few towards the end of the range as in Figure 15.2. The variation in the speed of onset of symptoms is influenced by all sorts of factors, such as:

- dose of organism or toxin consumed
- amount of other food consumed and thus the dilution and speed of passage through the gut
- individual susceptibility.

The organism causing the illness can be identified from the clinical picture and/or laboratory samples and then, knowing the incubation period, the approximate time at which all of the victims were infected and the meal at which the organisms were consumed pinpointed (see Figure 15.2). Sampling of leftovers or circumstantial evidence can then identify the responsible food and hopefully the unsafe practice that led to the outbreak.

Board (1983) gives an illustrative case history of an outbreak of food poisoning amongst the passengers and crew of a charter flight. More than half of the passengers on this flight developed food poisoning, a few at the end of the flight and large numbers at the airport within two hours of landing. The clinical picture (the symptoms, the rapid onset and short duration) indicated that the illness was probably due to ingestion of toxin from *S. aureus*. The time distribution of cases indicated that the breakfast served on the plane 90 minutes before landing was the likely source of the illness, and samples of

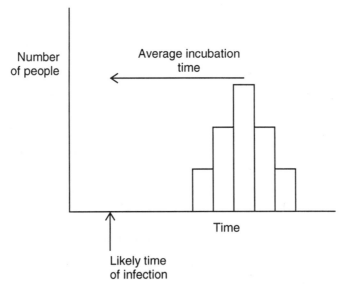

Number of people | Average incubation time

Time

Likely time of infection

Figure 15.2 Theoretical time distribution of first experiencing food poisoning symptoms after infection

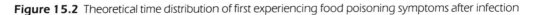

uneaten breakfasts confirmed the presence of this organism in the ham omelette. The food was found to have been contaminated by infected sores on the hands of one of the cooks at the catering company that had supplied the breakfasts to the airline. A long time (three days) had elapsed between the initial preparation of the food and its eventual serving to the passengers, and the food had not been kept cool for much of the time between preparation and serving.

If no food samples are available for analysis, then the responsible food can often be implicated by calculation of **attack rates**. All of those participating in the meal identified as the point of infection are asked to complete a questionnaire about which foods they consumed and whether they became ill. The attack rate is the percentage of persons becoming ill. For each food the percentage of those who became ill is calculated for those who did and those who did not consume that food, i.e. the **food specific attack rates**. A statistically significantly higher attack rate for those consuming a particular food as compared to those not consuming it, indicates that it was the likely source of the infection. In the example in Table 15.2, then eating food A significantly increased the attack rate whilst eating food B significantly reduced it; A and B were

alternative choices on the menu. It would thus seem almost certain that food A was the source of the infection.

If the temporal distribution of people reporting symptoms does not follow the bell-shaped model shown in Figure 15.2 (e.g. if there are multiple peaks or the number of new cases plateaus rather than dies away), then this indicates person-to-person spread or a continuing source of infection, e.g. a processing fault, an infected food handler or continuing use of a contaminated ingredient. Knowing the range of incubation times for the causative organism and identifying what all of the victims were doing (and eating) within the window of time when infection is predicted to have occurred, it should be possible to identify a common factor, e.g. all victims ate a particular processed food or ate at a particular place during the period when they were likely to have become infected.

A review of some common food poisoning organisms and foodborne illnesses

The *Salmonellae*

Many different types of the *Salmonella* group are responsible not only for common food poisoning but also for the more

Table 15.2 Food specific attack rates for persons present at a social function identified as the point of infection for an outbreak of food poisoning. After: Hobbs and Roberts (1993)

Food	Ate			Did not eat		
	ill	not ill	attack rate (%)	ill	not ill	attack rate (%)
A	30	131	19	0	51	0*
B	0	27	0	30	154	16*
C	8	49	14	21	125	14
D	21	95	18	9	84	10
E	8	69	10	22	107	17
F	13	60	18	17	121	12

* statistically significant difference between the attack rates of those who did and did not consume that particular food.

serious food and water borne illnesses, typhoid and paratyphoid. The common food poisoning organisms usually need in excess of 100 000 bacteria to represent an infective dose. These latter organisms produce diarrhoea, stomach pain, vomiting and fever about 12–48 hours after ingestion, and the illness lasts for between one and seven days. Intensive farming methods mean that all raw meat, poultry, eggs and raw milk should be regarded as potentially contaminated with these organisms. These organisms grow at temperatures between 6 and 46°C. They are relatively heat sensitive and are killed slowly at 60°C and very rapidly at 75°C. They are not tolerant of very acid conditions, i.e. pH less than 4.5.

Meat and especially poultry have long been regarded as foods with a high potential to cause *Salmonella* food poisoning, but in recent years the contamination of eggs with *Salmonellae* has been a major cause for concern in the UK. Many thousands of hens have been slaughtered in an apparently unsuccessful attempt to eradicate these organisms from the laying flock. Eggs have a number of natural barriers that tend to reduce the risk of bacterial entry, but they are sold in millions; even if only a very small proportion are contaminated, this can represent, in absolute terms, a large number of potentially infected meals. Eggs also have a number of systems that inhibit bacterial growth (bacteriostatic systems) by making nutrients unavailable to the bacteria. The likelihood of a single fresh egg containing an infective dose for a healthy adult is thus low. Well-cooked eggs should represent no hazard at all, and Britons are currently advised to eat only well-cooked eggs. Any potential hazard from eggs is increased very significantly if uncooked egg is added to other foods, e.g. mayonnaise or cheesecake and then the mixture stored under conditions that allow bacterial proliferation, e.g. at room temperature.

C. perfringens (also C. welchii)

This organism has a high infective dose of between a hundred and a thousand million organisms. Illness is due to a toxin produced within the gut when the organism forms spores. The disease has an incubation period of 8–12 hours and lasts for up to 24 hours; symptoms are diarrhoea and abdominal pain but not usually either vomiting or fever. The organism grows at temperatures of up to 53°C and the spores need temperatures of 100°C to kill them. Food poisoning from this organism is usually associated with meat and poultry consumption and the organism is of widespread distribution in the gut of animals and people and also in soil and dust. When food is inadequately cooked these organisms may continue to grow during the initial heating of the food, they will survive at temperatures of 60°C and then continue to grow during the cooling phase; the organism grows very rapidly at temperature towards the top end of its tolerable range.

S. aureus

The illness caused by this organism is due to a toxin present in food where this organism has grown. Greater than five million bacteria are usually regarded as necessary to produce enough toxin to evoke illness. The symptoms are vomiting, diarrhoea, abdominal pain but without fever; symptoms are rapid in onset (2–6 hours) and of short duration (6–24 h). The organism is heat sensitive; it grows within the range 8–46°C and is killed at temperatures in excess of 60°C but the toxin, once formed in food, is very heat stable and may not be eliminated by further heat treatment or irradiation of the food.

Food handlers are an important source of contamination. Many people carry the organism in their nasal passages, and this can lead to contamination of hands and thence food; infected lesions on the hands may contain this organism. The organism needs foods rich in protein to produce toxin, but it is comparatively tolerant of high salt and sugar concentrations, e.g. as found in ham or custard. *S. aureus* does not compete well with other bacteria present in raw food, but if essentially sterile, cooked food is then contaminated by the handler and, without any competition, the organism is able to grow even in foods with relatively high salt or sugar contents.

B. cereus

This organism is commonly found in soil and thus upon vegetables. It grows in starchy foods and, in the UK and US, poisoning due to this organism is usually associated with consumption of rice. The organism produces heat resistant spores which may survive cooking of rice. If the cooked rice, containing viable spores, is stored at temperatures that permit growth of the organism (7–49°C) then an infective dose will accumulate. Boiling rice in bulk and then storing it at room temperature prior to flash frying, e.g. in Chinese restaurants is a common scenario for food poisoning due to this organism. The resultant illness is acute in onset (1–16 hours) and of short duration (6–24 hours) and it is caused by toxins produced by the organism in the food. An infective dose is in excess of 100 000 organisms in the food; the symptoms depend upon the particular toxin involved, but may include diarrhoea, abdominal pain, nausea or vomiting.

C. botulinum

This organism grows under anaerobic conditions in low-acid foods. Tinned or bottled meats, fish or vegetables (but not acidic fruit) are potential sources of illness. The organism is killed by oxygen and thus the storage of these foods in airtight containers allows growth; the organism may also occasionally grow deep within non-tinned flesh foods or meat products. Commercial canning processes involve a heat treatment that is specifically designed to ensure that all of the heat stable spores of this organism are killed: the so-called **botulinum cook**. Cured meats and meat products contain nitrate, nitrite and salt which are effective in preventing growth of this organism, and the addition of these preservatives is legally required in the UK for meat products like sausages. Home canning or bottling of vegetables results in significant numbers of cases of botulism in the US each year because the heat treatment is insufficient to kill the *Clostridia* spores. The very rare cases in the UK have usually been traced to occasional rogue tins of imported meat or fish, e.g. after heat treatment contaminated water might be sucked into the cooling can through a damaged seam. The most recent UK outbreak in 1989 was traced to a tin of nut puree that was used to flavour yoghurt. In the US, honey is regarded as a potential source of small amounts of toxin, and so honey is not recommended for young children.

The organism produces an extremely potent toxin within the food; this toxin is destroyed by heat so danger foods are those eaten unheated (e.g. tinned salmon or corned beef) or those that are only warmed. The toxin, although a protein, is absorbed from the gut and affects the nervous system, blocking the release of the important nerve transmitter acetylcholine. A dry mouth, blurred vision and gradual paralysis are the symptoms, and death may result from paralysis of the respiratory muscles. In those victims who survive, recovery may take several months. The incubation period is normally 18–36 hours. This organism is included, even though rarely producing illness in the UK because the symptoms are frequently fatal and because the imperative to avoid contamination of food with this organism has had a great influence on food processing practices.

The Campylobacter

The *Campylobacter* were only recognised as a general source of foodborne disease in 1977; the organisms do not grow readily upon normal laboratory media and therefore suitable methods needed to be developed for their identification. From being almost totally ignored as a cause of food poisoning 20 years ago, this organism is now reckoned to be the most common cause of acute bacterial gastro-enteritis in the UK with around 30 000 cases recognised each year (Cooke, 1991). The illness has a relatively long incubation period (two to ten days) and it produces a quite severe and prolonged illness – initially flu-like symptoms and abdominal pain which last for one to two days followed by profuse, sometimes bloody, diarrhoea lasting for one to three days. It may take a week or more for complete recovery. The organism may contaminate water, unpasteurised milk, meat and poultry, and it may reside in the intestines of domestic animals. The organism has a low infective dose, and thus is potentially transmissible through water, through the hands of children playing with or near domestic animals, or even from person to person. Chicken and meat that has been inadequately cooked on garden barbecues has been blamed for many cases in the UK. The organism has a high optimum growth temperature but is killed at temperature similar to those required to kill the *Salmonellae*.

L. monocytogenes

Chilling of food has been a traditional method of storing food: it reduces both microbial growth and the rate of chemical deterioration. An enormous range of chilled foods are now available in supermarkets, e.g. fresh meat and fish, cheese, cooked meals, sandwiches, pies etc. Such foods are susceptible to the development of infective doses of pathogenic bacteria that continue to grow slowly at low temperatures. Small variations in temperature within the low range (0–8°C) or just above it, can have marked effects on the rate at which these low temperature organisms grow. Strict temperature control

is therefore of great importance in ensuring safe storage of chilled foods. For foods that are to be eaten without further cooking, or just re-warming, then current UK legislation requires that they be stored below 5°C, e.g. cook-chill ready meals, sandwiches, cured meat and fish.

The organism *L. monocytogenes* is one of these low temperature organisms that has attracted much media and public attention in the UK and US in the last few years. This organism will grow slowly at temperatures as low as 1°C and it will tolerate a salt concentration of 10% and a pH down to 5.2. Soft cheeses and pate which have a relatively long shelf life, are considered to be at particular risk from this organism. Its presence has been reported in many cook-chill ready meals and it is likely to survive the mild re-heating in a microwave oven recommended for many of these foods.

The organism causes a disease known as listeriosis in vulnerable groups like the elderly, infants, pregnant women and the immunodeficient, although it does not usually cause illness in healthy people. Symptoms range from those resembling mild flu to severe septicaemia and occasionally meningitis; if infection occurs during pregnancy then abortion, foetal abnormality or neonatal death may result. In the UK, pregnant women are currently advised to avoid those foods that are liable to harbour *Listeria* (e.g. pate and soft cheese made with unpasteurised milk) and to thoroughly re-heat cook-chill foods. Increased use of chilling led to an increase in recorded cases of listeriosis from around 25 per year in the early 1970s to around 300 per year by 1988. In 1988 there were 26 deaths of newborn babies, 52 total deaths and 11 abortions caused by listeriosis. In the 1990s, due to increased awareness and increased measures to prevent it, recorded cases of listeriosis have fallen to just over 100 cases per year (Cooke, 1991). The rise in the prominence of listeriosis with increased use of food chilling is a good illustration of how changing eating habits and processing methods can lead to changes in the prominence of different types of food poisoning organisms.

Bovine spongiform encephalopathy

Bovine spongiform encephalopathy (BSE), often called "Mad Cow Disease", is not a bacterial disease or even one that is clearly borne via human food, but it has attracted great media attention in recent years and engendered great public concern about the safety of British beef. Infected cattle show changes in behaviour, they become excitable, aggressive and easily panicked; they show abnormalities in gait and a tendency to fall. The disease first broke out in 1985, and it has so far resulted in the death or slaughter of over 120 000 infected cattle. The symptoms and the "spongiform" lesions in the brains of affected animals resemble those of other spongiform encephalopathies, which are all inevitably fatal. Other examples of spongiform encephalopathies are:

- the disease **scrapie** in sheep (and goats) – endemic in the British sheep flock since the 18th century and estimated to affect as many as 35–70 00 British sheep annually
- the rare human disease **Creutzfeld-Jacob disease (CJD)** which is responsible for around 30–40 deaths annually in the UK
- and, the disease **Kuru** associated with cannibalism in Papua New Guinea (particularly consumption of infected human brain tissue).

These diseases are thought to be caused by an unidentified transmissible agent or agents that are smaller and more resistant to destruction than viruses. These mysterious "organisms" have been termed **prions,** and they are not destroyed by processes that normally destroy nucleic acids. Nucleic acids are normally considered to be essential for the viability of all life forms, and they are the infective component of known viruses.

It is thought that BSE was introduced into British cattle, and the dairy herd in particular, when cattle were fed sheep offal that had been insufficiently heat-treated to destroy the scrapie agent. Re-cycling of infected cattle offal may then have contributed to its spread. The practice of feeding offal to cattle was outlawed in Britain in July 1988, and all affected cattle are slaughtered and their carcasses incinerated. The expectation is that these measures will result in a decline in the number of new cases of the disease (running at 1000 per week in 1992) and elimination of the disease in cattle once all of the previously-infected animals die out. The average incubation period for BSE in cattle is thought to be over four years. A much more pessimistic scenario would envisage the disease being transmitted vertically (from cow to calf) and horizontally (from cow to cow) through the cattle herd, as becoming endemic in the cattle herd as scrapie is in the sheep flock. Vertical transmission of scrapie from ewe to lamb does occur. At the time of writing (March 1994) there are some encouraging signs: new cases are now running at more than 20% below last year's levels; and, the compensation paid for slaughtered animals has been reduced to reflect the increasing age of affected cattle.

There has been speculation that CJD might be due to the scrapie agent, and thus that current cases of this disease in humans might originate from eating contaminated sheep meat. Scrapie has been endemic in British sheep for centuries, but CJD is extremely rare and is apparently no more common amongst those likely to be exposed to infected sheep carcasses, e.g. butchers, shepherds and slaughterhouse workers. However, the assumption that the disease has been transmitted across species (sheep to cow) by a dietary route has led to obvious concern that eating meat from infected animals could infect people, especially if they eat tissue with a high load of the infective agent, e.g. brain, thymus, spleen and lymph nodes. Measures have been taken in Britain to prevent these "high load" cattle tissues from entering the human food chain.

Some people have apparently been infected with CJD by injection of contaminated human brain material (e.g. growth hormone extracted from the brains of cadavers). The incubation period in these cases seems to average around 20 years, and so it will be many years before any strong evidence of increased rates of the human disease due to eating contaminated beef would be expected to show up; there were still only 30 cases of CJD in Britain in 1992. BSE reviewed by Symonds, 1990.

Food processing

Some general pros and cons of food processing

This term covers a multitude of processes to which food may be subjected; they may be traditional or modern, take place in the home, catering unit or factory. Unless one eats only raw, home-grown foods, then it is impossible to avoid some processing. It would be impossible to feed a large urban industrial society without some commercial processing of foods. For example, around 50% of the value of all food purchases in the UK are frozen or chilled. Processing includes cooking, smoking, drying, freezing, pasteurising, canning, irradiation, etc.

Processing of foods, particularly preparation of ready-to-eat foods "adds value" to the ingredients and increases their commercial potential for retailers and processors. Food processors and retailers represent some of the most commercially successful businesses in developed countries; this high profitability has tended to politicise food processing issues, sometimes to the detriment of constructive critical debate. The term "processed food" is often used to convey very negative connotations about modern food and

food suppliers, but it is such an all-embracing term, covering foods across the whole spectrum of composition, that its use in this way is unhelpful and probably warns of the prejudice or political motivation of the critic. Each processed food should be judged on its own merits and should be considered within the context of the whole diet rather than purely in isolation.

Commercial processing of food has a number of objectives, in addition, to the obvious commercial ones, such as:

1 It increases the shelf-life of foods and thus increases availability, reduces waste and may reduce the cost of food.
2 By destroying or preventing the growth of pathogens, processing lowers the risk of foodborne diseases.
3 It can increase the palatability of foods.
4 Processing enables new varieties of foods to be created.
5 Commercially prepared food, reduces the time that individuals need to spend on food preparation. Even those unable or unwilling to spend much time on food preparation can eat an interesting and varied diet.

Commercial processing usually, but not always, has some negative effects on the nutrient content of the unprepared food. These losses may be very similar or even less than those involved in home preparation of food. These losses are often not very significant in the diets of North Americans and Western Europeans who, in the main, have ample intakes of the essential nutrients. In many cases the nutrient content of processed foods (e.g. vitamins in frozen vegetables) may actually be higher than stale versions of the same food bought "fresh". It is often argued that food processors encourage people to consume foods high in fat, sugar and salt but low in complex carbohydrate and thus are partly responsible for the increased prevalence of the diseases of industrialisation. It seems probable, however, that even without the encouragement of food processors, our natural inclination to consume such a diet would have prevailed. Commercial processors and retailers provide what they can sell; they have, for example, been quick to recognise the commercial opportunities offered by the demand for "healthy foods". Many highly processed foods have a very healthy image, e.g. some margarines and low-fat spreads, some breakfast cereals, low-fat salad dressings, low-fat yoghurts, low-calorie drinks and certain meat-substitutes of vegetable or microbial origin.

Specific processing methods

Canning

This is a very good method for the long-term preservation of food. The food is maintained in sealed containers and thus protected from oxidative deterioration or growth of aerobic microorganisms. The food is subjected to a vigorous heat treatment after canning that is designed to ensure that there is no practical possibility that even heat-resistant bacterial spores will survive. The so-called botulinum cook ensures the destruction of all spores of the potentially lethal toxin-producing, anaerobic organism *C botulinum*. If commercially canned food is consumed soon after opening, then there is negligible risk of it being associated with food poisoning.

Pasteurisation

Mild heat is applied to a food; this is sufficient to destroy likely pathogenic bacteria and to reduce the number of spoilage organisms without impairing the food itself. It is usually associated with milk, but other food such as liquid egg, liquid ice cream mix and honey may be pasteurised. Pasteurisation of milk traditionally involved holding it at 63°C for 30 minutes – this was designed to ensure the destruction of the organism responsible for tuberculosis but it also kills *Salmonellae* and the other heat-sensitive pathogens usually found in milk. The same result can be achieved by the modern **high temperature short time** method in which the milk is raised to 72°C for 15 seconds.

Ultra high temperature (UHT) treatment

Once again this is usually associated with milk, but is also applied to other foods. Traditionally, milk was sterilised milk by heating it to temperatures of 105–110°C for 20–40 minutes. This severe heating results in marked chemical changes in the milk that impairs its flavour, appearance, smell and nutrient content. The UHT method relies upon the principle that the rate of chemical reactions only doubles with a 10°C rise in temperature, whereas the rate of bacterial killing increases about ten-fold. Thus full sterilisation can be achieved by holding the milk at 135°C for two seconds with little chemical change in the milk. Two seconds at 135°C has approximately the same bacterial killing effect as 33 minutes at 105°C, but results in chemical changes equivalent to only 16 seconds at this temperature. After UHT treatment, the milk is placed aseptically into sterile containers and will keep for up to six months. Chemical deterioration rather than microbial spoilage limits the duration of storage of UHT products.

Cook chill processing

With the cook chill process, foods are cooked separately as they would be in the home kitchen. Bacterial cells will be killed by this process, but spores will survive. The food is then chilled rapidly to temperatures below 5°C to minimise growth of the surviving spore-forming bacteria. The food is then divided into portions and packaged. Rigorous standards of hygiene are required during this portioning and packaging stage to prevent re-contamination with spoilage and food poisoning organisms. Most cook chill foods have a maximum permitted shelf life of six to eight days partly, because of the difficulty of preventing contamination by the ubiquitous *Pseudomonas* group of spoilage organisms. The introduction of cook chill foods into hospitals is an area of particular concern because vulnerable groups are concentrated in them: pregnant women and infants in maternity units; those whose immune systems have been suppressed by disease (e.g. AIDS patients) or by treatment (e.g. transplant patients treated with immunosuppressant drugs); and, more generally, those weakened by injury, disease or old age. Transplant units use irradiation as a means of ensuring the bacterial safety of foods fed to immunosuppressed patients.

Food irradiation

Irradiation involves exposing food to ionising radiation which can either be X-rays or more usually gamma rays emitted from a radioactive source such as cobalt-60 (reviewed by Hawthorn, 1989). There is no contact between the radioactive source and the food and so, the irradiated food does not itself become radioactive. The irradiation of food is not a new idea, its potential was recognised and demonstrated more than 75 years ago. It is only in recent years, however, that the widespread application of irradiation in food processing has become economically viable because of the widespread availability of gamma emitters like cobalt-60. Many countries have now approved the use of irradiation for some categories of foods.

In the USA, irradiation is classified with the food additives because it causes chemical changes in food. Its use is permitted upon a wide range of foods including onions, potatoes, herbs and spices, nuts and seeds, wheat, fish, poultry and meat. Irradiated food must be clearly labelled as having been irradiated.

In the UK prior to 1990, irradiation was forbidden for all foods with the exception of herbs and spices. At the beginning of 1991 this ban was withdrawn and irradiation of a wide range of foods is now permitted in properly licensed centres, e.g. fruit, vegetables, cereals, fish, shellfish and poultry may all now be legally irradiated in the UK.

The effects of irradiation on the food vary according to the dose used (see Figure 15.3).

Some of these changes are used to extend the shelf-life of foods through the inhibition of sprouting, delay in ripening and reduction in the numbers of spoilage organisms.

The killing of insect pests reduces losses and damage to food from this cause and reduces the need to fumigate with chemical insecticides.

The elimination of food poisoning organisms should reduce the risks of food poisoning, and sterilisation of food by irradiation may be particularly useful in ensuring the safety of food intended for immunosuppressed patients.

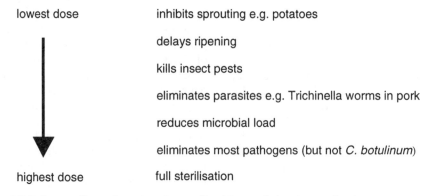

lowest dose — inhibits sprouting e.g. potatoes

delays ripening

kills insect pests

eliminates parasites e.g. Trichinella worms in pork

reduces microbial load

eliminates most pathogens (but not *C. botulinum*)

highest dose — full sterilisation

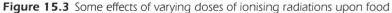

Figure 15.3 Some effects of varying doses of ionising radiations upon food

Despite these apparent advantages of food irradiation, its introduction has been vigorously opposed by certain pressure groups within the UK. It has been suggested that the full effects of irradiation are not yet well enough understood to be totally confident of its safety.

Some potential problems of irradiated foods:

1 The ionising radiation induces certain chemical changes within the food; it increases free radical production and certain chemical species known as **radiolytes** (see Chapter 10 for a discussion of free radicals and antioxidants). There is natural concern that these chemical changes may have detrimental effects on health, although it must be added that all processing methods produce some chemical changes in food, e.g. smoking and barbecuing lead to production of small amounts of potentially carcinogenic chemicals in food. The chemical changes induced in food by irradiation are less than those produced by heat processing. The low level of chemical change induced by irradiation is illustrated by the extreme difficulty in chemically identifying whether or not a food sample has been irradiated.

2 Some bacterial and fungal toxins will not be destroyed by irradiation, so, if irradiation is used to compensate for earlier poor hygiene, then food poisoning from these toxins may result.

3 At the doses usually used on foods, spores will survive and may later grow in the food. Irradiation is known to increase mutation rates; conceivably, new and dangerous mutants of microorganisms might be produced in food.

4 At high doses, e.g. those required to achieve sterilisation, there may be distinct adverse effects on the palatability of the food and major losses of some nutrients such as thiamin and vitamin E.

5 There is concern about the safety of workers at establishments where food irradiation takes place. This suggests a clear need to regulate and licence facilities for food irradiation.

The chemical safety of food

Overview of chemical hazards in food

Potential sources of chemical hazard in food:

1 *Food additives* – Chemicals that are deliberately added to food during processing.
2 *Natural toxicants* – Compounds naturally present in the food that may have toxic effects.
3 *Contaminants* – Substances that are incidentally or inadvertently added to foods during agricultural production, storage or processing, e.g. residues of drugs given to food animals, pesticide or fertiliser residues, contaminants leeching into food from packaging or containers, fungal toxins.

One dilemma that increasingly faces those trying to ensure the chemical safety of food is to decide at what level in the food the presence of any particular chemical substance represents a real hazard to consumers. Total absence of all traces of potentially hazardous chemicals from all foods is, and always has been, an impossible ideal. Almost every chemical, including most nutrients, are toxic if the dose is high enough. More substances are being subjected to rigorous safety tests which usually involve exposing animals to high doses of the chemical for prolonged periods; many chemicals that are ubiquitous in our environment can thus be shown to have toxic potential. Analytical procedures are also becoming increasingly sophisticated and sensitive, making it possible to detect infinitesimally small amounts of potentially hazardous chemicals in foods. This combination of factors, especially when distorted by popular journalists, can lead to the impression that the chemical hazards in our food are increasing at an alarming rate. At least some of this apparent increase in chemical danger from food is artefact caused by increased awareness of the potential hazards of chemicals and an increased ability to detect small amounts of these chemicals.

In a report by the Institute of Food Technologists (IFT, 1975), the panel distinguish between **toxic** which they define as "being inherently capable of producing injury when tested by itself" and **hazard** defined as "being likely to produce injury under the circumstances of exposure" as in food. Food naturally contains thousands of toxic substances, including many nutrients, but very few of these represent real hazard. For example, the average US consumer ingests around 10 000 mg of **solanine** from potatoes each year; enough of this atropine-like alkaloid to kill him/her if consumed in a single dose. The same average US consumer ingests about 40 mg of lethal hydrogen cyanide in his/her annual 1.85 pounds of lima beans and 14 mg of arsenic from seafood.

Most natural toxins are present in low concentrations in natural foods, and they do not usually accumulate. They are usually metabolised and/or excreted by a variety of mechanisms which are also involved in the disposal of ingested man-made chemicals like food additives, drugs and residues of agricultural chemicals. There are a variety of mechanisms and sites through which the different toxicants induce their effect; generally the effects of small amounts of individual toxicants are unlikely to be additive; 1% of a toxic dose of 100 different toxins almost certainly will not produce ill-effects (IFT, 1975).

Natural toxicants and contaminants

Circumstances that may increase chemical hazard

The chances of toxic potential becoming real hazard is likely to be increased if there is exaggerated consumption of one food for a prolonged period. This is true whether the toxin is naturally present, a contaminant or a deliberate additive; this is yet one more reason for encouraging diversity in the diet. Examples of natural toxicants in food producing serious illness may occur when abnormally high amounts of a particular food are consumed. The plant *Lathyrus sativa* has been widely grown in Asia and North Africa and the seeds (chick peas or khesari dhal) regularly consumed. However, during very dry seasons it was consumed in very large quantities because the plant is very drought resistant. When consumed in very large quantities it can produce a severe disease of the spinal cord, **lathyrism** which can lead to permanent paralysis. When only small quantities of chick peas are consumed as part of a mixed diet, they do not constitute a hazard and are nutritious.

Chemical hazard from food may arise if individual susceptibility causes increased sensitivity to a particular toxin. The common broad bean *Vicia faba* contains a substance that causes haemolysis (red cell breakdown). This can lead to a severe anaemia called **favism** in those who are genetically susceptible because they are deficient in a particular enzyme (glucose 6 phosphate dehydrogenase). As many as 35% of some Mediterranean peoples and 10% of American blacks have this particular genetic deficiency. Vomiting, abdominal pain and fever are the acute symptoms; jaundice and dark coloured urine may occur as a result of the haemolysis, with eventual severe anaemia a possibility.

Traditional methods of preparing, processing and selecting foods often minimises any potential hazard they may represent. Cassava is one of the most important staple foods for millions of people in the tropics; it may, for example, provide up to 60% of the calorific intake in Nigeria. Cassava contains certain alkaloids that release cyanide when acted upon by an enzyme in the cassava. The traditional method of preparing cassava involves peeling and soaking for several days, during which time most of the cyanide is lost due to fermentation. Cases of sometimes fatal cyanide poisoning are associated with inadequate processing of the cassava (particularly shortening of the fermentation time) and increased use of lower quality "bitter" cassava which has a higher cyanide content (see Akintowa and Tunawashe, 1992). As another example, polar bear liver contains toxic concentrations of retinol; Eskimos avoided eating the liver, but unwary polar explorers have been poisoned by eating it.

Some natural toxicants in "Western" diets

Few natural toxicants are thought to represent significant hazards to Western consumers. In her analysis of over a thousand recorded outbreaks of food poisoning in England and Wales, Roberts (1982) found that 54 outbreaks (about 5%) were due to chemical toxicity – 47 due to **scrombotoxin** from fish and seven from a **haemagglutinin** in red kidney beans. Some potential natural chemical hazards in food:

1 Scrombotoxic poisoning is caused by heat-stable toxins liberated by the action of bacteria upon fish protein during spoilage. The toxin is thus produced by bacterial action but is not in itself a bacterial toxin. Symptoms occur shortly after eating the contaminated fish and include a peppery taste in the mouth, flushing of the face and neck, sweating and sometimes nausea and diarrhoea. Almost all of the outbreaks investigated by Roberts were associated with contaminated processed fish.

2 Eating raw red kidney beans leads to short-lasting symptoms of nausea, vomiting and diarrhoea. These symptoms are thought to be due to a toxin that causes red cells to agglutinate (stick together), a haemagglutinin – the symptoms are probably due to damage to intestinal cells caused by this toxin. The haemagglutinin is destroyed by vigorous boiling, but it may persist if the beans are cooked by prolonged gentle heating in a slow cooker. These beans should always be subjected to ten minutes of vigorous boiling before being eaten. Roberts (1982) found that all of the outbreaks she investigated were due to eating the beans in an uncooked or undercooked state. As a general rule, raw or undercooked beans should not be eaten as they contain several mildly toxic factors and factors that interfere with the proper digestion of protein.

3 Some cheeses contain the substance **tyramine** which can cause a rise in blood pressure. This may be dangerous for those taking certain anti-depressant drugs because they sensitise the individual to the effects of tyramine.

4 Solanine is an atropine-like substance found in potatoes. In high enough doses it will cause headache, vomiting and diarrhoea and may perhaps even result in circulatory collapse and neurological disturbances. Levels of solanine in potatoes are rarely enough to produce illness, and established outbreaks of potato poisoning are rare.

5 Many species of Brassicae (cabbage family) contain goitrogens, chemicals that induce goitre. These do not represent a real hazard at levels of consumption normally found in industrialised countries.

6 Mussels that have ingested the plankton species *Gonyaulux tamarensis* may contain hazardous amounts of a heat stable neurotoxin – **saxitoxin**. At certain times the sea may turn red, "red

tides", due to large numbers of *Gonyaulux* in the water. These red tides may occasionally occur even off the coasts of Britain and the US, and at such times it is dangerous to eat mussels.

7 Some fungi produce toxic chemicals, **mycotoxins**. Some mycotoxins represent a hazard to the inexperienced gatherer of wild fungi, and some fungal toxins are deliberately consumed because they contain hallucinogenic agents. Moulds also grow upon many foods that will not support the growth of bacteria – they are more tolerant of low water activity and low pH than bacteria. Dry foods like nuts and bread, sugary foods like jam (jelly) and salty foods like cheese may all go mouldy. Several of the toxins produced by moulds are potent carcinogens. **Aflatoxins** produced by *Aspergillus flavus* cause liver damage and lead to liver cancer in animal studies. Mouldy nuts would be a likely source of aflatoxin in the US and UK. Mouldy grain is likely to contain the toxin **ergot,** and this has caused serious outbreaks of poisoning in the past and still does in some countries, a condition referred to as St Vitus' Dance. Mouldy food should therefore be regarded as potentially hazardous and should be discarded. The detection of small amounts of the mycotoxin **patulin** in some brands of apple juice has recently achieved great publicity in the UK.

Mould growth is deliberately encouraged in the production of some foods like blue cheese and mould ripened cheese – these are not thought to represent hazard at usual levels of consumption.

Residues of agricultural chemicals

Expert opinion is that the residues of agricultural chemicals in foods represent no significant hazard to consumers when current regulations are adhered to. These assurances have been insufficient to convince a significant minority of the population who are willing to pay considerably higher prices for **organic produce** that has been grown without the aid of modern agricultural chemicals. These consumers are also willing to accept the less than perfect appearance of their fruits and vegetables that organic farming practices sometimes produce. Many producers and suppliers have been quick to recognise the commercial opportunities afforded by this new market. One would hesitate to say anything that would discourage this minority from exercising their right to choose food grown in this way, but the practicability of supplying the whole population with organic food is doubtful.

Food additives

Uses

Chemicals are deliberately added to food for a variety of purposes, such as:

1 as processing aids, e.g. emulsifiers, flour improvers and anti-caking agents
2 to improve the sensory appeal of foods, e.g. colours and flavours
3 to prevent the growth of food poisoning and spoilage organisms, e.g. nitrites and nitrates in meat products
4 to inhibit the growth of moulds, e.g. propionic acid or vinegar in bread
5 to inhibit the chemical deterioration of foods, e.g. antioxidants like vitamins C and E
6 to improve the nutritional value of foods, e.g. vitamins and/or minerals added to bread, breakfast cereals and drinks.

Some arguments against the use of food additives

1 They are dangerous chemicals *per se*, in particular, chronic exposure to them will lead to increased cancer risk.

2 They can be used to disguise faulty or inferior products and thus deceive the consumer, e.g. do colourings, flavourings, and emulsifiers disguise the high-fat and low-grade meat used in some meat products?
3 Even generally safe additives may trigger adverse reactions in some individuals, e.g. allergy to the yellow food colourant tartrazine and to sulphites (sulphur dioxide) used to preserve many foods.
4 Preservatives can be used by manufacturers to compensate for poor hygiene.
5 Many of the cosmetic additives are unnecessary or perhaps even imposed upon the consumer by food producers and retailers.

Some counter arguments:

Additives performing the preservative roles on the above list (3, 4 and 5) are a necessity if large urban populations are to be supplied with a variety of safe, nutritious and affordable foods. Traditional preservatives have long been used for these purposes, e.g. salt, sugar, woodsmoke, vinegar, alcohol, nitrites/nitrates. When evaluating the safety of modern preservatives or when judging the merits of foods claiming to be "free from all artificial preservatives" it should be borne in mind that most of these traditional preservatives have been implicated in disease, e.g. salt has been linked to hypertension, nitrites lead to the generation of potentially carcinogenic nitrosamines and small amounts of potential carcinogens can be detected in some smoked foods.

Some additives are essential as processing aids or otherwise necessary for the manufacture of a considerable number of supermarket foods. Some of these foods are considered to be important in helping consumers to comply with current nutrition education guidelines, e.g. emulsifiers and stabilisers in the production of many "reduced fat" products, anti-caking agents in the manufacture of many powders that are to be instantly rehydrated like coffee whitener, artificial sweeteners in the production of many "low calorie" or "reduced sugar" foods.

The additives that are most vulnerable to criticism are those that serve cosmetic purposes, i.e. that are there to enhance the appearance or palatability of the food. These may even be claimed to be doing a positive disservice to Western consumers by encouraging overconsumption and obesity. If a purely scientific model of food function is used, then appearance and palatability of food could almost be regarded as a decadent irrelevance. Few people would, however really want to regard positive sensory appeal of food as an optional extra.

Food additive regulation

Different countries have differing regulations governing the use of food additives, but the common purposes of such regulations are to ensure that they are used safely, effectively, honestly and in the minimum amounts necessary to achieve their objectives.

The **Food and Drug Administration (FDA)** regulates the use of food additives in America. In order to get approval to use a new additive, a manufacturer is required to provide evidence that the additive is effective, safe and can be detected and measured in the final product. The approval of the additive is then considered after a public hearing at which experts testify for and against the use of the additive. Additives that were in use before this procedure was adopted were put onto a list of substances **generally recognised as safe (GRAS)**. The GRAS list is subject to a continuing process of review and revision. More than 30 years ago, Congress approved the so-called **Delaney clause** "no additive shall be deemed to be safe if it is found to induce cancer when ingested by man or animal". This requirement is now regarded as unreasonable absolute in its prohibition, and the FDA deems additives to be safe if the risk of human cancer is less than one in a million. Saccharin is a permitted sweetener in the US despite being reported to cause cancer when administered in very large doses to animals, i.e. although shown to be toxic it is not thought to represent a hazard to the US consumer.

In the UK, the responsibility for regulating the use of food additives lies with the **Ministry of Agriculture Fisheries and Food (MAFF)**. A **Food Advisory Committee** decides whether any proposed new additive or new usage of an existing additive is necessary. This committee is comprised of a wide variety of interested persons including academics, consumer representatives, food industry representatives and public analysts. Grounds for necessity would be factors like: increased shelf-life of a product; reduced cost; an improved product for the consumer; necessity for the manufacture of a new product or for the introduction of a new manufacturing process. Once need has been established, then evidence must be presented to an expert **Committee on Toxicology** that assesses the safety of the additive. Existing additives may be referred to this committee for safety review.

E numbers, have been used to designate many food additives in Britain, and the rest of the EC. They were introduced as part of efforts to harmonise legislation within the EC and to overcome language barriers. They were originally envisaged as ensuring consumer confidence, i.e. if an additive had an E number, then the consumer could be totally assured of its safety. In reality however, the effect was quite the opposite, E numbers on food labels evoke suspicion and have been used to epitomise everything that is unwholesome about "modern, adulterated and artificial food".

Testing the safety of food additives

There are four potential sources of information which might assist in evaluating the safety of food additives, namely:

1. human experiments
2. human epidemiology
3. *in vitro* tests
4. animal experiments.

The major concern relating to the safety of food additives is that life-time exposure to an additive may increase the risk of human cancer. Human experiments are inevitably either short term or small scale; such experiments can be of no real use in identifying even relatively large increases in cancer risk due to particular additives. Neither can epidemiology be expected to pinpoint harmful effects of individual additives. Epidemiology involves relating exposure to changes in disease rates; yet we are all exposed to hundreds of additives in amounts that would be difficult to quantify on an individual basis, and even on a "worse-case scenario" the increased cancer rate due to the additive is likely to be small. It proved difficult to show convincingly with epidemiological methods that smoking causes lung cancer even though the association is thought to be strong, the level of exposure is relatively easy to establish and there is an identifiable, matched but unexposed population.

In vitro tests involve the use of isolated mammalian cells or microorganisms. The best established of these tests are those, like the **Ames test**, that use the ability of compounds to cause mutation in bacteria as an indicator of their likely carcinogenicity in mammals. Mutagenesis, carcinogenesis and teratogenesis (causing foetal abnormalities) may all be caused by damage to the genetic material DNA. Such tests are a useful way of screening out some potential carcinogens or teratogens and thus in reducing the number of compounds that need to undergo full animal testing. *In vitro* tests are, however, not able to provide positive assurance that a compound or one of its metabolites is going to be safe in higher animals. Such tests are, in any case, validated by comparison of the mutagenic effects of chemicals with their carcinogenic effect when used in animal tests.

Animal tests upon food additives can be categorised under four main headings: acute and subacute toxicity tests; absorption, distribution, metabolism and excretion tests; teratogenicity tests; and, long-term carcinogenicity tests.

1 *Acute and subacute toxicity tests* – These tests seek to establish just how much of the additive is required to produce acute toxic and fatal effects. In the subacute tests, animals are exposed to very high doses for three months; tissues are examined microscopically at autopsy for signs of damage.

2 *Absorption, distribution, metabolism and excretion tests* – These seek to establish how much of the additive is absorbed, where it goes after absorption, how it is chemically processed after absorption and how quickly it is excreted. Such studies can give important pointers as to the dangers likely to be associated with consumption of the additive, for example:

- if the compound is not absorbed from the gut, then any adverse effects are likely to be confined to the gut
- if a water soluble substance is absorbed and then excreted unchanged in the urine, then the bladder is the likely danger organ if the substance is carcinogenic
- if the substance is absorbed but only slowly excreted or metabolised, then it will tend to accumulate – chronic low intakes may lead to build up of high levels
- if the substance is metabolised, then metabolites need to be identified and their potential toxicity also needs to be assessed

- if substances are absorbed and detoxified in the liver, and then excreted in the bile or urine, then the liver may be likely to be affected if the compound is carcinogenic.

3 *Teratogenicity testing* – This involves feeding large amounts of the compound to pregnant animals to see if the compound causes birth defects or in any way harms the developing foetuses.

4 *Long-term carcinogenicity testing* – This usually involves exposing test animals to relatively high doses of the additive over the whole life span; their tumour rates are then compared to those of control animals who, apart from lack of exposure to the additive, have been maintained under identical conditions. Such controlled experiments mean that experimenters are able to confidently attribute any increased tumour rate in the test group to the carcinogenic effect of the additive. There are a number of potential criticisms of these tests, such as:

- Substances that are not carcinogenic in laboratory animals may be carcinogenic in people.
- The controlled conditions of testing are very different to those of use. In the tests, genetically homogeneous animals are used; animals are usually fed single additives and are not usually exposed to other chemicals (e.g. drugs, cigarette smoke or alcohol), animals are also maintained on defined laboratory diets. In use, the additive will be fed to genetically diverse people – perhaps only certain genotypes will be sensitive to its toxic effects. In use, there is the possibility that the additive may only become toxic if it interacts with other chemicals or perhaps it becomes harmful under particular dietary or environmental conditions, e.g. deficiency of antioxidant vitamins or minerals.

- Laboratory animals have relatively high background tumour rates. This means that relatively large increases in tumour rate due to the additive will be needed if they are to be detected with the comparatively small numbers of animals used in the tests, i.e. the signal (increase due to additive) must be large to detect it against the background noise (spontaneous tumours not due to additive and occurring randomly in both groups). Thus these tests may be insensitive indicators of carcinogenicity and even small increases in risk can be significant if hundreds of millions of people are to be exposed.

Safety testing of additives depends very much upon animal experiments because they are the only practical methods available. In order to try and ensure safety in use, despite the potential flaws discussed, wide safety margins are used. A **no effect level** is identified in animal experiments, i.e. a dose of lifetime exposure that produces no detectable effects in any species used. This no effect level is then divided by a safety factor (usually 100) to determine an **acceptable daily intake** for people. It is, of course, difficult to predict individual intakes of additives and the difficulty of converting dosages between species of different sizes has already been discussed in Chapter 3.

Additives are very thoroughly tested; many substances naturally present in foods would probably fail such tests, but the inevitable flaws in the testing procedures do suggest the need to use the minimum effective amounts and for there to be a continuing critical review of which additives are to continue to be recognised as safe. Millstone (1986) gives a critical review of food additive regulation and testing from a UK perspective.

Appendix

Variations on a theme

This short section is intended to show how varying the components of a meal can bring about big changes in composition without changing the basic meal structure; sometimes even quite marginal selection changes can bring about relatively large compositional changes. Tables A.1, A.2 and A.3 each show five variations upon a particular meal theme, i.e. a toast and cereal breakfast; a picnic lunch; and a meat, potato and vegetable dinner. These meals have been arbitrarily selected with the sole intention of producing big compositional variations within the given theme and the choice of compositional criteria for display is also fairly arbitrary; there is no intention to suggest which meals are better or healthier or to influence the future choices of the reader. Note for example in Table A.1 the three-fold variation in sugar content, the eleven-fold difference in fibre content, the large variation in P:S values and the substantial variations in calcium and vitamin A contents of the five meals. Note in Table A.2 the large variation in energy density,

the big variation in the contributions of fat and carbohydrate to total calories, and the very large variations in fibre, calcium, vitamin A and vitamin C contents. Note in Table A.3 the large differences in total energy, protein, saturated fat, salt and iron contents of the five meals.

Davies and Dickerson (1991) have been used as a guide to portion sizes. The analysis was performed using computer software with a 1990 American database and so some values may vary slightly from those generated with a British database. The values for composition should, in any case, be regarded as general indicators rather than precise measurements.

This exercise has been used as the basis for undergraduate practical classes and mini projects; students have been asked to analyse given meals and also to devise variations upon themes of their own choosing. The exercise can be extended, for example, by adding in different compositional criteria, by costing the various options or by setting compositional targets within a given theme. The nutritional "value for money" of the different options can be calculated e.g. kcal/penny. The costs can be compared under different circumstances, for example: when using small shops or major supermarkets; when buying small individual packages or large economy packs; or, when buying cheapest or dearest brands. Anyone who has access to food composition software can spend an entertaining hour or two playing around with their own variations. Given time and patience, it is also possible to do it with printed food tables. I have found this to be a very useful and entertaining way of giving students a "feel" for the composition of different foods and which foods are major contributors of particular nutrients to the diet: an educational, nutrition computer game!

Table A.1 Variation 1 – the toast and cereal breakfast

Meal 1 – Cornflakes (25 g) with whole milk and 1 tsp sugar; orange juice (200 ml); cup of coffee with whole milk and 1 tsp sugar; two toasted pop tarts.
Meal 2 – Cornflakes with whole milk and sugar; orange juice; cup of coffee with whole milk and sugar; two slices of white toast (75 g) with two 5 g pats butter and jam (20 g).
Meal 3 – Cornflakes with semi-skimmed (2%) milk and sugar; orange juice; cup of coffee with semi-skimmed milk; two slices of wholemeal toast (70 g) with two 5 g pats soft margarine and jam.
Meal 4 – All Bran with semi-skimmed milk; orange juice; cup of coffee with semi-skimmed milk; two slices of wholemeal toast with butter and jam.
Meal 5 – Two Shredded Wheat with semi-skimmed milk and sugar; half grapefruit with 1 tsp sugar; cup of coffee with semi-skimmed milk; two slices of wholemeal toast with soft margarine.

Nutritional parameter	Meal number				
	1	2	3	4	5
Energy (kcal)	734	640	571	567	560
Weight food (g)	493	490	480	495	405
% calories from:					
Fat	21	22	21	20	21
Carbohydrate	72	69	69	67	67
Protein	7	9	11	13	12
Sugars (g)	60	51	46	47	18
Sat. fat (g)	7	9	4	7	4
P:S ratio	0.2	0.2	1.3	0.2	1.3
Cholesterol (mg)	20	43	11	33	11
Fibre (g)	2	2	9	22	13
Salt (g)	2.3	2.2	2.2	2.7	1.4
Calcium (mg)	404	292	275	311	288
Vitamin A µg RE	517	489	561	793	195
β-carotene µg RE	144	49	49	48	13

Table A.2 The picnic lunch

Meal 1 – Four slices of white bread (150 g) filled with butter (two 5 g pats) cheese (60 g) and 1 tbsp. coleslaw.
Meal 2 – Four slices of white bread filled with butter, ham (60 g) and coleslaw.
Meal 3 – Four slices of wholemeal bread (140 g) filled with soft margarine (two 5 g pats), cheese and tomato.
Meal 4 – Four slices of wholemeal bread filled with cheese and tomato; one apple; one banana.
Meal 5 – Four slices wholemeal bread filled with soft margarine, ham and tomato; one apple; one banana.

Nutritional	Meal number				
parameter	1	2	3	4	5
Energy (kcal)	780	616	677	791	700
Weight food (g)	236	236	333	575	585
% calories from:					
Fat	44	31	41	27	20
Carbohydrate	41	53	41	57	65
Protein	15	16	17	15	15
Saturated fat (g)	20	8	15	14	3
P:S ratio	0.3	0.6	0.4	0.2	1.7
Cholesterol (mg)	90	56	63	63	28
Fibre (g)	2	2	18	24	24
Salt (g)	3.4	4.7	3.2	2.9	4.4
Calcium (mg)	617	189	583	596	170
Vitamin C (mg)	0	16	22	40	56
Vitamin A					
μg RE	267	85	429	337	263
β-carotene					
μg RE	21	9	160	167	164

Table A.3 A meat, potato and vegetable dinner

Meal 1 – Fast food outlet: quarter pound cheeseburger; large french fries; mixed salad
with mayonnaise (16 g).
Meal 2 – Fast food outlet: quarter pound hamburger; small french fries; mixed salad with
oil and vinegar dressing (9 g).
Meal 3 – Half pound sirloin steak (external fat removed); jacket potato (140 g) with soft
margarine (10 g); mixed salad with with oil and vinegar dressing.
Meal 4 – Half pound sirloin steak (with external fat removed); mashed potatoes
(170 g mashed with milk and margarine); broccoli; gravy (from granules).
Meal 5 – One roast chicken leg (skin removed); boiled potatoes; broccoli; gravy
(from granules).

Nutritional parameter	Meal number				
	1	2	3	4	5
Energy (kcal)	1029	702	767	680	357
Weight food (g)	515	426	521	524	440
% calories from:					
Fat	52	50	38	37	21
Carbohydrate	34	33	22	20	44
Protein	14	17	40	43	35
Saturated fat (g)	22	14	11	10	2
P:S ratio	0.3	0.3	0.6	0.3	0.9
Cholesterol (mg)	139	95	181	184	89
Fibre (g)	3	3	6	7	7
Salt (g)	3.9	2.0	0.8	2.5	2.0
Calcium (mg)	335	170	61	121	76
Iron (mg)	5.5	5	8.8	7.1	2.4
Vitamin C (mg)	42	36	42	48	51
Vitamin A μg RE	167	150	272	227	198
β-carotene μg RE	150	150	159	180	180

Glossary

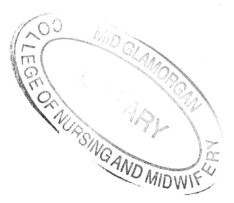

Acceptable daily intake – the daily intake of a food additive judged to be safe for lifetime consumption.

Acculturation – the cultural changes that occur when two cultures interact e.g. when immigrants adopt the cultural practices of the indigenous majority.

Activity diary – system for measuring the activity level. A detailed diary is kept of activities in each time block (say 5min) of the measurement period. Energy expenditure can be crudely estimated from the assumed energy costs of the individual activities.

Aerobic capacity – the capacity of the cardiopulmonary system to supply oxygen to the tissues, one definition of fitness. Can be measured by the vO_2 max., the PWC_{max}, or the PWC_{170}.

Alpha(α)-amylase – starch digesting enzyme present in saliva and pancreatic juice.

Alpha(α)-tocopherol – major dietary form of vitamin E.

Ames test – a test that assesses the carcinogenic potential of a chemical from its tendency to cause mutation in bacteria.

Amino acids – the units that make up proteins. They have an amino group (NH_2) and a carboxyl or acid group ($COOH$).

Amylose – a starch with the sugar residues in unbranched chains.

Amylopectin – the greater part of dietary starch with the sugar residues in branched chains.

Anaemia – low concentration of haemoglobin in blood. **Iron deficiency anaemia** – characterised by small red blood cells (**microcytic anaemia**). Anaemia due to folic acid or vitamin B_{12} deficiency is characterised by large unstable red cells (**macrocytic anaemia**); called **megaloblastic anaemia** after the immature red cell precursors, megaloblasts, in the bone marrow.

Anorexia Nervosa – a potentially fatal, psychological disease principally seen in adolescent girls. Characterised by an obsessive desire to be thin and self starvation.

Anthropometric assessment – assessing nutritional status from anthropometric measurements.

Anthropometry – human measurement, measurements of weight and body dimensions.

Appetite – the hedonistic desire to eat.

Appestat – notional system that monitors and maintains body energy stores by regulating the feeding drive, analagous to a thermostat regulating temperature.

Arachidonic acid, 20:4$_{\omega 6}$ – fatty acid of the ω-6 series; precursor of the eicosanoids.

Attack rates – in food poisoning, the proportion of people who become ill after exposure to a food poisoning "incident". **Food specific attack rate** – the proportion of people eating a particular food who become ill.

ATP, adenosine triphosphate – important short term intracellular energy store. Energy released during the metabolism of foodstuffs is "trapped" as ATP. ATP energy drives synthetic and other energy requiring cellular processes.

Available carbohydrate – sugars and starches, the digestible carbohydrates. Non starch polysaccharides, indigestible by gut enzymes, are the **unavailable carbohydrate**.

Balance – difference between intake and losses of a nutrient. If intake exceeds losses – **positive balance;** if losses exceed intake – **negative balance**. Note particularly **energy balance** and **nitrogen balance**.

Behaviour therapy – psychological approach to the treatment of, for example, obesity. Subjects modify behaviour to avoid situations that trigger inappropriate eating behaviour and reward appropriate behaviours, e.g. taking exercise.

Beriberi – deficiency disease due to lack of thiamin.

"Best before" – date marked on UK foods that are unlikely to become microbiologically unsafe but whose eating qualities may have deteriorated by this time.

Beta(β)-oxidation – process in which fatty acids are metabolised to acetyl coenzyme A in the mitochondria.

Bifidus factor – substance in breast milk that stimulates the growth of certain *lactobacilli*.

Blind challenge – diagnostic procedure used to confirm food intolerance. The subject is offered foods that do and do not contain the suspected cause but is unaware of which is which.

BMI, Body mass index – the weight in kilogrammes divided by the height in metres squared. Used as an indicator of overweight or obesity. Ideal range for adults – 20–25 kg/m^2.

Bomb calorimeter – device for measuring the heat released when food is burned; a crude indication of its dietary energy value.

Botulism – rare but potentially fatal form of food poisoning caused by the toxin of *Clostridium botulinum*. Causes paralysis, including the respiratory muscles.

Botulinum cook – vigorous heat treatment applied to canned foods to ensure the destruction of spores of *Clostridium botulinum*.

Bran – outer layer of the cereal grain containing most of the fibre (NSP); may be removed during milling. White flour has had the bran removed but in wholemeal flour it remains.

Brown adipose tissue (BAT) or brown fat – literally adipose tissue that appears brown. Prominent in small mammals and babies where it is the principal site of non shivering thermogenesis. Postulated as a site for luxoskonsumption or diet-induced thermogenesis.

BSE, bovine spongiform encephalopathy – a disease of cattle, one of a group of fatal degenerative brain infections that result in "spongiform lesions" in the brain. Other spongiform encephalopathies are: **scrapie** in sheep and goats; **kuru**, associated with cannibalism in New Guinea; and, **Creutzfeld-Jacob disease, CJD** which causes about 30 deaths each year in the UK.

Bulimia – an eating disorder. Characterised by alternating periods of fasting and binging.

C-terminal – the end of a protein that has a free carboxyl group.

Cancer cachexia – weight loss associated with malignant disease.

Carbohydrate loading – training and dietary regimens that attempt to boost muscle glycogen stores.

Casein – a milk protein, the dominant protein in cow milk.

Casein dominant formula – infant formula with casein as the dominant protein.

Case-control study – type of epidemiological study. Cases of a disease are matched with unaffected controls and the diet of the two groups compared. Differences may suggest the cause of the disease.

Beta(β)-carotene – a plant pigment found in many coloured fruits and vegetables; acts as a vitamin A precursor.

Catalase – iron containing enzyme involved in free radical disposal.

Centile – hundredths of the population e.g. the fifth centile for height would be the height below which would be found 5% of a population. Note also **quintile** (division into fifths), **quartile** (division into quarters) and **tertile** (divided into thirds).

Chemical score – a measure of protein quality. Amount of the limiting amino acid in a gram of test protein as a percentage of that in a gram of reference protein e.g. egg.

Cholecalciferol – vitamin D_3.

Chylomicrons – triglyceride-rich lipoproteins found in plasma after feeding. The form in which absorbed fat is transported away from the gut.

Chronic renal failure – progressive loss of renal function associated with uraemia. Low protein diets give symptomatic relief of uraemia and may slow down progression of the disease.

Coeliac disease – allergy to the wheat protein, gluten, causing damage to the absorptive surface of the gut. Characterised by malabsorption, various gastointestinal symptoms and malnutrition.

Coenzyme/cofactor – non protein substance needed for an enzyme to function; many are derivatives of vitamins.

Colostrum – protein and antibody rich fluid secreted from the breast in very early lactation.

COMA, Committee on Medical Aspects of Food Policy – a committee within the UK Department of Health. Produces many important nutrition and food-related reports.

Committee on Toxicology, COT – UK committee that advises upon the safety of food additives.

Confounding variable – an epidemiological term. An association between a dietary variable and a disease may be an artefact caused because both test variables are influenced by a third "confounding" variable, e.g. a relationship between alcohol intake and lung cancer might be because smoking causes lung cancer and smokers drink more alcohol than non-smokers.

Cohort study – type of epidemiological study. Measurements are recorded on a sample or cohort of people and these measurements related to subsequent mortality or morbidity.

Collagen – the most abundant protein in the human body. A key structural component of muscle, bone, heart muscle and connective tissue.

Complete proteins – proteins with good amounts of all the essential amino acids, e.g. most animal and legume proteins.

Contaminants – chemicals that are incidentally or accidentally added to foods, e.g. residues of agricultural chemicals.

Cretinism – a condition in young children caused by undersecretion of thyroid hormones e.g. in iodine deficiency. Physical and mental development can be severely impaired.

Cultural relativism – the opposite of ethnocentrism, trying to regard all different cultural practices as normal.

Cultural superfood – a food that has acquired a cultural significance that goes beyond its purely nutritional or dietary importance, e.g. rice in Japan.

Cystic fibrosis – inherited disease that results in progressive fibrosis and loss of function of the lungs and pancreas. Failure of pancreatic secretion reduces digestion and absorption of fat and protein and poor fat soluble vitamin absorption.

Death rate – crude death rate is the number of deaths per year per 1000 people in the population. **Age-specific death rate** is the number of deaths of people within a specified age range per year per 1000 people in that age range. May also be for a specified cause.

Deficiency disease – a disease caused by lack of a nutrient.

Delaney clause – passed by the US Congress "no additive shall be deemed to be safe if it is found to induce cancer when ingested by man or animal". Nowadays regarded as unreasonably absolute in its prohibitions.

Dermatitis herpetiformis – form of coeliac disease that presents as a chronic skin disorder.

Diet-heart hypothesis – the suggestion that high dietary saturated fat increases LDL-cholesterol leading to increased atherosclerosis and ultimately increased risk of coronary heart disease.

Diabetes mellitus – disease caused by lack of the pancreatic hormone insulin. Characterised by high blood glucose, glucose loss in urine and, in severe cases, ketosis. Severe diabetes, **insulin dependent diabetes mellitus (IDDM)**, usually presents in childhood and requires insulin replacement; the milder form **non insulin dependent diabetes mellitus (NIDDM)** presents in middle or old age and does not require insulin.

Diabetic nephropathy – progressive loss of renal function associated with diabetes.

Diabetic retinopathy – progressive degeneration of the retina that may cause blindness in diabetics.

Dietary fibre – plant material in the diet that resists digestion by human gut enzymes, "roughage". Essentially synonymous with non starch polysaccharide.

1,25 dihydroxycholecalciferol, 1,25 DHCC – hormone produced in the kidney from vitamin D. Stimulates the production of proteins necessary for the active absorption of calcium in gut and kidney.

Discretionary salt – salt that is added during home cooking of food or at the table.

Decayed, missing and filled teeth, (DMF) – a measure of dental health, usually of children.

Double blind trial – clinical trial using real and placebo treatments where neither the subject nor operator knows which is which until the trial is completed.

Doubly-labelled-water-method – method of estimating the long-term energy expenditure of free living subjects. Subjects are given water labelled with both the heavy isotopes of oxygen and hydrogen. Labelled oxygen is lost as both CO_2 and water whereas hydrogen is lost only as water. The difference between the rate of loss of oxygen and hydrogen can thus be used to estimate CO_2 output and therefore energy expenditure.

Dietary reference values (DRVs) (UK) – a general term to cover all dietary standards. It includes the RNI (listed separately), the **estimated average requirement (EAR),** and the **lower reference nutrient intake (LRNI)** – the estimated requirement of people with a particularly low need for the nutrient. Where data is limited, a **safe intake** is given.

Delayed-type cutaneous hypersensitivity (DTH) – functional test of cell-mediated immune function. Antigen is injected into the skin and a reaction occurs after several hours delay e.g. the **Mantoux reaction** to a cutaneous tuberculin injection.

Dual-centre hypothesis – the notion that feeding is regulated by two centres within the hypothalamus. A spontaeously active **feeding centre** in the lateral hypothalamus that is periodically inhibited by a **satiety centre** in the ventromedial hypothalamus.

E numbers – a European system of designating food additives by number.

Eicosanoids – a group of locally acting regulatory molecules synthesised from essential fatty acids, e.g. **prostaglandins, thromboxanes** and **prostacyclins**.

Elemental diet – diet composed of purified nutrients, e.g. in the diagnosis of food allergy.

Endergonic reaction – chemical reaction that absorbs energy.

Energy density – amount of energy per unit weight of food, e.g. kcal/g

Energy equivalent of oxygen – the energy expended when one litre of oxygen is consumed by a subject. Varies according to the mix of substrates being metabolised (around 4.8 kcal/l [20kJ/l]).

Enzymes – proteins that speed up cellular reactions. All cellular reactions are "catalysed" by specific enzymes.

Erythrocyte glutathione reductase activation coefficient (EGRAC) – biochemical indicator of riboflavin status. Derived from one of the erythrocyte enzyme activation tests used to assess vitamin status. The extent to which the enzyme is activated by addition of an excess of vitamin-derived coenzyme is inversely related to the vitamin status of the donor.

Endurance – the maximum duration that one is able to sustain an activity. Training increases the endurance of particular muscle groups and the cardiopulmonary system.

Enteral feeding – feeding via the gut, e.g. using a nasogastric tube.

Entero-hepatic circulation – re-absorption and return to the liver of substances secreted in the bile, e.g. bile acids.

EPA, eicosapentaenoic acid, $20:5_{\omega 3}$ – fatty acid of the ω-3 series. With **DHA, docosahexaenoic, $22:6_{\omega 3}$** the "active ingredients" of fish oils.

Essential amino acids – those amino acids that are essential in the diet because they cannot be made by transamination.

Essential fatty acids – polyunsaturated fatty acids that must be provided in the diet. They serve structural functions and are the precursors of the eicosanoids.

Ethnocentrism – the tendency to regard one's own cultural practices as the norm and others as inferior or wrong.

Exergonic reaction – chemical reaction that releases energy.

Factorial calculation – an apparently logical prediction, of say nutrient needs by taking into account a series of factors, e.g. predicting the additional calcium needs of pregnant women from the rate of calcium accumulation during pregnancy and the assumed efficiency of calcium absorption in the gut.

Flavin adenine dinucleotide and flavin mononucleotide FAD, FMN, – prosthetic groups derived from riboflavin, important as hydrogen acceptors/donators in several cellular oxidation/reduction reactions.

Familial hypercholesteraemia – inherited condition characterised by very high serum LDL-cholesterol. The defect is in the LDL receptor and is associated with increased risk of heart disease.

Fat cell theory – the proposal that overfeeding in childhood permanently increases susceptibility to obesity by increasing the number of fat cells.

Fat soluble vitamins – th lipid soluble vitamins, i.e. A, D, E and K.

Fatty acids – the major components of fats. Made up of a hydrocarbon chain and a terminal carboxyl or acid group (COOH). If no double bonds in the hydrocarbon chain – **saturated**, one double bond – **monounsaturated**, more than one – **polyunsaturated**.

Favism – a haemolytic anaemia that may result from eating broad beans. Around 30% of Mediterranean people and 10% of black Americans may be susceptible.

Food and Drug Administration (FDA) – the US department responsible for food and drug regulation.

Feeding centre – see dual-centre hypothesis.

Ferritin – an iron protein complex, the principal storage form of iron in the body.

Fitness – conditioning brought about by exercise; often defined as aerobic capacity but could include all physical and mental effects of training.

Flavoproteins – enzymes with FAD or FMN prosthetic groups.

Flexibility – joint mobility. The range of movement that can be safely and comfortably achieved.

Foetal alcohol syndrome (FAS) – a syndrome of children born to mothers who consume excess alcohol during pregnancy.

Food additives – chemicals deliberately added to food, e.g. preservatives, colours, flavourings etc.

Food Advisory Committee, FAC – UK committee that advises upon the necessity for food additives.

Food allergy – intolerance to a food that involves an abnormal immunological reaction.

Food balance sheets – population method of estimating food intake. The food available for human consumption is estimated and then expressed on a *per capita* basis.

Foodborne disease – a disease that can be transmitted via food. Includes both food poisoning and diseases like typhoid and cholera where there is no need for the organism to grow in the food.

Food groups – dividing foods up into groups or categories according to their nutrient contents. Selecting from each group should ensure nutritional adequacy, e.g. the **four food group plan**: the meat group; the fruit and vegetable group; the milk group; and, the cereal group.

Food guide pyramid – a visual guide to food selection. A development of the four food group plan but additionally indicates the ideal proportions from the different groups to meet current dietary guidelines.

Food intolerance – "a reproducible, unpleasant (i.e. adverse) reaction to a specific food or ingredient which is not psychologically based".

Fractional catabolic rate – the proportion of the total body pool of a nutrient that is catabolised each day, e.g. around 3% of body vitamin C is broken down each day.

Food poisoning – illness, usually acute gastroenteritis, caused by ingestion of food in which there has been active growth of bacteria.

Free radicals – highly reactive chemical species produced as a by-product of oxidative processes in cells. Free radical damage has been implicated in the aetiology of many diseases including cancer and atherosclerosis.

Galactosaemia – inherited condition in which galactose cannot be metabolised and accumulates in the blood. Sufferers must avoid lactose, milk sugar.

Gatekeeper – someone who effectively controls the food choices of others. Wives and mothers have traditionally been family gatekeepers but also describes catering managers in institutions.

Gas liquid chromatography (GLC) – a separation technique, e.g. of fatty acids or fat soluble vitamins.

Gluconeogenesis – the synthesis of glucose, e.g. from amino acids.

Glucostatic theory – the notion that sensors (e.g. in the ventromedial hypothalamus) modulate the feeding drive in response blood glucose concentration.

Glutathione peroxidase – selenium containing enzyme involved in free radical disposal.

Glutathione reductase – flavoprotein enzyme involved in free radical disposal.

Gluten – a protein in wheat.

Glycogen – form of starch stored in the liver and muscles of animals.

Glycosylated – having reacted abnormally with glucose. Proteins become glycosylated due to hyperglycaemia in diabetics. Glycosylation may cause some of the long term problems of diabetes e.g. diabetic retinopathy and nephropathy.

Goitre – swelling of the thyroid gland, e.g. due to lack of dietary iodine.

Gold thioglucose – chemical that produces permanent obesity in mice by damaging the ventromedial region of the hypothalamus – see dual-centre hypothesis.

Generally recognised as safe (GRAS) – a list of permitted food additives whose use became widespread before current regulatory procedures were established.

Haemagglutinin – substance that causes red blood cells to clump together. Found in red kidney beans; causes vomiting and diarrhoea if undercooked beans are eaten.

Haemoglobin – iron containing pigment in blood that transports oxygen.

Hartnup disease – rare inherited disorder with symptoms of pellagra. Caused by failure to absorb tryptophan and responds to niacin therapy.

Hazard – "being likely to produce injury under the circumstances of exposure," e.g. as in food c.f. toxic.

High density lipoprotein (HDL) – a blood lipoprotein. Carries cholesterol from the tissues to the liver. Negatively associated with risk of heart disease.

Heat stroke – combination of hyperthermia and dehydration that may affect endurance athletes.

Hexose – a six carbon sugar e.g. glucose, fructose or galactose.

High temperature-short time – modern method of pasteurisation that exposes food to a higher temperature than traditional pasteurisation but for a much shorter time.

Hot and cold – traditional food classification system, widely used in China, India and South America.

24 hour recall – retrospective method of estimating food intake. Subjects recall and quantify everything eaten and drunk in the previous 24 hours. Note also **diet histories** where an interviewer tries to obtain a detailed assessment of the subject's habitual intake and self administered **food frequency questionnaires**.

Hormone replacement therapy (HRT) – oestrogen administered to postmenopausal women when natural production of sex hormones ceases.

Hunger – the physiological drive or need to eat.

Hydrogenated vegetable oils – margarine and solid vegetable-based shortening. Vegetable oil that has been treated with hydrogen to solidify it.

Hydroxyapatite – the crystalline, calcium phosphate material of bones.

Hydroxyl radical – a free radical.

Hypernatraemic dehydration – literally, dehydration with high blood sodium concentration. Associated with high sodium infant formulae prior to 1976 in the UK.

Immunoglobulin (Ig) – antibodies. **IgA** protects mucosal surfaces, **IgG** is the main circulating antibody and **IgE** the fraction associated with allergic responses.

Incidence – the number of new cases of a disease occurring within a specified time period.

Incomplete proteins – proteins deficient in one or more essential amino acids.

Infective dose – the number of microorganisms that must be ingested to provoke illness.

Irradiation – of food. Exposing food to ionising radiation in order to delay ripening, inhibit sprouting, kill insect pests or kill spoilage and pathogenic organisms.

Isomers – chemicals that have the same set of atoms but whose spatial arrangement is different.

Isomerisation – changing the isomeric form.

Joule – The Standard International unit of energy: "the energy expended when a mass of 1 kg is moved through a distance of 1 m by a force of 1 newton". **Kilojoule (kJ)** = 1000 joules; **megajoule (MJ)** = a million joules; 4.2 kJ = 1 kcal.

Kcal, kilocalorie – widely used in nutrition as the unit of energy "the heat required to raise the temperature of a litre of water by 1°C". 1 kcal = 4.2 kJ. Calorie and kcal often used as synonyms.

Keshan disease – a degeneration of heart muscle seen in parts of China and attributed to selenium deficiency.

Ketone bodies – substances produced from fatty acids and used as alternative brain substrates during starvation – β-hydroxybutyrate, acetoacetic acid and acetone.

Ketosis – toxic accumulation of ketone bodies, e.g. in diabetes.

Krebs cycle – the core pathway of oxidative metabolism in mitochondria. Activated acetate feeds in and carbon dioxide, ATP and reduced coenzymes (e.g. $NADH_2$) are the products.

Kwashiorkor – one manifestation of protein energy malnutrition in children. Often oedema, swollen liver and subcutaneous fat is still present. Traditionally attributed to primary protein deficiency, now widely considered to be a manifestation of simple starvation.

Lactose – milk sugar, disaccharide of glucose and galactose.

Lactose intolerance – an inability to digest lactose found in many adult populations; milk consumption causes diarrhoea and gas production.

Lathyrism – a severe disease of the spinal cord caused by eating very large amounts of chick peas (*Lathyrus sativa*).

Low density lipoprotein (LDL) – a blood lipoprotein. Rich in cholesterol and the form in which cholesterol is transported to the tissues. High LDL is associated with increased risk of heart disease.

LDL-receptor – receptor that binds to LDL and removes it from the blood. 75% of LDL-receptors are in the liver.

Limiting amino acid – the essential amino acid present in the lowest amount relative to requirement. It can limit the extent to which other amino acids can be used for protein synthesis.

Lipase – a fat digesting enzyme, e.g. in pancreatic juice.

Lipoprotein lipase – an enzyme in capillaries that hydrolyses fat in lipoproteins prior to absorption into the cell.

Lipoproteins – lipid/protein complexes. Fats are transported in blood as lipoproteins.

Lipostatic theory – the notion that body fat level is regulated by it having a modulating effect upon the feeding drive.

Listeriosis – foodborne disease caused by *Listeria monocytogenes*. Can cause miscarriage, stillbirth or neonatal death. Associated with chilled foods like pate, cheese made with raw milk and chilled ready meals.

Low birth weight (LBW) – of babies. Birth weight under 2.5 kg. Associated with increased risk of perinatal mortality and morbidity.

Luxoskonsumption – an adaptive increase in metabolic rate in response to overfeeding – diet-induced thermogenesis.

Mid-arm circumference (MAC) – circumference of the mid part of the upper arm. Anthropometric indicator of nutritional status, used in Third World children and bedridden hospital patients who cannot be weighed.

Mid-arm muscle circumference (MAMC) – a measure of lean body mass = MAC – [π × triceps skinfold].

Ministry of Agriculture, Fisheries and Food, (UK). **(MAFF)**

Marasmus – one manifestation of protein energy malnutrition in children. Affected children are emaciated; attributed to simple energy deficit.

Metabolic rate – rate of body energy expenditure. May be measured directly as the heat output in a **whole body calorimeter** or indirectly from the rate of oxygen consumption using: a **static spirometer; Max Planck respirometer**; analysis of expired air collected in a **Douglas bag**; or, analysis of expired air of subject in a **respiration chamber**.

Metabolic response to injury – changes in metabolism that follow mechanical or disease "injury". A period of reduced metabolism, shock or **ebb,** followed by a longer period of increased metabolism and protein breakdown, **flow.**

Metabolisable energy – the "available energy" from a food after allowing for faecal loss of unabsorbed material and urinary loss of nitrogenous compounds from incomplete oxidation of protein.

Mitochondria – subcellular particles; the site of oxidative metabolism.

Mutual supplementation of proteins – compensation for deficit of an essential amino acid in one dietary protein by excess in another.

Mycotoxins – toxic substances produced by fungi or moulds, e.g. **aflatoxins** (mouldy nuts), **patulin** (apples or apple juice) and **ergot** (mouldy grain). Some are known carcinogens.

Myelin – the fatty sheath around many nerve fibres.

Myoglobin – a pigment similar to haemoglobin found in muscle.

N-terminal – the end of a protein with a free amino group.

National Advisory Committee on Nutrition Education (NACNE) – an *ad hoc* group who in 1983 produced the most influential series of nutrition education guidelines in the UK.

Nicotine adenine dinucleotide (NAD) – hydrogen acceptor molecule produced from niacin. A coenzyme in numerous oxidation/reduction reactions. Re-oxidation of reduced NAD in oxidative phosphorylation yields most of the ATP from the oxidation of foodstuffs.

NADP – a phosphorylated derivative of NAD that usually acts as a hydrogen donor, e.g. in fat synthesis.

National Food Survey – an example of a **household survey**. An annual survey of the household food purchases of a representative sample of UK households. Provides information about regional and class differences in food purchasing and national dietary trends.

Natural toxicants – toxic substances naturally present in food that may occasionally represent a hazard to the consumer.

Niacin equivalents – way of expressing the niacin content of food. Includes both niacin and niacin produced endogenously from the amino acid tryptophan.

Niacytin – the bound form of niacin in many cereals. In this form it is unavailable to humans.

Night blindness – impaired vision at low light intensity. Early sign of vitamin A deficiency.

No effect level – intake of additive that produces no adverse effects in animal tests.

Non-milk extrinsic sugars – added dietary sugars, i.e. all the sugars other than those naturally in fruits, vegetables and milk.

Non-starch polysaccharide (NSP) – dietary polysaccharides other than starch. Indigestible by human gut enzymes and thus they make up the bulk of dietary fibre.

Normal distribution – even distribution of individual values for a variable around the mean value. Most individual values are close to the mean and the further away from the mean the lower the frequency of individuals becomes. Results in a bell-shaped curve when a frequency distribution is plotted.

Net protein utilisation (NPU) – a measure of protein quality. The percentage of nitrogen retained when a protein (or diet) is fed at amounts that do not satisfy an animals total protein needs. Losses are corrected for those on a protein-free diet.

National Research Council (NRC) – a group that has produced several important reports relating to food and nutrition in the US. Under the auspices of the National Academy of Sciences.

Neural Tube Defects (NTD) – a group of birth defects, e.g. spina bifida.

Nutrient density – the amount of a nutrient per kcal or per kJ. Indicates the value of a food as a source of the nutrient; when applied to diets indicates the likely adequacy of that diet for the nutrient.

Nutritional supplements – concentrated nutrient sources, usually given in liquid form to boost the intakes of patients.

Nutrition team – specialist group in a hospital charged with supervising the nutritional management of problem patients, e.g. those on TPN. May include physicians, dietitians, nutrition nurse specialists, pharmacists and sometimes speech therapists.

Odds ratio – indirect measure of relative risk in case-control studies "the odds of case exposure divided by the odds of control exposure".

Oil of evening primrose – source of gamma-linolenic acid ($18:3_{\omega 6}$). Widely taken as a dietary supplement.

Omega(ω)-3 fatty acids – polyunsaturated fatty acids where the first double bond is between carbons 3 and 4. The predominant polyunsaturates in many fish oils, a few vegetable oils have good amounts e.g. walnut oil, soya oil and rapeseed (canola) oil.

Omega(ω)-6 fatty acids – polyunsaturated fatty acids where the first double bond lies between carbons 6 and 7. The predominant polyunsaturates in most vegetable oils.

Organic produce – food produced without the aid of agricultural chemicals.

Osteomalacia – disease of adults caused by lack of vitamin D.

Osteoporosis – a progressive loss of bone matrix and mineral making bones liable to fracture, especially in postmenopausal women.

Oxidative phosphorylation – the re-oxidation of reduced coenzymes in the mitochondria with oxygen. This process produces the bulk of the ATP in aerobic metabolism.

Parenteral feeding – intravenous feeding.

Pasteurisation – mild heat treatment of foods that kills likely pathogens without impairing palatability or nutrient content, e.g. pasteurised milk.

Peak bone mass – the maximum bone mass reached by adults in their thirties. After this bone mass starts to decline.

Pellagra – deficiency disease due to lack niacin.

Pentose phosphate pathway – a metabolic pathway that produces ribose for nucleic acid synthesis and reduced NADP for processes like fatty acid synthesis.

Protein energy malnutrition (PEM) – general term used to cover undernutrition due to lack of energy or protein or both. Encompasses kwashiorkor and marasmus.

Peptidases – enzymes in protein digestion that hydrolyse peptide bonds in small proteins (peptides).

Peptide bond – bonds that link amino acids together in proteins. An amino group of one amino acid is linked to the carboxyl group of another.

Pernicious anaemia – autoimmune disease. Failure to produce **intrinsic factor** in the stomach, necessary for vitamin B_{12} absorption. Symptoms are severe megaloblastic anaemia and **combined subacute degeneration of the spinal cord** leading to progressive paralysis.

Phospholipids – lipids containing a phosphate moiety. Important components of membranes.

Phenylketonuria (PKU) – inherited disease in which there is inability to metabolise the amino acid phenylalanine. Intake of phenylalanine must be strictly controlled to avoid severe mental retardation.

Phylloquinone – the major dietary form of vitamin K.

Placebo – dummy treatment that enables the psychological effects of treatment to be distinguished from the physiological effects.

Plaque – a sticky mixture of food residue, bacteria and bacterial polysaccharides that adheres to teeth.

Pre-eclampsia – hypertension of pregnancy.

Prevalence – number of cases of a disease at any point in time; depends both upon the prevalence and the duration of the illness.

Prions – unidentified, virus-like infective agents responsible for causing BSE and the other spongiform encephalopathies.

Proline hydroxylase – a vitamin C dependent enzyme vital for collagen formation.

Prosthetic group – a non protein moiety that is tightly bound to an enzyme an is necessary for it to function.

Prostaglandins – see eicosanoids.

Proteases – enzymes involved in protein digestion. Break proteins into smaller peptide fragments by hydrolysing peptide bonds.

Protein efficiency ratio – a measure of the quality of dietary protein. If growing rats are fed restricted protein diets with other nutrients in excess, then this is the grams of body weight gain per gram of protein consumed.

Protein gap – the notional gap between world protein requirements and supplies that disappeared as estimates of human protein requirements were revised downwards.

Protein turnover – the total amount of protein broken down and re-synthesised in a day.

Prothrombin time – a functional test of prothrombin level in blood used as a measure of vitamin K status.

PWC$_{170}$ – work load at which pulse rate reaches 170 beats per minute. A measure of aerobic fitness.

PWC$_{max}$ – work load at maximum heart rate. A measure of aerobic fitness.

Radiolytes – short-lived chemicals produced in foods by irradiation.

Recommended dietary allowance (RDA) (US) – the suggested average daily intake of a nutrient for healthy people in a population. Equivalent to the UK RNI, represents the estimated requirement of those people with a particularly high need for the nutrient. The energy RDA is the best estimate of average requirement.

Relative risk – an epidemiological term. Ratio of the number of cases per 1000 in an exposed population to those in an unexposed population e.g. the ratio of deaths per 1000 in smokers v non smokers.

Retinol – vitamin A.

Retinol equivalents – the way of expressing vitamin A content: 1 mg retinol or 6 mg carotene = 1 mg retinol equivalents.

Retinopathy of prematurity – blindness in newborn babies caused by exposure to high oxygen concentrations. Believed to result from free radical damage.

Rhodopsin – light sensitive pigment in the rods of the retina. Contains a derivative of vitamin A, **11 *cis* retinal**. All visual pigments are based upon 11 cis retinal.

Rickets – disease of children caused by lack of vitamin D.

Respiratory quotient (RQ) – ratio of CO_2 produced to oxygen consumed. Varies according to the substrates being oxidised and can indicate the mix of substrates being oxidised by a subject.

Reliability – the technical accuracy or repeatability of a measurement (c.f. **validity**).

Saccharide – a sugar. Note **mono**saccharide (comprised of one sugar unit), **di**saccharide (two units), **oligo**saccharide (a few) and **poly**saccharide (many).

Satiety centre – see dual-centre hypothesis.

Satiety signals – physiological signals that induce satiation, e.g. high blood glucose and stomach fullness.

Saxitoxin – a plankton neurotoxin that may cause poisoning if mussels are eaten at times when this red plankton is abundant in the sea, "red tides".

Scrombotoxin – a toxin produced in spoiled fish by the action of bacteria upon fish protein.

Scurvy – deficiency disease due to lack of vitamin C.

Skin sensitivity tests – used in the identification of (food) allergens. Suspected allergens are injected into the skin and the extent of the skin reaction used to indicate sensitivity.

Solanine – poisonous alkaloid found in small amounts in potatoes.

Soluble fibre/non-starch polysaccharide (NSP) – that part of the dietary fibre that forms gums or gels when mixed with water, c.f. **insoluble fibre/NSP** that part which is insoluble in water like cellulose.

Spoilage – deterioration in the appearance or palatability of food caused by the action of spoilage bacteria.

Standard deviation (SD) – a statistical term that describes the distribution of individual values around the mean in a normal distribution. Approximately 95% of individual values lie within two SD either side of the mean.

Standard mortality ratio (SMR) – way of comparing death rates in populations of differing age structures "the ratio of actual deaths in test population to those predicted assuming it had the same age-specific death rates as a reference population".

Specific activity – amount of activity per unit weight, e.g. the amount of radioactivity per mg of labelled substance or the amount of enzyme activity/mg of protein.

Sugar-fat-seesaw – the tendency for fat and sugar intakes of affluent individuals to be inversely related, i.e. low fat diets tend to be high sugar and vice versa.

Superoxide radical – a free radical.

Superoxide dismutase – zinc containing enzyme that disposes of superoxide free radicals.

Taurine – an amino acid. Not used in protein synthesis and can be made from cysteine. Present in large amounts in breast milk and may be essential for babies.

Thermic effect of feeding/postpandial thermogenesis – short-term increase in metabolic rate (thermogenesis) that follows feeding. Due to energy expended in digestion, absorption etc. c.f. diet-induced thermogenesis that usually refers to the longer-term adaptive response to overfeeding.

Thermogenesis – literally heat generation. Metabolic heat generation may be increased by exercise (**exercise induced thermogenesis**), eating (**diet induced thermogenesis**), drugs (**drug induced thermogenesis**) and by cold stress (either shivering or **non-shivering thermogenesis**).

Thyrotropin – pituitary hormone that stimulates release of **thyroxine** and **triiodothyronine** from the thyroid gland.

Toxic – "being inherently capable of producing injury when tested by itself" c.f. hazard.

Total parenteral nutrition (TPN) – fed wholly by infusion into a large vein.

Trans **fatty acids** – isomeric form of unsaturated fatty acids in which the hydrogen atoms around a double bond are on opposite sides c.f. most natural fatty acids where they are on the same side (cis isomer). Major sources are hydrogenated vegetable oils.

Transferrin – protein in plasma that transports iron. Level of **transferrin saturation** with iron is a measure of iron status.

Transamination – the transfer of an amino group (NH_2) from one amino acid to produce another.

Transit time – time taken for ingested material to pass through the gut. Fibre/NSP decreases transit time.

Traveller's diarrhoea – gastroenteritis experienced by traveller's. Often caused by *E. coli* bacteria from contaminated water to which the traveller has low immunity.

Triglyceride – principal form of fat in the diet and adipose tissue. Composed of glycerol and three fatty acids.

Tyramine – substance found in some foods (e.g. cheese) that causes a dangerous rise in blood pressure in people taking certain anti-depressant drugs.

Ultra High Temperature (UHT) – sterilisation by exposing food (e.g. milk) to very high temperatures for very short times, induces much less chemical change than traditional methods.

Uraemia – high blood urea concentration, seen in renal failure, leads to symptoms that include nausea, anorexia, headache and drowsiness.

USDA – United States Department of Agriculture.

"Use by" – date marked on foods in the UK to indicate when they are are likely to become microbiologically unsafe.

Validity – the likelihood that a measurement is a true measure of what one is intending to measure c.f. reliability e.g. a biochemical index of nutritional status could be very precise (high reliability) but not truly indicate nutritional status (low validity).

Vegetarian – one who eats only food of vegetable origin. A **vegan** avoids all animal foods. The prefixes **lacto-**(milk), **ovo-**(eggs) and **pesco-**(fish) are used if some animal foods are used.

Very low calorie diets – preparations designed to contain very few calories but adequate amounts of other nutrients, used in obesity treatment.

Very low density lipoprotein (VLDL) – a triglyceride-rich blood lipoprotein. Transports endogenously produced fat to adipose tissue.

vO₂ max. – the oxygen uptake when exercising maximally, the capacity of the cardiopulmonary system to deliver oxygen tissues. One definition of fitness.

Waist:hip ratio – ratio of waist circumference to that at the hip. Indicator of the level of health risk of obesity, high value considered undesirable.

The **"Wall"** – state of exhaustion in endurance athletes when muscle glycogen reserves are depleted.

Water soluble vitamins – vitamins that are soluble in water i.e. the B and C vitamins.

Weaning – process of transferring infants from breast milk or infant formula onto a solid diet.

Weighed inventory – prospective method of measuring food intake. Subjects weigh and record everything consumed. Household measures rather than weighing may be used.

Wernicke-Korsakoff syndrome – neurological manifestations of thiamin deficiency; often associated with alcoholism.

Whey – a milk protein, the dominant protein in human milk.

Whey dominant formula – infant formula with whey as the major protein.

World Health Organisation (WHO) – the "health department" of the United Nations.

Xerophthalmia – literally dry eyes. Covers all the ocular manifestations of vitamin A deficiency that range from drying and thickening of the conjunctiva through to ulceration/rupture of the cornea and permanent blindness.

References

Akintonwa, A. and Tunwashe, O.L. 1992 Fatal cyanide poisoning from cassava-based meal. *Human and Experimental Toxicology* 11, 47–49

Allied Dunbar National Fitness Survey. 1992 *A report on activity patterns and fitness levels.* London: Sports Council. (Brief summary in Groom, 1993b)

Altschul, A.M. 1965 *Proteins their chemistry and politics.* New York: Basic Books Inc.

Anon. 1984 Marine oils and platelet function in man. *Nutrition Reviews* 42, 189–191

Anon. 1980 Preventing iron deficiency. *Lancet* i, 1117–1118

Armstrong, N., Balding, J., Gentle, P. and Kirby, B. 1990 Physical activity among 11 to 16-year-old British children. *British Medical Journal* 301, 203–205

Ashwell, M. 1992 The BNF Task Force Report on unsaturated fatty acids. *British Nutrition Foundation Nutrition Bulletin* 17, 160–163

Ashwell, M. 1993 Trans in transition. *British Nutrition Foundation Nutrition Bulletin* 18, 150–153

Baker, E.M., Hodges, R.E., Hood, J., Sauberlich, H.E., March, S.C. and Canham, J.E. 1971 Metabolism of ^{14}C- and ^{3}H-labeled L-ascorbic acid in human scurvy. *The American Journal of Clinical Nutrition* 24, 444–454

Barker, D.J.P. and Rose, G. 1990 *Epidemiology in medical practice.* 4th edn. Edinburgh: Churchill Livingstone

Bavly, S. 1966 Changes in food habits in Israel. *The Journal of the American Dietetic Association* 48, 488–495

Bender, D.A. 1983 Effects of a dietary excess of leucine on tryptophan metabolism in the rat: a mechanism for the pellagragenic action of leucine. *British Journal of Nutrition* 50, 25–32

Berry, C.S. 1988 Resistant starch – a controversial component of dietary fibre. *British Nutrition Foundation Nutrition Bulletin* 13, 141–152

Bignall, J. 1993 Decline in sudden infant deaths. *Lancet* 341, 887

Bingham, S.A. 1990 Mechanisms and experimental and epidemiological evidence relating dietary fibre (non starch polysaccharides) and starch to protection against large bowel cancer. *The Proceedings of the Nutrition Society* 49, 153–171

Binns, N.M. 1992 Sugar myths. In *Nutrition and the consumer.* ed. Walker, A.F. and Rolls, B.A. London: Elsevier Applied Science. 161–181

Bistrian, B.R., Blackburn, G.L., Hallowell, E. and Heddle, R. 1974 Protein status of general surgical patients. *Journal of the American Medical Association* 230, 858–860

Blair, S.N., Kohl, H.W., Paffenbarger, R.S., Clark, D.G., Cooper, K.H. and Gibbons, L.W. 1989 Physical fitness and all cause mortality. A prospective study of healthy men and women. *Journal of the American Medical Association* 262, 2395–2401

Blundell, J.E. and Burley, V.J. 1987 Satiation, satiety and the action of dietary fibre on food intake. *International Journal of Obesity* 11 supp. 1, 9–25

BMA 1950 British Medical Association. *Report of the committee on nutrition.* London: British Medical Association

Board, R.G. 1983 *A modern introduction to food microbiology.* Oxford: Blackwell Scientific Publications

Bogert, L.J., Briggs, G.M. and Calloway, D.H. 1973 *Nutrition and physical fitness.* 9th edn. Philadelphia: Saunders

Brobeck, J.R. 1974 Energy balance and food intake. In *Medical physiology* 13th edn. vol 2. ed. Mountcastle, V.B. Saint Louis: The C.V. Mosby Company

Brown, M.S. and Goldstein, J.L. 1984 How LDL receptors influence cholesterol and atherosclerosis. *Scientific American* 251(5), 52–60

Bryan, F.L. 1978 Factors that contribute to outbreaks of foodborne disease. *Journal of Food Protection*, 41, 816–827

Burkitt, D.P. 1971 Epidemiology of cancer of the colon and rectum. *Cancer* 28, 3–13

Burr, M.L., Fehily, A.M., Gilbert, J.F., Rogers, S., Holliday, R.M., Sweetnam, P.M., Elwood, P.C. and Deadman, N.M. 1991 Effects of changes in fat, fish and fibre intakes on death and myocardial infarction: Diet and reinfarction trial (DART). *Lancet* ii, 757–761

Carlson, E., Kipps, M., Lockie, A. and Thomson, J. 1985 A comparative evaluation of vegan, vegetarian and omnivore diets. *Journal of Plant Foods* 6, 89–100

Chandra, R.K. 1993 Nutrition and the immune system. *Proceedings of the Nutrition Society* 52, 77–84

Chesher, 1990 Changes in the nutritional content of household food supplies during the 1980s. In *Household food consumption and expenditure.* Annual report of the National Food Survey Committee. London: HMSO

Church, M. 1979 Dietary factors in malnutrition: quality and quantity of diet in relation to child development. *Proceedings of the Nutrition Society* 38, 41–49

Coghlan, A. 1991 Europe's search for the winning diet. *New Scientist* 30 November, 29–33

COMA 1984 Committee on Medical Aspects of Food Policy. *Diet and cardiovascular disease.* Report on health and social subjects No. 28. London: HMSO

COMA 1988 Committee on Medical Aspects of Food Policy. *Present day practice in infant feeding: third report.* Report on health and social subjects No. 32. London: HMSO

COMA 1989a Committee on Medical Aspects of Food Policy. *Report of the panel on dietary sugars and human disease.* Report on health and social subjects No. 37. London: HMSO

COMA 1989b Committee on Medical Aspects of Food Policy. *The diets of British schoolchildren.* Report on health and social subjects No. 36. London: HMSO

COMA 1991 Committee on Medical Aspects of Food Policy. *Dietary reference values for food energy and nutrients for the United Kingdom.* Report on health and social subjects No. 41. London: HMSO

COMA 1992 Committee on Medical Aspects of Food Policy. *The nutrition of elderly people.* Report on health and social subjects No. 43. London: HMSO

Conning, D. 1991 *Antioxidant nutrients in health and disease.* Briefing paper 25. London: The British Nutrition Foundation

Cooke, E.M. 1991 Epidemiology of foodborne illness: UK. In *Foodborne illness. A Lancet review.* ed. Waites, W.M. and Arbuthnott, J.P. London: Edward Arnold.

Cooper, C. and Eastell, R. 1993 Bone gain and loss in premenopausal women. *British Medical Journal* 306, 1357–1358

Coutts, J. 1979 The dietary management of phenylketonuria. *Proceedings of the Nutrition Society* 38, 315–320

Cramer, D.M., Harlow, B.L., Willett, W.C., Welch, W.R., Bell, D., Scully, R.E., Ng, W.G. and Knapp, R.C. 1989 Galactose consumption and metabolism in relation to risk of ovarian cancer. *Lancet* ii, 66–71

Creagan, E.T., Moertel, C.G., O'Fallon, M.J., Schutt, A.J., O'Connell, M.J., Rubin, J. and Frytak, S. 1979 Failure of high-dose vitamin C to benefit patients with advanced cancer. *New England Journal of Medicine* 301, 687–690

Crouse, J.R. 1989 Gender, lipoproteins, diet, and cardiovascular risk. *Lancet* i, 318–320

Cummings, S.R., Kelsey, J.L., Nevitt, M.C. and O'Dowd, K.J. 1985 Epidemiology of osteoporosis and osteoporotic fractures. *Epidemiologic Reviews* 7, 178–208

Cuthbertson, D.P. 1980 Historical approach. (Introduction to a symposium on surgery and nutrition). *Proceedings of the Nutrition Society* 39, 101–105

Davidson, S. and Passmore, R. 1963 *Human nutrition and dietetics*. 2nd edn. Edinburgh: Livingstone

Davies, J. and Dickerson, J.W.T. 1991 *Nutrient content of food portions*. Cambridge: Royal Society of Chemistry

Davies, J.N.P. 1964 The decline of pellagra in the United States. *Lancet* ii, 195–196

Debenham, K. 1992 Nutrition for specific disease conditions. In *Nutrition and the consumer*. ed Walker, A.F. and Rolls, B.A. London: Elsevier Applied Science. 249–270

Debons, A.F., Krimsky, I., Maayan, M.L., Fani, K. and Jimenez, L.A. 1977 The goldthioglucose obesity syndrome. *Federation Proceedings of the Federation of American Societies for Experimental Biology* 36, 143–147

Denman, A.M. 1979 Nature and diagnosis of food allergy. *Proceedings of the Nutrition Society* 38, 391–402

DH 1992a Department of Health. *The health of the nation. A strategy for health in England*. London: HMSO

DH 1992b Department of Health Expert Advisory Group. *Folic acid and prevention of neural tube defects*. London: Department of Health. (Briefly summarised in Halliday 1992)

DH 1992c Department of Health. *The health of elderly people: an epidemiological overview*. Central health monitoring unit epidemiological overview series, volume 1. London: HMSO

DH 1993 Department of Health. *Report of the Chief Medical Officer's Expert Group on the sleeping position of infants and cot death*. London: HMSO

DHHS 1992 Department of Health and Human Services. *Healthy people 2000*. Boston: Jones and Bartlett Publishers Inc.

DHSS 1969 Department of Health and Social Security. *Recommended intakes of nutrients for the United Kingdom*. Report on public health and medical subjects No. 120. London: HMSO

DHSS 1972 Department of Health and Social Security. *A nutrition survey of the elderly*. Report on health and social subjects No. 3. London: HMSO

DHSS 1979 Department of Health and Social Security. *Nutrition and health in old age*. Report on health and social subjects No. 16. London: HMSO

Diplock, A.T. 1991 Antioxidant nutrients and disease prevention: an overview. *American Journal of Clinical Nutrition* 53, 189S–193S

Dodge, J.A. 1992 Nutrition in cystic fibrosis: a historical overview. *Proceedings of the Nutrition Society* 51, 225–235

Dunnigan, M.G. 1993 The problem with cholesterol. *British Medical Journal* 306, 1355–1356

Durnin, J.V.G.A. 1992 In *Nutrition and physical activity*. ed Norgan, N.G. Cambridge: Cambridge University Press

Durnin, J.V.G.A. and Womersley, J. 1974 Body fat assessed from total body density and its estimation from skinfold thickness: measurements on 481 men and women aged 16 to 72 years. *British Journal of Nutrition* 32, 77–97

Dwyer, T., Ponsonby, L.B., Newman, N.M. and Gibbons, C.E. 1991 Prospective cohort study of prone sleeping position and sudden infant death syndrome. *Lancet* 337, 1244–1247

Dyerberg, J. and Bang, H.O. 1979 Haemostatic function and platelet polyunsaturated fatty acids in Eskimos. *Lancet* ii, 433–435

Easterbrook, P.J., Berlin, J.A., Gopalan, R. and Matthews, D.R. 1992 Publication bias in clinical research. *Lancet* 337, 867–872

Eastwood, M. and Eastwood, M. 1988 Nutrition and diets for endurance runners. *British Nutrition Foundation Nutrition Bulletin* 13, 93–100

Eklund, H., Finnstrom, O., Gunnarskog, J., Kallen, B. and Larsson, Y. 1993 Administration of vitamin K to newborn infants and childhood cancer. *British Medical Journal* 307, 89–91

Elliot, D.L. and Goldberg, L. 1985 Nutrition and exercise. *Medical Clinics of North America* 69, 71–82

Engelberg, H. 1992 Low serum cholesterol and suicide. *Lancet* 339, 727–729

Engelberts, A.C. and de Jonge, G.A. 1990 Choice of sleeping position for infants: possible association with cot death. *Archives of Disease in Childhood* 65, 462–467

Fabry, P. 1969 *Feeding patterns and nutritional adaptations*. London: Butterworths

FDA 1992 Food and Drug Administration. The new food label. *FDA Backgrounder* 92–4, 1–9

Fieldhouse, P. 1986 *Food and nutrition: customs and culture*. London: Croom Helm

Flynn, A. and Connolly, J.F. 1989 Nutrition for athletes. *British Nutrition Foundation Nutrition Bulletin* 14, 163–173

Frantz, I.D. and Moore, R.B. 1969 The sterol hypothesis in atherogenesis. *American Journal of Medicine* 46, 684–690

Frost, C.D., Law, M.R. and Wald, N.J. 1991 By how much does dietary salt reduction lower blood pressure? II – Analysis of observational data within populations. *British Medical Journal* 302, 815–818

Fujita, Y. 1992 Nutritional requirements of the elderly: a Japanese view. *Nutrition Reviews* 50, 449–453

Garrow, J.S. 1992 The management of obesity. Another view. *International Journal of Obesity* 16(suppl 2), S59–S63

Garrow, J.S. 1993 Composition of the body. In Garrow, J.S. and James, W.P.T. eds. *Human nutrition and dietetics. 9th edn.* Edinburgh: Churchill Livingstone. pp.12–23

Garrow, J.S. and James, W.P.T. 1993 *Human nutrition and dietetics. 9th edn.* Edinburgh: Churchill Livingstone

Gilbert, S. 1986 *Pathology of eating. Psychology and treatment.* London: Routledge and Kegan Paul

Gleibermann, L. 1973 Blood pressure and dietary salt in human populations. *Ecology of Food and Nutrition* 2, 143–156

Gold, R.M. 1973 Hypothalamic obesity: the myth of the ventromedial nucleus. *Science* 182, 488–490

Golding, J., Greenwood, R., Birmingham, K. and Mott, M. 1992 Childhood cancer: intramuscular vitamin K, and pethidine given during labour. *British Medical Journal* 305, 341–345

Gounelle de Pontanel, H. 1972 Chairman's opening address. In *Proteins from hydrocarbons. The proceedings of the 1972 symposium at Aix-en-Provence.* London: Academic Press pp.1–2

Gregory, J., Foster, K., Tyler, H. and Wiseman, M. 1990 *The dietary and nutritional survey of British adults.* London: HMSO

Groom, H. 1993a What price a healthy diet? *The British Nutrition Foundation Nutrition Bulletin* 18, 104–109

Groom, H. 1993b How fit is our nation? *The British Nutrition Foundation Nutrition Bulletin* 18, 8–10

Groom, H. and Ashwell, M. *Nutritional aspects of fish.* London: British Nutrition Foundation

Group 1994 The Alpha-Tocopherol, Beta Carotene Cancer Prevention Study Group. The effect of vitamin E and Beta Carotene on the incidence of lung cancer and other cancer in male smokers. *New England Journal of Medicine* 330, 1029–1035

Hallas, T.J. and Walker, A.F. 1992 Vegetarianism: the healthy alternative? In *Nutrition and the consumer.* ed. Walker, A.F. and Rolls, B.A. London: Elsevier Applied Science. pp. 211–247

Halliday, A. 1993 Folic acid and neural tube defects. *British Nutrition Foundation Nutrition Bulletin* 18, 96–99

Halliday, A. and Ashwell, M. 1991a *Non–starch polysaccharides. Briefing paper 22.* London: British Nutrition Foundation

Halliday, A. and Ashwell, M. 1991b *Calcium. Briefing paper 24.* London: British Nutrition Foundation

Hamilton, E.M.N., Whitney, E.N. and Sizer, F.S. 1991 *Nutrition. Concepts and controversies. 5th edn.* St. Paul, MN: West Publishing Company

Harris, M.B. 1983 Eating habits, restraint, knowledge and attitudes toward obesity. *International Journal of Obesity* 7, 271–286

Hausberger, F.X. and Volz, J.E. 1984 Feeding in infancy, adipose tissue cellularity and obesity. *Physiology and Behaviour* 33, 81–88

Hawthorn, J. 1989 Safety and wholesomeness of irradiated foods. *British Nutrition Foundation Nutrition Bulletin* 14, 150–162

Hayden, R.M. and Allen, G.J. 1984 Relationship between aerobic exercise, anxiety, and depression: convergent validation by knowledgeable informants. *Journal of Sports Medicine* 24, 69–74

Hazel, T. and Southgate, D.A.T. 1985 Trends in the consumption of red meat and poultry – nutritional implications. *British Nutrition Foundation Nutrition Bulletin* 10, 104–117

HEA 1994 Health Education Authority. *The balance of good health.* London: Health Education Authority

Health and Fitness 1993 A supplement to *Chemist and Druggist,* 13 March 1993

Hegsted, D.M. (1986) Calcium and osteoporosis. *Journal of Nutrition,* 116, 2316–2319

Hervey, G.R. and Tobin, G. 1983 Luxuskonsumption, diet-induced thermogenesis and brown fat: a critical review. *Clinical Science* 64, 7–18

Hetzel, B.S. 1993 Iodine deficiency disorders. In Garrow, J.S. and James, W.P.T. eds. *Human nutrition and dietetics. 9th edn.* Edinburgh: Churchill Livingstone. pp.534–555

Hill, G.L., Blackett, R.L., Pickford, I., Burkinshaw, L., Young, G.A., Warren, J.V., Schorah, C.J. and Morgan, D.B. 1977 Malnutrition in surgical patients. An unrecognised problem. *Lancet* i, 689–692

Hirsch, J. and Han, P.W. (1969) Cellularity of rat adipose tissue: effects of growth, starvation and obesity. *Journal of Lipid Research* 10, 77–82

Hobbs, B.C. and Roberts, D. 1993 *Food poisoning and food hygiene.* 6th. edn. London: Edward Arnold

Hull, D. 1992 Vitamin K and childhood cancer. *British Medical Journal* 305, 326–327

Hulley, S.B., Walsh, J.M.B. and Newman, T.B. 1992 Health policy on blood cholesterol time to change directions. *Circulation* 86, 1026–1029

IFT 1975 A report by the Institute of Food Technologists' Expert Panel on Food Safety and Nutrition and the Committee on Public Information. Naturally occurring toxicants in foods. *Food Technology* 29(3), 67–72

Isles, C.G., Hole, D.J., Gillis, C.R., Hawthorne, V.M. and Lever, A.F. 1989 Plasma cholesterol, coronary heart disease, and cancer in the Renfrew and Paisley survey. *British Medical Journal* 298, 920–924

Jacob, M. 1993 Legislation. In Hobbs, B.C. and Roberts, D. 1993 *Food poisoning and food hygiene.* 6th. edn. London: Edward Arnold. pp. 280–302

Jacobs, D., Blackburn, H., Higgins, M., Reed, D., Iso, H., Mcmillan, G., Neaton, J., Nelson, J., Potter, J., Rifkind, B., Rossouw, J., Shekelle, R. and Yusuf, S. 1992 Report of the conference on low blood cholesterol: mortality associations. *Circulation* 86, 1046–1059

Jacobson, M.S. 1987 Cholesterol oxides in Indian Ghee: possible cause of unexplained high risk of atherosclerosis in Indian immigrant populations. *Lancet* ii, 656–658

James, W.P.T., Ralph, A. and Sanchez–Castillo, C.P. 1987 The dominance of salt in manufactured food in the sodium intake of affluent societies. *Lancet* i, 426–428

Jarjou, L.M.A., Prentice, A., Sawo, Y., Darboe, S., Day, K., Paul, A.A. and Fairweather-Tait, S. 1994 Changes in the diet of Mandinka women in The Gambia between 1978–79 and 1990–91: consequences for calcium intakes. *Proceedings of the Nutrition Society* In press

Jelliffe, D.B. 1966 *The assessment of nutritional status of the community.* WHO monograph series No. 53. New York: WHO. (summarised in Passmore and Eastwood, 1986)

Jelliffe, D.B. 1967 Parallel food classifications in developing and industrialised countries. *The American Journal of Clinical Nutrition* 20, 279–281

Johnell, O., Gullberg, B., Allander, E. Janis, J.A. and the MEDOS study group. 1992 The apparent incidence of hip fracture in Europe: a study of national register sources. *Osteoporosis International* 2, 298–302

Jones, A. 1974 *World protein resources.* Lancaster, England: Medical and Technical Publishing Company

Joossens, J.V. and Geboers, J. 1981 Nutrition and gastric cancer. *Proceedings of the Nutrition Society* 40, 37–46

Kanarek, R.B. and Hirsch, E. 1977 Dietary-induced overeating in experimental animals. *Federation Proceedings of the American Society for Experimental Biology* 36, 154–158

Keen, H. and Thomas, B. Diabetes mellitus. In *Nutrition in the clinical management of disease.* ed. Dickerson, J.W.T. and Lee, H.A. London: Edward Arnold. pp. 167–190

Keys, A., Anderson, J.T. and Grande, F. 1959 Serum cholesterol in man: diet fat and intrinsic responsiveness. *Circulation* 19, 201–204

Keys, A., Anderson, J.T. and Grande, F. 1965a Serum cholesterol responses to changes in the diet. I. Iodine value of dietary fat versus 2S-P. *Metabolism* 14, 747–758

Keys, A., Anderson, J.T. and Grande, F. 1965b Serum cholesterol responses to changes in the diet. II. The effect of cholesterol in the diet. *Metabolism* 14, 759

Keys, A., Brozek, J., Henschel, A., Mickelson, O. and Taylor, H.L. 1950 *The biology of human starvation.* Minneapolis: University of Minnesota Press

KFC 1992 King's Fund Centre *A positive approach to nutrition as treatment.* London: King's Fund Centre

Knittle, J.L. and Hirsch, J. 1969 Effect of early nutrition on the development of rat epididymal fat pads: cellularity and metabolism. *Journal of Clinical Investigation* 47, 2091–2098

Kremer, J.M., Bigauoette, J., Mickalek, A.V., Timchalk, M.A., Lininger, L., Rynes, R.I., Huyck, C., Zieminski, J. and Bartholomew, L.E. 1985 Effects of manipulation of dietary fatty acids on clinical manifestation of rheumatoid arthritis. *Lancet* i, 184–187

Kromhout, D. 1990 n–3 fatty acids and coronary heart disease: epidemiology from Eskimos to Western populations. *British Nutrition Foundation Nutrition Bulletin* 15, 93–102

Kune, G.A., Kune, S. and Watson, L.F. 1993 Perceived religiousness is protective for colorectal cancer: data from the Melbourne Colorectal Cancer Study. *Journal of the Royal Society of Medicine* 86, 645–647

Laurent, C. 1993 Private function? *Nursing Times* 89(47), 14–15

Law, M.R., Frost, C.D. and Wald, N.J. 1991a By how much does dietary salt reduction lower blood pressure? I – Analysis of observational data among populations. *British Medical Journal* 302, 811–815

Law, M.R., Frost, C.D. and Wald, N.J. 1991b By how much does dietary salt reduction lower blood pressure? III – Analysis of data from trials of salt reduction. *British Medical Journal* 302, 819–824

Lee, H.A. 1988 The nutritional management of renal disease. In *Nutrition in the clinical management of disease.* ed. Dickerson, J.W.T. and Lee, H.A. London: Edward Arnold. pp. 262–279

Leeds, A.R. 1979 The dietary management of diabetes in adults. *Proceedings of the Nutrition Society* 38, 365–371

Leichter, I., Margulies, J.Y., Weinreb, A., Mizrahi, J. Robin, G.C., Conforty, B., Makin, M. and Bloch, B. 1982 The relationship between bone density, mineral content, and mechanical strength in the femoral neck. *Clinical Orthopaedics and Related Research* 163, 272–281

Lennard, T.W.J. and Browell, D.A. 1993 The immunological effects of trauma. *Proceedings of the Nutrition Society* 52, 85–90

Leon, D.A. 1985 Physical activity levels and coronary heart disease: analysis of epidemiologic and supporting studies. *Medical Clinics of North America* 69, 3–19

Leon, D.A. 1993 Failed or misleading adjustment for confounding. *Lancet* 342, 479–481

Locatelli, F., Alberti, D., Graziani, G., Buccianti, G., Redaelli, B., Giangrande, A. and the Northern Italian Cooperative Study group 1991 Prospective, randomised, multicentre trial of the effect of protein restriction on progression of chronic renal insufficiency. *Lancet* 337, 1299–1304

Lock, S. 1977 Iron deficiency anaemia in the UK. In *Getting the most out of food, No. 12.* London: Van den Berghs and Jurgens Ltd

McColl, K. 1988 The sugar–fat "seesaw". *The British Nutrition Foundation Nutrition Bulletin* 13, 114–118

MacGregor, G.A., Markandu, N., Best, F., Elder, F., Cam, J., Sagnella, G.A. and Squires, M. 1982 Double-blind random crossover of moderate sodium restriction in essential hypertension. *Lancet* i, 351–355

McClaren, D.S. 1974 The great protein fiasco. *Lancet* ii, 93–96

McCormick, J. and Skrabanek, P. 1988 Coronary heart disease is not preventable by population interventions. *Lancet* i, 839–841

McGill, H.C. 1979 The relationship of dietary cholesterol to serum cholesterol concentration and to atherosclerosis in man. *The American Journal of Clinical Nutrition* 32, 2664–2702

McKeigue, P.M., Marmot, M.G., Adelstein, A.M., Hunt, S.P., Shipley, M.J., Butler, S.M., Riemersma, R.A. and Turner, P.R. 1985 Diet and risk factors for coronary heart disease in Asians in northwest London. *Lancet* ii, 1086–1089

McKeigue, P.M., Shah, B. and Marmot, M.G. 1991 Relation of central obesity and insulin resistance with high diabetes prevalence and cardiovascular risk in South Asians. *Lancet* 337, 382–386

McWhirter, J.P. and Pennington, C.R. 1994 Incidence and recognition of malnutrition in hospital. *British Medical Journal* 308, 945–948

MAFF 1993 Ministry of Agriculture Fisheries and Food *The National Food Survey 1992.* Annual report of the National Food Survey committee. London: HMSO

MAFF 1991 Ministry of Agriculture Fisheries and Food. *Fifty years of the National Food Survey 1940–1990.* Ed. Slater, J.M. London: HMSO

Maiman, L.A., Wang, V.L., Becker, M.H., Finlay, J. and Simonson, M. 1979 Attitudes towards obesity and the obese among professionals. *Journal of the American Dietetic Association,* 74(3), 331–336

Manson, J.E., Colditz, G.A., Stampfer, M.J., Willett, W.C., Rosner, B., Monson, R.R., Speizer, F.E. and Hennekens, C.H. 1990 A prospective study of obesity and coronary heart disease in women. *New England Journal of Medicine* 322, 882–889

Marsh, A.G., Sanchez, T.V., Michelsen, O., Chaffee, F.L. and Fagal, S.M. 1988 Vegetarian lifestyle and bone mineral density. *American Journal of Clinical Nutrition* 48, 837–841

Maslow, A.H. 1943 A theory of human motivation. *Psychological Reviews* 50, 370–396

Mattson, F.H. and Grundy, S.M. 1985 Comparison of effects of dietary saturated, monounsaturated and polyunsaturated fatty acids on plasma lipids and lipoproteins in man. *Journal of Lipid Research* 26, 194–202

Mayer, J. 1956 Appetite and obesity. *Scientific American* 195(5), 108–116

Mayer, J. 1960 The obese hyperglycaemic syndrome of mice as an example of "metabolic" obesity. *American Journal of Clinical Nutrition* 8, 712–718

Mayer, J. 1968 *Overweight: causes, cost and control.* Engelwood Cliffs, New Jersey: Prentice Hall

Mensink, R.P. and Katan, M.J. 1990 Effect of dietary trans fatty acids on high-density and low-density lipoprotein cholesterol levels in healthy subjects. *The New England Journal of Medicine* 323, 439–445

Miller, D.S. 1979a Non-genetic models of obesity. In *Animal models of obesity*. ed. Festing, M.W.F. London: Macmillan. pp. 131–140

Miller, D.S. 1979b Prevalence of nutritional problems in the world. *Proceedings of the Nutrition Society* 38, 197–205

Miller, D.S. and Payne, P.R. 1962 Weight-maintenance and food intake. *Journal of Nutrition* 78, 255–262

Miller, D.S. and Payne, P.R. 1969 Assessment of protein requirements by nitrogen balance. *Proceedings of the Nutrition Society* 28, 225–234

Millstone, E. 1985 Food additive regulation in the UK. *Food Policy* 10, 237–252

Mitchell, E.B. 1988 Food intolerance. In *Nutrition in the clinical management of disease*. ed. Dickerson, J.W.T. and Lee, H.A. London: Edward Arnold. pp. 374–391

Morgan, J.B. 1988 Nutrition for and during pregnancy. In *Nutrition in the clinical management of disease. 2nd edition*. ed. Dickerson, J.W.T. and Lee, H.A. London: Edward Arnold. pp. 1–29

Morris, J.N., Everitt, M.G., Pollard, R., Chave, S.P.W. and Semmence, A.M. 1980 Vigorous exercise in leisure-time: protection against coronary heart disease. *Lancet* ii, 1207–1210

MRC 1991 The MRC Vitamin Study Group. Prevention of neural tube defects: results of the Medical Research Council Vitamin Study. *Lancet* 338, 131–137

MRFIT 1982 Multiple Risk Factor Intervention Trial Research Group. Multiple risk factor intervention trial. *Journal of the American Medical Association* 248, 1465–1477

NACNE 1983 The National Advisory Committee on Nutrition Education. *A discussion paper on proposals for nutritional guidelines for health education in Britain*. London: Health Education Council

Naismith, D.J. 1980 Maternal nutrition and the outcome of pregnancy – a critical appraisal. *Proceedings of the Nutrition Society* 39, 1–11

Neaton, J.D., Blackburn, H., Jacobs, D., Kuller, L., Lee, D-J., Sherwin, R., Shih, J., Stamler, J. and Wentworth, D. 1992 *Archives of Internal Medicine* 152, 1490–1500

Newton, D.J., Clark, R.G. and Woods, H.F. 1980 The nutritional fate of the undernourished surgical patient in convalescence. *Proceedings of the Nutrition Society* 39, 141–148

NRC 1943 National Research Council. *Recommended dietary allowances*. 1st edn. Washington D.C.: National Academy of Sciences

NRC 1989a National Research Council. *Recommended dietary allowances*. 10th edn. Washington D.C.: National Academy of Sciences

NRC 1989b National Research Council. Diet and health: implications for reducing chronic disease risk. *Nutrition Reviews* 47, 142–149

Nutrition Society 1988 Stable isotopic methods for measuring energy expenditure. *Proceedings of the Nutrition Society* 47, 195–268. (Symposium proceedings)

Oliver, M.F. 1981 Diet and coronary heart disease. *British Medical Bulletin* 37, 49–58

Oliver, M.F. 1991 Might treatment of hypercholesteraemia increase non-cardiac mortality? *Lancet* 337, 1529–1531

Paffenbarger, R.S., Hyde, R.T., Wing, A.L. and Hsieh, C-C. 1986 Physical activity, all-cause mortality, and longevity of college alumni. *New England Journal of Medicine* 314, 605–613

Passim, H. and Bennett, J.W. 1943 *Social progress and dietary change*. National Research Council Bulletin 108. Washington DC: National Research Council. (summarised in Fieldhouse, 1986)

Passmore, R. and Eastwood, M.A. 1986 *Human nutrition and dietetics*. 8th edn. Edinburgh: Churchill Livingstone

Paul, A.A. and Southgate, D.A.T. 1979 *The composition of foods. 4th edition*. HMSO: London

Pauling, L. 1972 *Vitamin C and the common cold*. London: Ballantine Books

Perkins, M.N., Rothwell, N.J., Stock, M.J. and Stone, T.W. 1981 Activation of brown adipose tissue thermogenesis by the ventromedial nucleus. *Nature, London* 289, 401–402

Peters, R.H., Wellman, P.J. and Gunian, M.W. 1979 Experimental obesity syndromes in rats: influence of diet palatability on maintenance of body weight. *Physiology and Behaviour* 23, 693–700

Peto, R., Doll, R., Buckley, J.D. and Sporn, M.B. 1981 Can dietary beta-carotene materially reduce human cancer rates? *Nature, London* 290, 201–208

Pocock, N.A., Eisman, J.A., Yeates, M.G., Sambrook, P.N. and Ebert, S. 1986 Physical fitness is a major determinant of femoral neck and lumbar spine bone mineral density. *Journal of Clinical Investigation* 78, 618–621

Poleman, T.T. 1975 World food: a perspective. *Science* 188, 510–518

Pomrehn, P.R., Wallace, R.B. and Burmeister, L.F. 1982 Ischemic heart disease mortality in Iowa farmers. *Journal of the American Medical Association* 248, 1073–1076

Pond, C. 1987 Fat and figures. *New Scientist* 4 June, 62–66

Poskitt, E.M.E. 1988 Childhood. In *Nutrition in the clinical management of disease*. ed. Dickerson, J.W.T. and Lee, H.A. London: Edward Arnold. pp. 30–68

Prentice, A., Laskey, M.A., Shaw, J., Hudson, G.J., Day, K.C., Jarjou, L.M.A., Dibba, B. and Paul, A.A. 1993 The calcium and phosphorus intakes of rural Gambian women during pregnancy and lactation. *British Journal of Nutrition* 69, 885–896

Prentice, A.M. 1989 Energy expenditure in human pregnancy. *British Nutrition Foundation Nutrition Bulletin* 14, 9–22

Ravnskov, U. 1992 Cholesterol lowering trials in coronary heart disease: frequency of citation and outcome. *British Medical Journal* 305, 15–19

Renaud, S. and de Lorgeril, M. 1992 Wine, alcohol, platelets and the French paradox for coronary heart disease. *Lancet* 339, 1523–1526

Richards, J.R. 1980 Current concepts in the metabolic responses to injury, infection and starvation. *Proceedings of the Nutrition Society* 39, 113–123

Riemersma, R.A., Wood, D.A., Macintyre, C.C.A., Elton, R.A., Fey, K.F. and Oliver, M.F. 1991 Risk of angina pectoris and plasma concentrations of vitamins A, C, and E and carotene. *Lancet* 337, 1–5

Rimm, E.B., Giovannucci, E.L., Willett, W.C., Colditz, G.A., Ascherio, A., Rosner, B. and Stampfer, M.J. 1991 Prospective study of alcohol consumption and risk of coronary disease in men. *Lancet* 338, 464–468

Rimm, E.B., Stampfer, M.J., Ascherio, A., Giovannucci, E., Colditz, G.A. and Willett, W.C. 1993 Vitamin E consumption and the risk of coronary heart disease in men. *New England Journal of Medicine* 328, 1450–1455

Rink, T.J. 1994 In search of a satiety factor. *Nature* 372, 406–407

Rivers, J.P.W. and Frankel, T.L. 1981 Essential fatty acid deficiency. *British Medical Bulletin* 37, 59–64

Roberts, D. 1982 Factors contributing to outbreaks of food poisoning in England and Wales 1970–1979. *Journal of Hygiene. Cambridge* 89, 491–498

Robertson, I., Glekin, B.M., Henderson, J.B., Lakhani, A. and Dunnigan, M.G. 1982 Nutritional deficiencies amongst ethnic minorities in the United Kingdom. *Proceedings of the Nutrition Society* 41, 243–256

Rolls, B.A. 1992 Calcium nutrition. In *Nutrition and the consumer*. ed. Walker, A.F. and Rolls, B.A. London: Elsevier Applied Science. pp. 69–95

Rolls, B.J., Rowe, E.A. and Rolls, E.T. 1982 How flavour and appearance affect human feeding. *Proceedings of the Nutrition Society* 41, 109–117

Rothwell, N.J. and Stock, M.J. 1979 A role for brown adipose tissue in diet-induced thermogenesis. *Nature*, London 281, 31–35

Rutishauser, I.H.E. 1992 Vitamin A and carotenoids in human nutrition. In *Nutrition and the consumer* ed. Walker, A.F. and Rolls, B.A. London: Elsevier Applied Science. pp.17–68

Ryder, C.J. 1991 UK food legislation. In: *Foodborne illness. A Lancet review.* ed. Waites, W.M. and Arbuthnott, J.P. London: Edward Arnold. pp. 44–52

Sanders, T.A.B. 1985 Influence of fish-oil supplements on man. *Proceedings of the Nutrition Society* 44, 391–397

Sanders, T.A.B. 1988 Growth and development of British vegan children. *American Journal of Clinical Nutrition* 48, 822–825

Sanders, T.A.B., Mistry, M. and Naismith, D.J. 1984 The influence of a maternal diet rich in linoleic acid on brain and retinal docosahexaenoic acid in the rat. *British Journal of Nutrition* 51, 57–66

Sanderson, F.H. 1975 The great food fumble. *Science* 188, 503–509

Schachter, S. 1968 Obesity and eating. *Science* 161, 751–756

Schachter, S. and Rodin, J. 1974 *Obese humans and rats.* New York: Halstead Press

Schutz, H.G., Rucker, M.H. and Russell, G.F. 1975 Food and food-use classification systems. *Food Technology.* 29(3), 50–64

Seidell, J.C. 1992 Regional obesity and health. *International Journal of Obesity* 16(suppl 2), S31–S34

Simopolous, A.P. 1991 Omega 3 fatty acids in health and disease and in growth and development. *American Journal of Clinical Nutrition* 54, 438–463

Simpson, H.C.R. 1981 High-carbohydrate, high-fibre diets for diabetics. *Proceedings of the Nutrition Society* 40, 219–225

Smith, G.D., Song, F. and Sheldon, T.A. 1993 Cholesterol lowering and mortality: the importance of considering initial level of risk. *British Medical Journal* 306, 1367–1373

Smith, R. 1987 Osteoporosis: cause and management. *British Medical Journal* 294, 329–332

Sorensen, T.I.A. 1992 Genetic aspects of obesity. *International Journal of Obesity* 16 (suppl 2), S27–S29

Spector, T.D., Cooper, C. and Fenton Lewis, A. 1990 Trends in admissions for hip fracture in England and Wales 1968–1985. *British Medical Journal* 300, 1173–1174

Stampfer, M.J., Hennekens, C.H., Manson, J.E., Colditz, G.A., Rosner, B. and Willett, W.C. 1993 Vitamin E consumption and the risk of coronary disease in women. *New England Journal of Medicine* 328, 1444–1449

Stock, M.J. 1992 Thermogenesis and energy balance. *International Journal of Obesity* 16 (suppl 2), S13–S16

Symonds, H. 1990 Observations on bovine spongiform encephalopathy. *British Nutrition Foundation Nutrition Bulletin* 15, 159–168

Tobian, L. 1979 Dietary salt (sodium) and hypertension. *American Journal of Clinical Nutrition* 32, 2659–2662

Todd, E. 1991 Epidemiology of foodborne illness: North America. In *Foodborne illness. A Lancet review.* ed. Waites, W.M. and Arbuthnott, J.P. London: Edward Arnold. pp. 9–15

Tompson, P., Salsbury, P.A., Adams, C. and Archer, D.L. 1991 US food legislation. In: *Foodborne illness. A Lancet review.* ed. Waites, W.M. and Arbuthnott, J.P. London: Edward Arnold. pp. 38–43

Tremblay, A., Plourde, G., Despres, J–P. and Bouchard, C. 1989 Impact of dietary fat content and fat oxidation on energy intake in humans. *American Journal of Clinical Nutrition* 49, 799–805

Trowell, H.C. 1954 Kwashiorkor. *Scientific American* 191(6), 46–50

USDA 1992 United States Department of Agriculture. *The food guide pyramid.* Home and garden bulletin number 252. Washington DC: United States Department of Agriculture

Wald, N., Idle, M., Boreham, J. and Bailey, A. 1980 Low serum-vitamin-A and subsequent risk of cancer. *Lancet* ii, 813–815

Walker, A.F. 1990 The contribution of weaning foods to protein-energy malnutrition. *Nutrition Research Reviews* 3, 25–47

Waterlow, J.C. 1979 Childhood malnutrition – the global problem. *Proceedings of the Nutrition Society* 38, 1–9

Waterlow, J.C., Cravioto, J. and Stephen, J.M.L. 1960 Protein malnutrition in man. *Advances in Protein Chemistry* 15, 131–238

Webb, G.P. 1989 The significance of protein in human nutrition. *Journal of Biological Education* 23(2), 119–124

Webb, G.P. 1990 A selective critique of animal experiments in human-orientated biological research. *Journal of Biological Education* 24(3), 191–197

Webb, G.P. 1991 Nutribland – the first fifteen years. *Nutrition News and Notes* issue 19, 6

Webb, G.P. 1992a A critical survey of methods used to investigate links between diet and disease. *Journal of Biological Education*, 26(4), 263–271

Webb, G.P. 1992b Viewpoint II: Small animals as models for studies on human nutrition. In *Nutrition and the consumer.* ed. Walker, A.F. and Rolls, B.A. London: Elsevier Applied Science. pp. 279–297

Webb, G.P. 1994 A survey of fifty years of dietary standards 1943–1993. *Journal of Biological Education* 28(1), 101–108

Webb, G.P. and Jakobson, M.E. 1980 Body fat of mice and men: a class exercise in theory or practice. *Journal of Biological Education* 14(4), 318–324

Wenkam, N.S. and Woolff R.J. 1970 A half century of changing food habits among Japanese in Hawaii. *The Journal of the American Dietetic Association* 57, 29–32

Wheeler, E. 1992 What determines food choice, and what does food choice determine? *The British Nutrition Foundation Nutrition Bulletin,* 17 (supplement 1), 65–73

Wheeler, E. and Tan, S.P. 1983 From concept to practice: food behaviour of Chinese immigrants in London. *Ecology of Food and Nutrition,* 13(1), 51–57

White, A., Freeth, S. and O'Brien, M. 1992 *Infant feeding 1990.* London: HMSO

White, A., Nicolaas, G., Foster, K., Browne, F. and Carey, S. 1993 *Health survey for England 1991* London: HMSO

Wickham, C.A.C., Walsh, K., Barker, D.J.P., Margetts, B.M., Morris, J. and Bruce, S.A. 1989 Dietary calcium, Physical activity, and risk of hip fracture: a prospective study. *British Medical Bulletin* 299, 889–892

Willett, W.C., Stampfer, M.J., Colditz, G.A., Rosner, B.A. and Speizer, F.E. 1990 Relation of meat, fat and fiber intake to the risk of colon cancer in a prospective study among women. *The New England Journal of Medicine* 323, 1664–1672

Willet, W.C., Stampfer, M.J., Manson, J.E., Colditz, G.A., Speizer, F.E., Rosner, B.A., Sampson, L.A. and Hennekens, C.H. 1993 Intake of *trans* fatty acids and risk of coronary heart disease among women. *Lancet* 341, 581–585

Williams, C.A. and Qureshi, B. 1988 Nutritional aspects of different dietary practices. In Dickerson, J.W.T. and Lee, H.A. (ed.) *Nutrition in the clinical management of disease*. London: Edward Arnold. pp. 422–439

Wohl, M.G. and Goodhart, R.S. 1968 *Modern nutrition in health and disease*. 4th ed. Philadelphia: Lea and Febiger

Wood, D.A., Riemersma, R.A., Butler, S., Thomson, M., Macintyre, C., Elton, R.A. and Oliver, M.F. 1987 Linoleic acid and eicosapentaenoic acid in adipose tissue and platelets and risk of coronary heart disease. *Lancet* i, 177–182

Wortman, S. 1976 Food and agriculture. *Scientific American* 235(3), 31–39

Yeung, D.L., Cheung, L.W.Y. and Sabry, J.H. 1973 The hot-cold food concept in Chinese culture and its application in a Canadian-Chinese community. *The Journal of the Canadian Dietetic Association*. 34, 197–203

Zhang, Y., Proenca, R., Maffei, M., Barone, M., Leopold, L. and Friedman, J.M. 1994 Positional cloning of the mouse obese gene and its human homologue. *Nature* 372, 425–432

Index